theclinics.com

CLINICS IN PLASTIC SURGERY

Lipoplasty

Guest Editor

LUIZ S. TOLEDO, MD

January 2006 • Volume 33 • Number 1

ELSEVIER
SAUNDERS

An imprint of Elsevier, Inc
PHILADELPHIA LONDON TORONTO MONTREAL SYDNEY TOKYO

W.B. SAUNDERS COMPANY
A Division of Elsevier Inc.

1600 John F. Kennedy Blvd., Suite 1800, Philadelphia, PA 19103-2899

http://www.theclinics.com

CLINICS IN PLASTIC SURGERY Volume 33, Number 1
January 2006 ISSN 0094-1298, ISBN 1-4160-3378-5

Editor: Sarah Barth

Clinics in Plastic Surgery (ISSN 0094-1298) is published quarterly by W.B. Saunders Company. Corporate and editorial offices: Elsevier Inc., 1600 John F. Kennedy Blvd., Suite 1800, Philadelphia, PA 19103-2899. Accounting and circulation offices: 6277 Sea Harbor Drive, Orlando, FL 32887-4800. Periodicals postage paid at Orlando, FL 32862, and additional mailing offices. Subscription prices are $260.00 per year for US individuals, $390.00 per year for US institutions, $130.00 per year for US students and residents, $295.00 per year for Canadian individuals, $445.00 per year for Canadian institutions, $315.00 per year for international individuals, $445.00 per year for international institutions, and $155.00 per year for Canadian and foreign students/residents. To receive student/resident rate, orders must be accompanied by name of affiliated institution, date of term, and the *signature* of program/residency coordinator on institution letterhead. Orders will be billed at individual rate until proof of status is received. Foreign air speed delivery is included in all *Clinics* subscription prices. All prices are subject to change without notice. POSTMASTER: Send address changes to *Clinics in Plastic Surgery*, W.B. Saunders Company, Periodicals Fulfillment, Orlando, FL 32887-4800. **Customer Service: 1-800-654-2452 (US). From outside of the US, call 1-407-345-4000.**

Clinics in Plastic Surgery is covered in *Current Contents, EMBASE/Excerpta Medica, Science Citation Index, Index Medicus, ASCA, and ISI/BIOMED.*

Printed in the United States of America.

LIPOPLASTY

GUEST EDITOR

LUIZ S. TOLEDO, MD
Plastic Surgeon in Private Practice; Professor of Postgraduate Education in Aesthetic Plastic Surgery–ISAPS, São Paulo, Brazil

CONTRIBUTORS

PRISCILA CHIARELLO DE SOUZA PINTO ABDALA, MD
Staff, Department of Plastic Surgery, Santa Cecília University, Brazil

MARGUERITE E. AITKEN, MD, MFA
Plastic Surgery Associates, PC, Grand Rapids, Michigan

JOSE ARROYAVE, BSc, MSc, TEM, SEM
Professor of Histology, Centro Internacional de Agricultura Tropical–Ciat Universidad Libre Facultad de Medicina, Cali, Columbia

JUAREZ M. AVELAR, MD
Head, Brazilian Scientific Institute of Aesthetic and Reconstructive Plastic Surgery; Plastic Surgeon, Alameda Gabriel, São Paulo, Brazil

WILLIAM CRIOLLO, BSc, MSc
Specialist in Cellular Cultures, Basic Science Department, Universidad del Valle, Cali, Colombia

ROBERT A. ERSEK, MD, FACS
Personique Surgery Center, Austin, Texas

J. WILLIAM FUTRELL, MD
Clinical Professor of Surgery, University of Pittsburgh; Adjunct Professor of Bioengineering, Carnegie-Mellon University, Pittsburgh, Pennsylvania

CARLO GASPERONI, MD
Professor of Aesthetic Surgery, Plastic Surgery, Specialization School of the Università Cattolica Del Sacro Cuore; Plastic Surgeon, Clinica Quisisana, Rome, Italy

PAOLO GASPERONI, MD
Plastic Surgeon, Clinica Quisisana, Rome, Italy

ROBERT G.W. GIRLING V
Personique Surgery Center, Austin, Texas

MARIA I. GUTIERREZ, MD, MSc, PhD
Epidemiology, Faculty of Medicine, Universidad del Valle, Cali, Colombia

OSCAR GUTIERREZ, MD, MSc
Assistant Professor of Basic Sciences, Faculty of Medicine, Universidad del Valle, Cali, Colombia

JOSEPH P. HUNSTAD, MD, FACS
The Hunstad Center, Charlotte, North Carolina

YVES GÉRARD ILLOUZ, MD
Associate Professor in Plastic and Aesthetic Surgery, Saint-Louis Hospital, Paris, France

CAROLINA ISAZA, MD, MSc
Professor, Faculty of Medicine, Department of Genetics, Universidad del Valle, Cali, Colombia

ADAM J. KATZ, MD
Assistant Professor of Plastic and Reconstructive Surgery, University of Virginia Health Sciences Center, Charlottesville, Virginia

RAMON LLULL, MD, PhD
Associate Professor, Department of Cell Biology, University of Barcelona Medical School, Barcelona, Spain

CHRISTOVAM MONTECINOS MACIEL, MD
Resident, Department of Plastic Surgery, Santa Cecilia University, Brazil

RAUL MAUAD, MD
Plastic Surgeon in Private Practice,
São Paulo, Brazil

MANUEL SANCHEZ MOSQUERA, MD
Specialist in Anesthesiology, Private Practice,
São Paulo, Brazil

RODRIGO NEIRA, MD
Professor of Plastic Surgery, Maxillofacial and Hand Surgery, Pontificia Universidad Javeriana, Cali, Colombia

ROY C. OGLE, PhD
Professor of Cell Biology, Professor of Plastic and Reconstructive Surgery, and Professor of Neurosurgery, University of Virginia Health Sciences Center, Charlottesville, Virginia

CLARA L. ORTIZ-NEIRA, MD
Assistant Professor, Pediatric Radiology, Alberta Children Hospital; Faculty of Medicine, University of Calgary, Calgary, Alberta, Canada

EWALDO BOLIVAR DE SOUZA PINTO, MD
Chief, Department of Plastic Surgery,
Santa Cecilia University, Brazil

HUGO RAMIREZ, VMD, MSc
Professor of Histology, Universidad Libre de Colombia, Bogata, Colombia

ÂNGELO REBELO, MD
Chairman, International Academy of Cosmetic Surgery; Plastic Surgeon; Clinical Director, Clinica Milénio, Lisbon, Portugal

FÁBIO LUÍS FERRARI REGATIERI, MD
Specialist in Anesthesiology, Private Practice,
São Paulo, Brazil

J. PETER RUBIN, MD
Assistant Professor of Plastic and Reconstructive Surgery, University of Pittsburgh, Pittsburgh, Pennsylvania

MARK A. SALISBURY, MD
Personique Surgery Center, Austin, Texas

FABIANA DE PAULA TURCHIARI DOS SANTOS, MD
Resident, Department of Plastic Surgery,
Santa Cecilia University, Brazil

EFRAIN SOLARTE, Dr, Rer, Nat, MSc
Professor, Faculty of Sciences, Department of Physics, Universidad del Valle, Cali, Colombia

RODRIGO PESSOA MARTELLO DE SOUZA, MD
Resident, Department of Plastic Surgery,
Santa Cecilia University, Brazil

SUNIL S. THOLPADY, MS, MD, PhD
Resident, Department of Plastic and Reconstructive Surgery, University of Virginia Health Sciences Center, Charlottesville, Virginia

LUIZ S. TOLEDO, MD
Plastic Surgeon in Private Practice; Professor of Postgraduate Education in Aesthetic Plastic Surgery–ISAPS, São Paulo, Brazil

LIPOPLASTY

Volume 33 • Number 1 • January 2006

Contents

FORTHCOMING ISSUES

April 2006

Abdominal Wall Reconstruction
Mimis Cohen, MD, *Guest Editor*

July 2006

Gluteal Augmentation
V. Leroy Young, MD, *Guest Editor*

October 2006

Noninvasive Facial Enhancement
David A. Jansen, MD, *Guest Editor*

RECENT ISSUES

October 2005

Challenges in Hand Surgery
Nancy McKee, MD, FRCS(C), FACS,
Guest Editor

July 2005

Microsurgical Reconstruction of the Head and Neck
Achilleas Thoma, MD, MSc, FRCS(C), FACS,
Guest Editor

April 2005

Surgical Management of Cutaneous Disease
Mark S. Granick, MD, *Guest Editor*

ELSEVIER
SAUNDERS

CLINICS IN PLASTIC SURGERY

Clin Plastic Surg 33 (2006) xi–xii

Preface
Lipoplasty

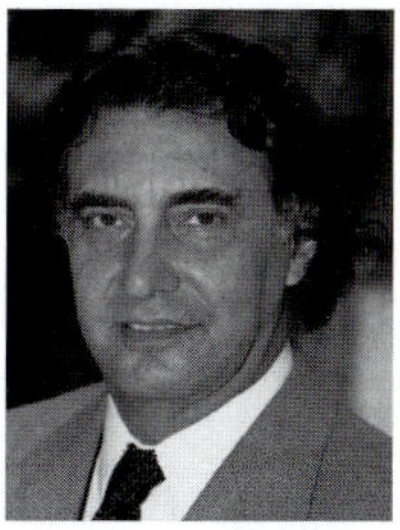

Luiz S. Toledo, MD
Guest Editor

Luiz S. Toledo, MD
Av. Brg. Luiz Antonio, 4442
São Paulo 01402-002, Brazil

E-mail address:
lstoledo@netpoint.com.br

It is an honor for me to be the Guest Editor of this issue of *Clinics in Plastic Surgery* devoted entirely to Lipoplasty—the surgical technique to treat the fat layer with aesthetic purpose. I would like to thank the Editors for putting their trust in my judgment. The first decade of my life as a doctor was in a world without liposuction. We were faced with difficult challenges then, having to indicate or not a vertical or circumferential thigh dermolipectomy on a 16-year-old young woman. We all knew then that these procedures represented a "gray area" in surgical decision making ("should I operate or not"), and that the benefits of such procedures were questionable. Many times, the resulting scar was not a good option to obtain a good-shaped leg in a young patient who would probably never be able to wear a bathing suit confidently in public.

Yves Gérard Illouz created liposuction, the technique to aspirate fat for aesthetic purpose. When he first showed the technique in Brazil in November 1980, it was clear to those of us who saw his presentation in Fortaleza that many things were going to change with this technique. At the time, liposuction was attacked by old professors, who compared it to other similar techniques, which curetted fat using small incisions, with terrible complications. When Illouz introduced liposuction in the United States at the ASPS Hawaii Congress of 1982, the technique found respect within the international plastic surgery community. Surgeons soon found out that Illouz's results were reproducible, and the technique became popular.

In 1985, Pierre Fournier modified liposuction and created liposculpture—the technique to aspirate and, if necessary, to inject fat with aesthetic purpose. Instead of the aspirator, he used syringes, creating the so-called liposculpture. As soon as these techniques became popular, modifications were made that improved and, in some cases, made the technique dangerous. In the first years, when surgeons were cautious and still learning its boundaries, liposuction produced great results. The problems began when some began testing the limits of the technique, not only by changing the instruments but by modifying the technique itself. Although many improvements were good, some of them brought many complications. Something had to change, limitations had to be established.

It became obvious that the limit of extracting 3 L of fat per surgery was wrong, because it completely left aside the fact that people vary in weight. Today, several countries have passed regulations specifying

0094-1298/06/$ – see front matter
doi:10.1016/j.cps.2005.09.004
plasticsurgery.theclinics.com

where the procedure should be performed and what percentage of the patient's weight can be removed in one stage. The Medical Council in Brazil has passed a regulation stating that lipoplasty is a surgical procedure, and can be performed only by doctors with surgical training. This is a step in the right direction, to demand better training of surgeons performing the technique.

The idea of producing this issue of *Clinics in Plastic Surgery* was to present some of the most influential ideas that have been introduced in lipoplasty by surgeons who have created or modified tactics, and who represent different facets in the field. I would like to thank them for a job well done. You will find here the state of the art of lipoplasty in the world. I hope you will enjoy it.

ELSEVIER
SAUNDERS

CLINICS IN PLASTIC SURGERY

Clin Plastic Surg 33 (2006) 1–11

Complications of Body Sculpture: Prevention and Treatment

Luiz S. Toledo, MD[a,*], Raul Mauad, MD[b]

In many countries, lipoplasty is the most frequently performed aesthetic procedure. It has been promoted as a safe, easy-to-learn, outpatient procedure. Currently there is even something called "lunch time" liposuction. Although plastic surgeons have developed safety measures to perform the technique, there are serious risks, including death at a rate of 1/5000 procedures [1]. We cannot forget that liposuction is also performed by dermatologists, aesthetic medicine practitioners, gynecologists, oral surgeons, and otolaryngologists in facilities that range from hospital operating rooms to small offices. Lipoplasty is ideally performed in an accredited facility with an anesthesiologist present at all times when the removal of more than 1 L of fat is planned. The facility should have a cardiac monitor, pulse oximeter, noninvasive blood pressure, defibrillator, intubation equipment, laryngeal mask, reanimation material, vasoactive drugs, support equipment, infusion pump, a gas central, and an aspirator. Refer to Box 1 for descriptions of the various aesthetic surgical procedures.

The American Society of Aesthetic Plastic Surgeons Lipoplasty Task Force established the main factors that increase risk in lipoplasty: (1) Injecting too much fluid and local anesthesia. (2) Removing too much fat. (3) Performing too many procedures during the same surgical act. (4) Performing the procedure for the wrong indication (eg, health problems). (5) Monitoring megaliposuction patients inadequately [2]. Safety measures in body contour procedures should avoid life-threatening complications and aesthetic complications [Boxes 2 and 3].

Dr. Mark Gorney, a past president of the ASAPS and medical director of The Doctors Company's (a physician-owned medical malpractice insurance provider in the United States), says that "in comparison with frequency of other Plastic Surgery procedures, liposuction only constitutes 3% of all plastic surgery claims. However it is by far the most expensive. The settlements or verdicts are always near policy limits. By the year 2000 the numbers of liposuction claims were climbing alarmingly. Worse yet, there were some fatal outcomes which are universally settled for policy limits [US$1 million]. By the end of that year we had counted 67 fatalities for the past 3 years nationwide." At that point Dr. Gorney addressed the ASAPS at the Boston meeting and convinced the society to limit the extracted fat to 5000 mL maximum. He also enforced that rule under threat of policy cancellation, and the mortalities dropped to zero the next

[a] Private Practice, Av. Brg. Luiz Antonio, 4442, São Paulo 01402-002, Brazil
[b] Private Practice, R. Manoel Cebrian Ferrer, 60, São Paulo 04023-070, Brazil
* Corresponding author.
E-mail address: lstoledo@netpoint.com.br (L.S. Toledo).

0094-1298/06/$ – see front matter doi:10.1016/j.cps.2005.08.001
plasticsurgery.theclinics.com

Box 1: Terminology

Lipoplasty is the surgical procedure used to treat and reshape adipose tissue.

Liposuction is the surgical procedure used to aspirate excess adipose tissue of the body for aesthetic purposes.

Liposculpture is the surgical procedure used to improve the contours of the body through aspiration or injection of fat obtained from the same person for aesthetic purposes.

year (M. Gorney, personal communication, 2004). We must remember that these numbers relate to board-certified plastic surgeons and do not include other doctor groups that perform liposuction.

A questionnaire was addressed to 600 members of the French Society of Plastic Reconstructive and Aesthetic Surgery [3]. The society received 112 replies and showed that out of 19,000 interventions, cosmetic surgical procedures represented 35% of the global surgical activity of French plastic surgeons. The most frequent interventions were liposuction (19%), breast augmentation (16%), blepharoplasty (14%), abdominoplasty (12%), mammaplasty (10%), facelift (10%), and rhinoplasty (8%). The techniques that registered more than 10% of problems were abdominoplasty and mammaplasty. The techniques with between 5% and 10% of problems were rhinoplasty, facelift, and breast augmentation, and the techniques with less than 5% of problems were liposuction and blepharoplasty. On average, the most frequent cosmetic surgical procedures give rise to 7% of complications.

Prevention and treatment of life-threatening complications

Prevention is better than treatment. The ideal situation involves a properly selected patient who is treated by a well-trained surgeon and anesthesiologist team who work in a fully equipped, certified, and accredited facility with a well-trained operating room and recovery room staff.

Box 2: Life-threatening complications

- Pulmonary embolism
- Hemorrhage
- Perforation
- Infection
- Lidocaine toxicity
- Epinephrine toxicity
- Third space fluid shifts
- Fat embolism syndrome

Box 3: Aesthetic complications

- Undercorrection: insufficient fat removal
- Overcorrection: excess fat removal
- Irregular fat removal with palpable and visible irregularities
- Edema
- Hematoma
- Seroma
- Local infection: insufficient sterilization, patient with low immunity
- Bad patient selection: a patient who needs skin resection treated with liposuction
- Cutaneous slough
- Hyperpigmentation, vasculopathies, permanent color changes in the skin

Pulmonary embolism

For the last 25 years, pulmonary embolism has been the main killer among patients who have undergone cosmetic surgery and has been responsible for one fourth of unavoidable deaths [4]. The remaining three fourths of perioperative complications are open to preventive or corrective intervention. Symptoms of pulmonary embolism include sudden, sharp chest pain, shortness of breath, chest pain that worsens with deep breathing or coughing, coughing up blood, tachycardia, sweating, and anxiety.

Pulmonary embolism should be prevented in patients with a higher risk of deep venous thrombosis. It is more likely to occur in patients who have an inherited condition that causes increased risk of clotting, patients who are immobile during surgery for more than 2 hours, patients who have a low blood flow in a deep vein or other medical conditions, such as varicose veins, and patients who are older than 60, under hormone therapy, and overweight. Prevention is ensured with monitoring, oxygen, and anticoagulants. Long procedures increase the risk of complications; the optimum length of surgery should not exceed 3 hours. Procedures longer than 2 hours with the patient in the same position require the use of compression boots or drug prevention of deep venous thrombosis. Liposuction patients in the same position for more than 2 hours also should have sequential compression massaging boots intraoperatively. Even early postoperative mobilization, elastic stockings, and compressive wound dressing might not prevent pulmonary embolism, however [5]. Drug prevention of deep venous thrombosis is Nadroparin, 7500 UI/d, or enoxieparin, 20 to 40 mg/d.

Hemorrhage, perforation, and infection

Hemorrhage, perforation, and infection are preventable through proper training of surgeons. Hemorrhage can occur perioperatively or postoperatively.

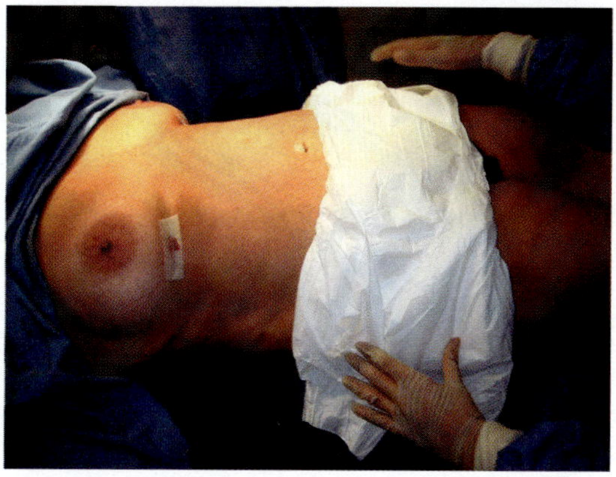

Fig. 1. Sterilized absorbent dressings are placed under a girdle for 24 hours.

It can be caused by major vessel perforation, coagulopathy, or simply a bad surgical technique. Liposuction is precise, and sometimes a device invented to ease the procedure for the surgeon can make it difficult to work with precision.

Extra care should be taken when using vibrating cannulas or power-assisted liposuction. If it seems easier to aspirate difficult areas, it is because with the vibration the cannula penetrates the hard and fibrotic tissues. A surgeon must be accustomed to the feel of the device to avoid perforation of the abdominal wall and organs. Vibrating cannulas are unnecessary but can be helpful in some difficult areas, as in the men's dorsal region, or when treating gynecomastia and secondary procedures with subcutaneous fibrosis. Seromas (1.4%) are always a possibility, however [6].

The internal ultrasound-assisted liposuction technique, which was popular in the 1990s, is still used by many surgeons. Its introduction in 1997 was received with great enthusiasm, but reports that

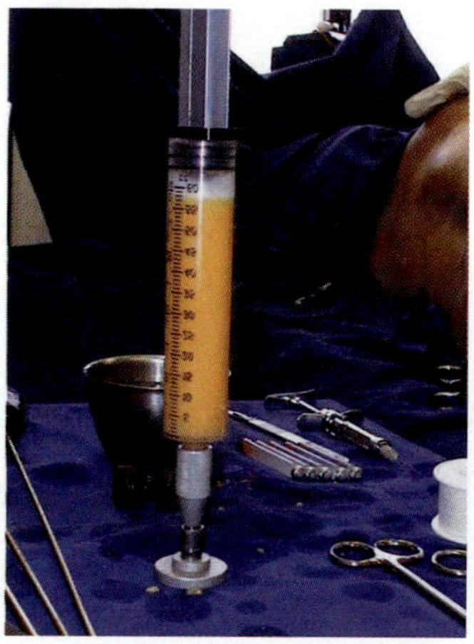

Fig. 2. Fat is saved in a 60-cc syringe with a decanting tip that allows transferring to a luer-lock syringe.

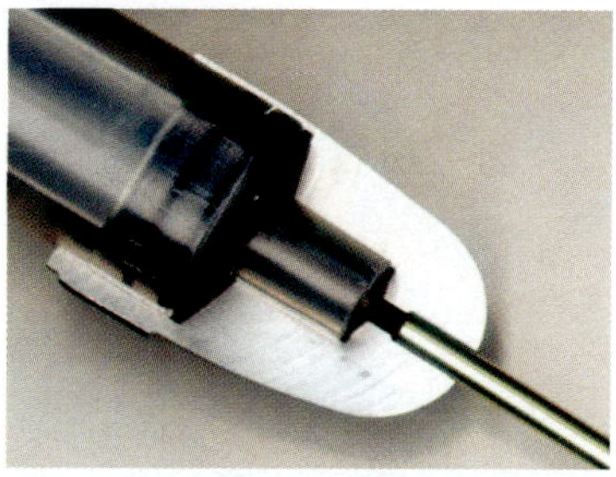

Fig. 3. A 60-cc Toomey-tip syringe is adapted to the Tulip cannula.

described the limitations and complications of ultrasound-assisted liposuction, such as burns and seroma formation [7], showed that the technique does not necessarily give better results, does not make it easier to aspirate, is not faster, is more traumatic, is less safe, and is more expensive. Ultrasound-assisted liposuction generates heat during liposuction that can burn the skin, subcutaneous tissue, and nerves, which increases the risk of bleeding and necrosis seroma formation. The cause of these complications was speculated to be a result of prolonged ultrasonic energy time. Consequently, some authors recommended limiting the amount of ultrasonic energy time per site and even complete avoidance of ultrasound-assisted liposuction in certain body areas [8].

Treating the abdominal wall without proper care can cause viscera perforation caused by misdirection of the cannula or bad positioning of the patient during surgery. One way to avoid this complication is to hyperextend the abdominal region, either by bending the table or placing a support under the patient's hips, so the tip of the cannula introduced in the pubic area tends to come up through the skin of the epigastrium rather than down and perforating the abdomen.

In more than 1000 procedures we have encountered one case of infection when performing suction alone. In more than 1000 procedures of fat injection we have had three cases of infection: one in the medial thigh and two in the buttocks. Infection can be avoided with total antisepsis and

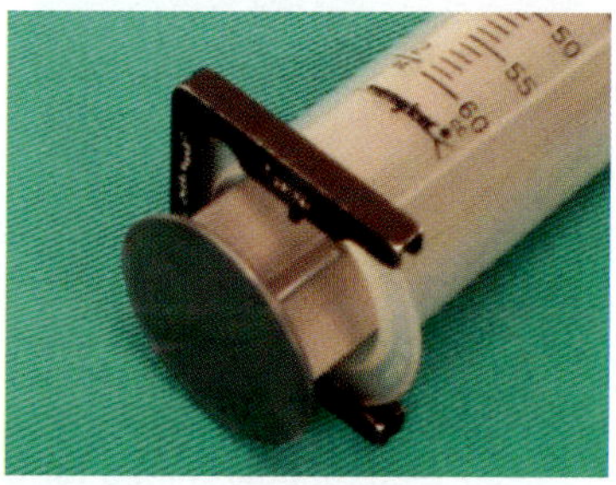

Fig. 4. The plunger lock maintains vacuum in the syringe.

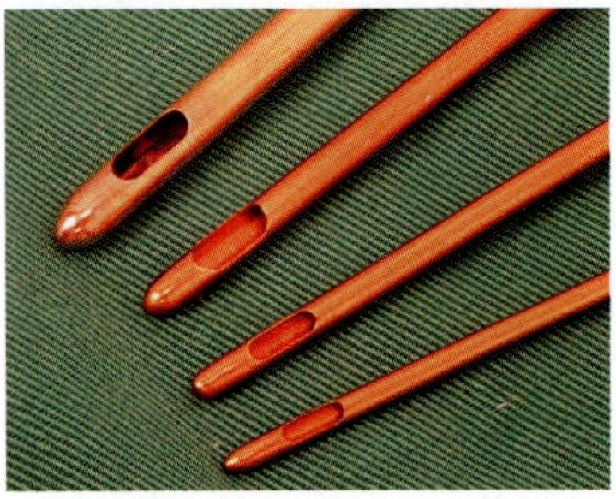

Fig. 5. Zirconium-fused cannulas provoke less friction during fat aspiration.

proper antibiotics. I use 2 g of intravenous cephalosporin intraoperatively, plus 1 g every 4 hours, a total of 8 g intravenously on the first day, and Azythromicin, 500 mg orally, for 3 days.

There are related cases of patients with skin and soft tissue infection after liposuction and liposculpture caused by rapidly growing mycobacteria after cosmetic liposuction and liposculpture [9]. Microorganisms were isolated from the purulent drainage and identified by routine microbiologic techniques. When infection occurs, patients exhibit signs of inflammation, microabscesses, and purulent wound drainage. Treatment includes surgical drainage and sometimes prolonged treatment with antibiotics. A patient who complains about pain disproportional to the surgical trauma can be exhibiting early signs of necrotizing fasciitis, however. If not recognized early and treated aggressively, the infection is often fatal [9]. Routine laboratory tests, contrast MRI, and biopsy can help with the diagnosis. Necrotizing fasciitis usually provokes widespread necrosis of the superficial and deep fascia, which is associated with severe systemic toxic reactions. The treatment involves radical débridement of the skin, subcutaneous tissue, fasciae, and sometimes muscle. Postoperative care involves antibiotics, artificial respiration, and skin grafting.

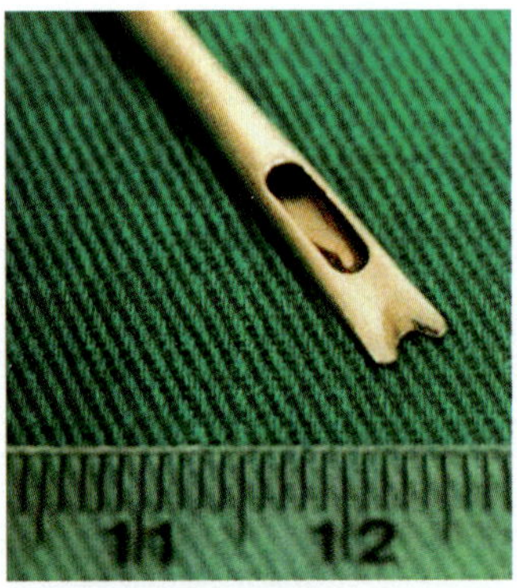

Fig. 6. The Toledo V-tip cannula is used for dissection, aspiration, and injection of fat.

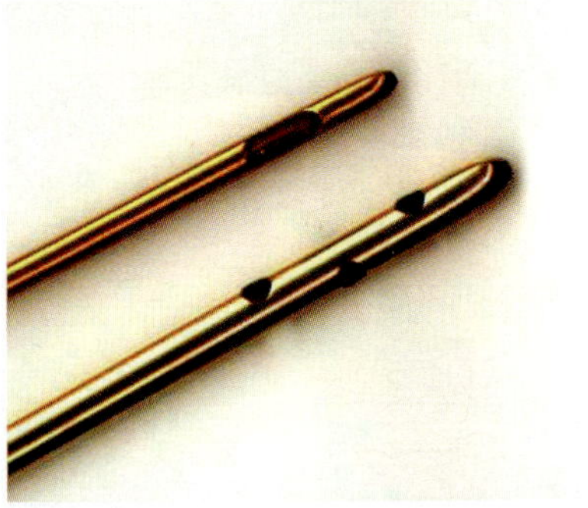

Fig. 7. The 3- and 4.6-mm gauge cannulas used for superficial and deep suction.

Lidocaine toxicity

The question "was this death attributable to lidocaine toxicity" remains unanswered because of lack of postmortem toxicology [4]. Because we prefer local anesthesia with sedation, however, we must be careful with the amount of lidocaine injected. We inject 1 mL of solution for each milliliter of aspirate removed. Excessive infiltration of wetting solution in a proportion of 3:1 can cause lidocaine toxicity, cardiotoxicity, convulsions, drug interaction, and overdose. The toxic blood level of lidocaine varies between 5 and 6 μg/mL. With 55 mg/kg, the maximum blood level of lidocaine reaches 1.9 μg/mL [10]. Our anesthesia solution is well within the safety limits. Pulmonary edema can be caused by overhydration after injection of too much tumescent fluid, intravenous fluid overload, and tumescent fluid absorption, combined with poor patient or drug monitoring. The peak of lidocaine absorption is 8 to 12 hours after injection. We should not liberate a patient too soon because the plasma levels may peak when the patient is at home.

Epinephrine toxicity

Epinephrine toxicity can provoke hypertension and tachycardia. It is undocumented and difficult to diagnose.

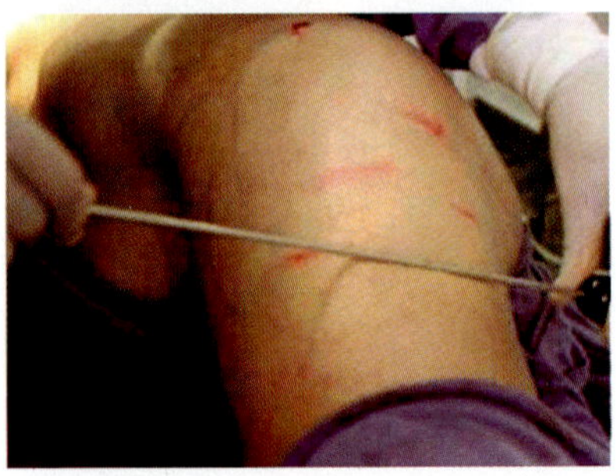

Fig. 8. The pizza roll in use. A steel bar passed on the wet skin helps to find irregularities.

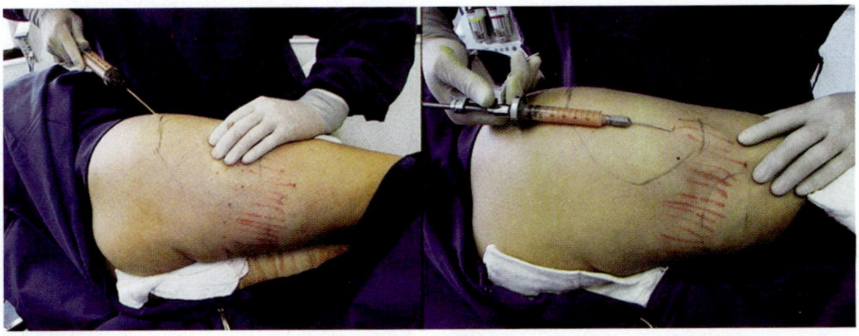

Fig. 9. Aspiration of fat from a localized fat deposit and injection into a depressed region.

Third space fluid shifts

Third space fluid shifts are caused by excessive fat aspiration and extensive subsurface "burn." The so-called mega-liposuction removes many liters of fat from a patient in a single procedure. Many doctors remove 8 or 10 L of fat or more. We limit the aspirate to less than 5% of the body weight and treat less than 30% of the body surface. We always can repeat the procedure to remove more fat. The local anesthesia solution is heated before the injection to 37°C because hypothermia alters the coagulation factors, increases bleeding, and can cause coagulopathy [11]. Hypothermia and postoperative shivering are reduced by heating every intravenous and subcutaneous fluid to 37°C. Hot air blankets peri- and postoperatively prevent hypothermia and avoid metabolic and blood composition changes, which lead to complications, such as infections, blood loss, heart attacks, and even death.

To remove up to 1 L of aspirate we use oral sedation with midazolan, 15 mg. For large procedures, intravenous sedation with midazolan, fentanyl, and propofol is preferred. The induction is done with Tenoxicam 20 mg, Cephalexin 2 g (plus 1 g every 4 hours, a total of 8 g), Dramin DL 10 mL (30 mg), Dipyrone 2 mL (1 g), Dexamethasone 4 mg, Meperidine 1.0 to 1.5 mg/kg. Maintenance with Midazolan 0.1 mg/kg – 0.3 mg/kg, Propofol 25 to 75 Âμg/kg/min, Fentanyl 1 to 5 Âμg/kg slowly. The local infiltration solution contains 20 cc 2% Lidocaine, 1 cc Adrenaline (1:1000), 500cc Ringer's Lactate, 5cc 3% sodium bicarbonate. This solution is injected slowly at a rate of 1:1 to 1.5:1, injecting 1 mL of fluid per milliliter of fat we estimate to aspirate. This proportion avoids pulmonary edema and lidocaine overdose. We know that the toxic blood level of lidocaine varies between 5 and 6 μg/mL. The safe dose of lidocaine is 55 mg/kg when using the tumescent technique with adrenaline [10]. With 55 mg/kg, the maximum blood level of lidocaine reaches only 1.9 μg/mL. With this technique the mean amount of blood per liter of aspirate is 10.5 ± 5.2 mL [12].

Fat embolism syndrome

Fat embolism syndrome is rare after liposuction [13]; only five cases have been reported [14–18]. Of these five cases, four patients survived. Only one patient underwent liposuction alone and not as a combined procedure, as described in the other

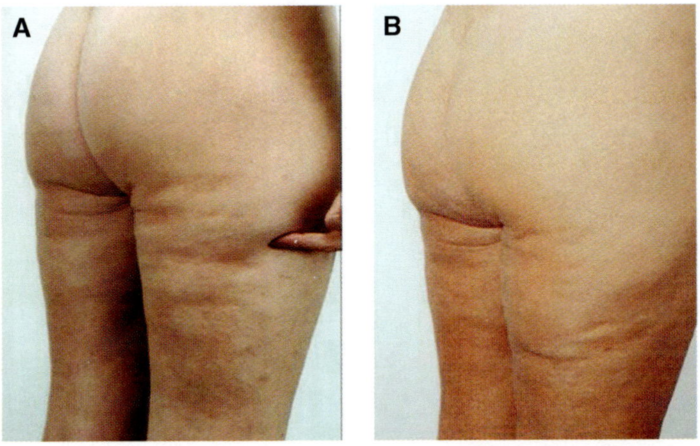

Fig. 10. Before (*A*) and 1 year after (*B*) the operation, which involved correction of depressions.

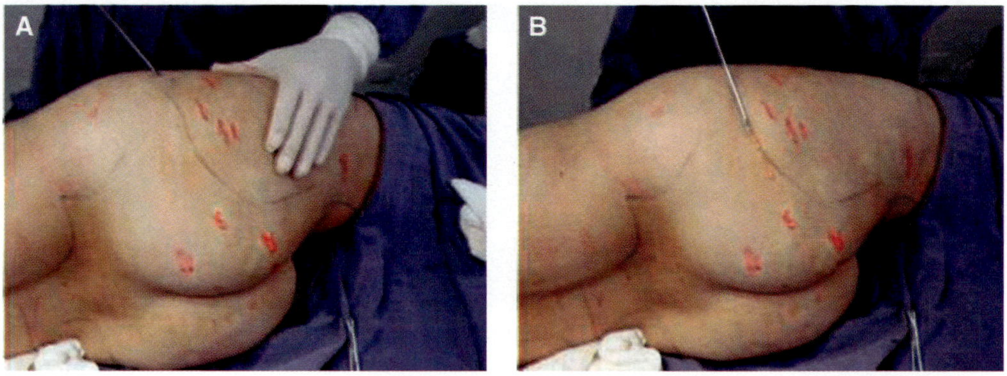

Fig. 11. (*A, B*) Breaking the fibrous adherences with the V-tip Toledo cannula and injecting fat.

case reports. According to some authors we should revise the concept that fat embolism syndrome after liposuction occurs only after long, combined procedures. They believe that the incidence of fat embolism syndrome after liposuction might be underestimated because this diagnosis is not systematically considered and because the clinical pattern of fat embolism syndrome often is not specific [19].

Aesthetic complications

Prevention is always better than treatment. The increasing number of liposuction procedures performed has led to a growing number of iatrogenic fat tissue deformities, and so the need for corrective procedures also has increased. In recent years several techniques have been developed. When a dissatisfied patient complains not to have changed much as a result of the procedure, it is important to have the preoperative records (weight and measurements and preoperative photographs.) Many patients with scoliosis have a deformity in the dorsal region that causes accumulation of fat more on one side than the other. They usually only note this difference after the procedure. Liposuction reduces the number of fixed fat cells in the treated area of the body. The fat cells that remain and fat cells in the untreated areas can still gain weight.

Photographing is of utmost importance as a guide for the surgeon during the surgery and for postoperative comparison. Some patients simply forget what they looked like before surgery. The difference can be seen when you show them comparable before-and-after pictures side by side. Many patients may feel that they have not changed, but when weighed after surgery, they are usually several kilograms lighter. Sometimes postoperative changes do not seem visible but can be shown in the change in measurements.

I prefer to conduct the consultation with computer imaging. It is better if a patient can visualize

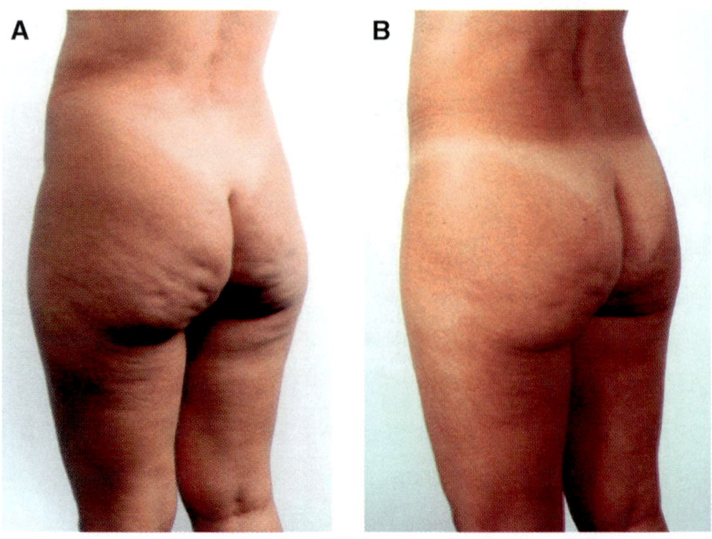

Fig. 12. Before (*A*) and 8 years after (*B*) liposculpture for treatment of superficial irregularities.

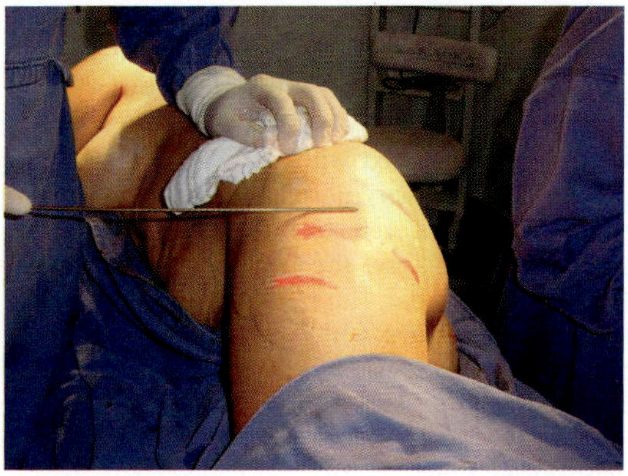

Fig. 13. The areas marked in red are depressed. Fat is aspirated or moved from the adjacent areas, and the surgeon mobilizes the fat layer to a uniform position.

what a surgeon can and cannot achieve, and the limits of surgical improvement are established preoperatively. I do not print the image or give a patient any guarantees of the result. The projected image includes the limitations of the surgeon and the technique. This type of consultation also helps to screen patients with unrealistic expectations.

The most common aesthetic complications are as follows: edema, ecchymosis, undercorrection, overcorrection, irregularities, seroma, hematoma, vasculopathy, cutaneous hyperpigmentation, and liquefied fat.

Edema and ecchymosis

Edema and ecchymosis can occur after almost every procedure and can be uncomfortable for a patient in the early postoperative period. We minimize edema and increase patient comfort by not suturing the liposuction incisions and applying sterilized absorbent dressings for the first 24 hours and providing manual lymphatic drainage in the early postoperative days [**Fig. 1**]. Ecchymosis is considered normal in the liposuction postoperative phase and should disappear 2 to 3 weeks after surgery. It can be minimized by compressive dressing of the treated areas.

The most common complications of lipoplasty are undercorrection (insufficient fat removal,) overcorrection (excessive fat removal), and irregular fat removal (with palpable and visible irregularities.) These aesthetic complications can be prevented by choosing the proper technique, a technique that allows precise measurement of the aspirated and injected amounts of fat. The normal liposuction aspirator vial is usually too big to measure the aspirated fat precisely, which can be important when treating pair adiposities. Even if the deformity is not even, it is better to know the exact amount of pure fat and

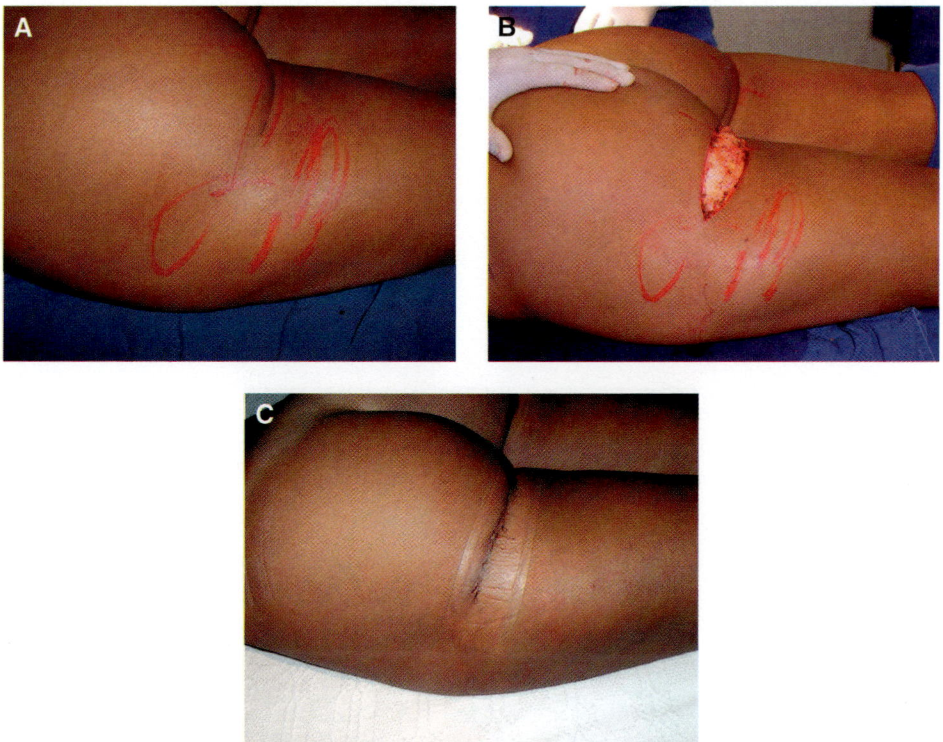

Fig. 14. (*A–C*) Skin resection can be the best option to treat a defect.

of total aspirate. This information is also important for medicolegal purposes. The use of the syringe method is one of the best techniques to help prevent uneven fat removal. Using a 60-mL Toomey-tip syringe, we always know the exact amount of aspiration and pure fat. Even when I do not plan to reinject fat I always harvest and keep a few syringes for possible immediate corrections [Fig. 2].

A member of the surgical crew keeps a map with the same markings as the patient and notes the amount of aspiration from each area. By keeping the preoperative photographs visible during surgery, we can check what the deformity looks like with the patient in the standing position. We can remove the same amount if both sides look the same or more from one area if it needs more treatment. Bad positioning of a patient on the operating table also can be the cause of irregularities. A patient who is not properly anesthetized is not calm during surgery, which may affect a surgeon's work [Figs. 3–7].

To treat undercorrection we must aspirate more fat. Overcorrection is often treated only with fat injection. The possible treatments for areas with irregularities include fat suction, fat injection, subcision, fat shifting or mobilization, and skin resection. Irregularities can be primary (eg, cellulite dimples) or iatrogenic (eg, liposuction sequelae), and they can be produced by aspirating fat irregularly from both fat layers (areolar and lamellar). To control the depth of aspiration, we use the outstretched hand—wetting the skin surface with an antiseptic solution—or the pinch test, which should be performed with dry skin. It is possible to observe skin irregularities by palpation or by changes of light reflex. An instrument devised to control regularity, the "pizza roll," which is a 1-cm-thick steel bar, can be passed on the wet skin to find irregularities, which can be corrected immediately with a fine cannula [Fig. 8]. Treatment consists in freeing the fibrous adherences, aspirating fat from the high areas, and injecting fat in the depressions [Figs. 9, 10].

Depressions are addressed by first freeing the fibrous adherences with the V-tip Toledo cannula and injecting fat. I obtain a 40% to 50% improvement on the skin irregularities, which is called subcision [Figs. 11, 12]. In many cases it is not necessary to inject fat, being sufficient only to perform fat shifting or fat mobilization. We use the Toledo V-tip cannula in the areas adjacent to the defect releasing the depression and mobilize the fat layer to a uniform position [Fig. 13]. There is a limit to skin retraction. Some patients prefer tight-looking skin, and if that can be achieved only by removing excess skin, it is better to perform a skin resection [Fig. 14].

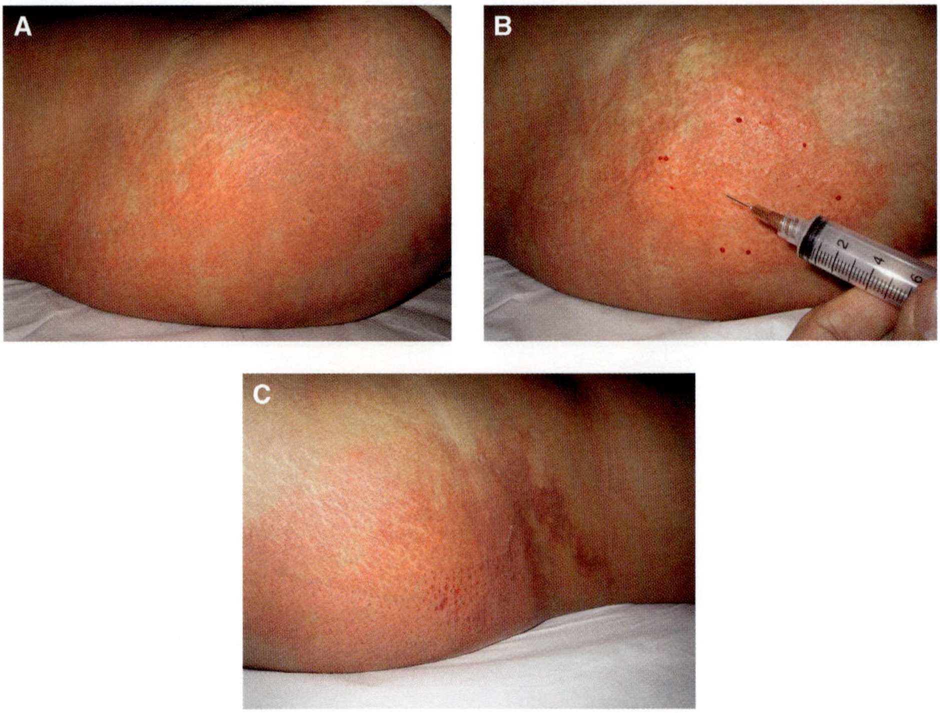

Fig. 15. (*A*) 24 hours after the operation, a vasculopathy on the right flank (*B*) was treated with intradermal injections of air. (*C*) One month after the operation with partial improvement.

Vasculopathy and cutaneous hyperpigmentation are usually connected. If we do not identify and treat the vasculopathy, it can produce cutaneous hyperpigmentation. In some cases it can be improved, but it can be permanent. The internal trauma provoked by the liposuction cannula can provoke skin sloughs that can result in skin discoloration or a more serious necrosis that will requires skin débridement. Vasculopathy sometimes may be difficult to identify. It starts postoperatively as an area of erythema that can be identified by digital pressure of the area. After a few weeks the area may become

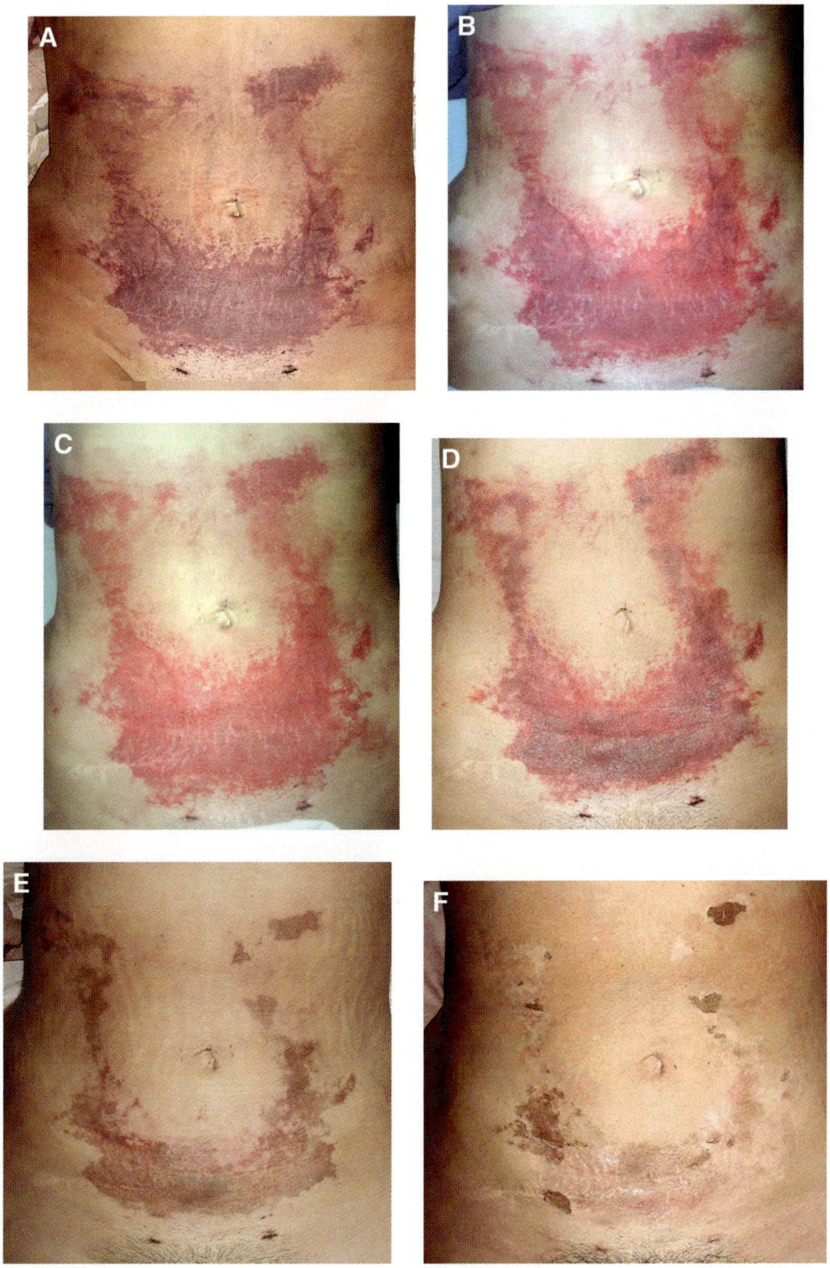

Fig. 16. (*A*) A 29-year-old patient 24 hours after lipoplasty, with aspiration of 8 L, with referred severe burning pain in the abdomen. (*B, C*) Patient at 36 hours after the operation, before (*B*) and after (*C*) the hyperbaric treatment. The patient at 6 days (*D*), 15 days (*E*), and 1 month (*F*) after the operation. Patient at 3 (*G*) and 6 (*H*) months after the operation. Hyperchromia was treated and has improved with 2% hydroquinone, Kojik acid, glycolic acid, and aloe vera. This patient received a total of 20 hyperbaric chamber sessions, one every 12 hours at 20 PSI for 60 minutes. (Courtesy of Dr. Carlos Alberto Guerrero, Cali, Colombia.)

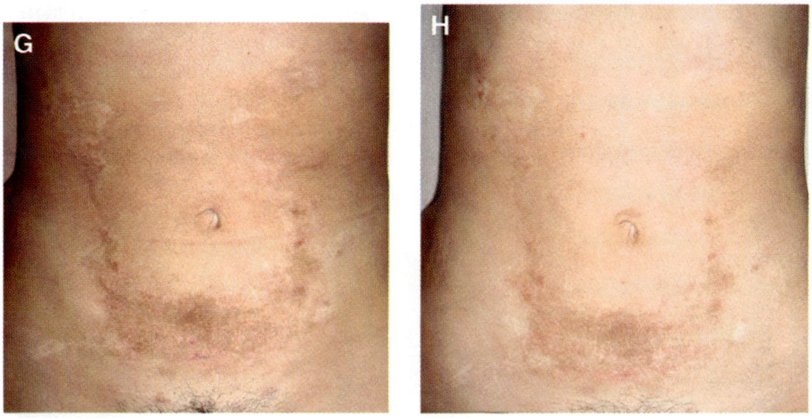

Fig. 16 (*continued*).

Box 4: Suggested steps for reducing and preventing complications of lipoplasty

- Ensure proper patient selection
- Ensure proper technique selection [21]
- Obtain preoperative examinations of the patient, including photographs, weight and measurements records, preoperative anamnesis, general information, and informed consent
- Determine how much surgery is contemplated and follow country and state regulations [22]
- Determine autologous blood/adequate blood bank availability
- Evaluate a patient's oxygenation, ventilation, circulation, and temperature continuously
- Control infiltrated volume intravenously and subcutaneously (37°C)
- Ensure complete sterilization and antibiotics
- Check patient position on the operating table
- Obtain patient photographs in the operating room
- Prevent deep venous thrombosis
- Ensure that laryngeal mask or intubation instruments are ready in the operating room
- Provide monitoring devices for patients in an outpatient setting (ie, pulse oximeters, disconnect alarms, continuous cardiac monitoring devices)
- Control duration of surgery
- Supply postoperative dressing and girdles with adequate compression
- Administer oxygen catheter when necessary for inpatients or temporary catheter for outpatients
- Provide adequate patient surveillance
- Schedule postoperative visit (on the day of and the first day after surgery)
- Educate patients that liposuction is not a treatment for obesity
- Take extra care with concomitant surgeries
- Have two people review the preparation of the anesthetic solution

hyperpigmented. The cause is probably the local trauma and consequent lack of oxygen at the capillary level.

Treatment can consist of five or six sessions in the hyperbaric chamber, but I also have treated it with intradermal injection of oxygen starting when I see the erythema [19]. The injections result in the immediate whitening of the area. I repeat the injections every other day for 1 to 2 weeks until the problem disappears or improves [Fig. 15]. Hyperbaric therapy can be used as prevention of or treatment of complications of lipoplasty [Fig. 16].

Summary

Box 4 provides a list of suggested steps to ensure the reduction and prevention of complications [20].

References

[1] Lehnhardt M, Homann HH, Druecke D, et al. No problem with liposuction? Chirurg 2003;74(9):808–14.

[2] Hughes CE. Reduction of lipoplasty risks and mortality: An ASAPS survey. Aesth Plast Surg 2001;21:120–7.

[3] Knipper P, Jauffret JL. Aesthetic snapshot: study about cosmetic surgical procedures and complications. Ann Chir Plast Esthet 2003;48(5):299–306.

[4] De Jong RH. Mega-dose lidocaine dangers seen in tumescent liposuction. Anesthesia Patient Safety Foundation Newsletter 1999;14(3):25–7.

[5] Richling N, Friedrich E, Deutinger M, et al. Surgical reduction of fat surplus leading to pulmonary embolism. Wien Klin Wochenschr 2004;116(24):854–7.

[6] Katz BE, Bruck MC, Felsenfeld L, et al. Power liposuction: a report on complications. Dermatol Surg 2003;29(9):925–7 [discussion 927].

[7] Topaz M. Possible long-term complications in

ultrasound-assisted lipoplasty induced by sonoluminescence, sonochemistry, and thermal effect. Aesthetic Surgery Journal 1998;18(1):19–24.
[8] Perez JA, van Tetering JP. Ultrasound-assisted lipoplasty: a review of over 350 consecutive cases using a two-stage technique. Aesthetic Plast Surg 2003;27(1):68–76.
[9] Nagelvoort RW, Hulstaert PF, Kon M, et al. Necrotising fasciitis and myositis as serious complications after liposuction. Ned Tijdschr Geneeskd 2002;146(50):2430–5.
[10] Ostad A, Kageyama N, Moy RL. Tumescent anesthesia with a lidocaine dose of 55 mg/kg is safe for liposuction. Dermatol Surg 1996;22(11): 921–7.
[11] Toledo LS, Regatieri FLF, Carneiro JDA. The effect of hypothermia on coagulation and its implications for infiltration in lipoplasty: a review. Aesthetic Surgery Journal 2001;21(1):40–4.
[12] Samdal F, Amland PF, Bugge JF. Blood loss during liposuction using the tumescent technique. Aesthetic Plast Surg 1994;18(2):157–60.
[13] Fourme T, Vieillard-Baron A, Loubieres Y, et al. Early fat embolism after liposuction. Anesthesiology 1998;89(3):782–4.
[14] Boezaart AP, Clinton CW, Braun S, et al. Fulminant adult respiratory distress syndrome after suction lipectomy. S Afr Med J 1990;78(11):693–5.
[15] Laub Jr DR, Laub DR. Fat embolism after liposuction: a case report and review of the literature. Ann Plast Surg 1990;2:48–52.
[16] Christman KD. Death following suction lipectomy and abdominoplasty. Plast Reconstr Surg 1986;78:428–30.
[17] Ross RM, Johnson GW. Fat embolism after liposuction. Chest 1988;93:1294–5.
[18] Abbes M, Bourgeon Y. Case report of fat embolism after dermolipectomy and liposuction. Ann Chir Plast Esthet 1989;34:160–1.
[19] Dillerud E. Abdominoplasty combined with suction lipoplasty: a study of complications, revisions, and risk factors in 487 cases. Ann Plast Surg 1990;25:48–53.
[20] Grazer FM. Body contouring. In: McCarthy JM, editor. Plastic surgery. Philadelphia: WB Saunders; 1990. p. 3964–4028.
[21] Siddiky SA, Malo AK, Wahab A, et al. Tulip liposuction in plastic surgery. Mymensingh Med J 2002;11(2):82–6.
[22] Tumescent Liposuction. Minnesota Department of Health. Available at: http://www.health.state.mn.us/htac/lipo.htm. Accessed May 2002.

ELSEVIER
SAUNDERS

CLINICS IN PLASTIC SURGERY

Clin Plastic Surg 33 (2006) 13–25

Liposuction: Techniques and Guidelines

Joseph P. Hunstad, MD, FACS[a,*], Marguerite E. Aitken, MD, MFA[b]

Schrudde first introduced the closed lipectomy, a sharp excisional technique using uterine curettes in the early 1970s [1]. Kesselring [2], and separately Fischer [3], conceived evacuating the fat also using sharp suction techniques. Although Fischer sharply separated the fat to be removed using a planotome, Kesselring connected suction to a double-bladed sharp curette for fat removal. He advocated minimal fluid, fat removal in layers and diffuse undermining of the areas being treated.

Illouz, however, in 1977, introduced the revolutionary concept of tunneling, rather than undermining, in a layered fashion using a blunt-tipped cannula [3]. The "wet technique" gained wide acceptance, rapidly growing in popularity in the United States through the efforts of Hetter, Grazer, and Teimourian [1]. Many improvements have been made to the technique since its inception, including changes to the injected fluid, cannulae design, ultrasonic liposuction, and power-assisted liposuction.

Early liposuction procedures saw careful selection of patients in whom good results could be anticipated. This included those with lipodystrophy or localized adiposity that could be removed easily with suctioning. As the field expanded and experience was gained over the ensuing years, more and more patients were considered appropriate candidates, including obese patients in whom large volumes of fat could be safely suctioned [4]. We find in the United States that it is unrealistic to expect every patient to be at their ideal body

[a] The Hunstad Center, 8605 Cliff Carmeron Drive, Suite 100, Charlotte, NC 28269, USA
[b] Plastic Surgery Associates, P.C., Grand Plaza Place, 220 Lyon Street NW, Suite 700, Grand Rapids, MI 49503, USA
* Corresponding author.
E-mail address: jph1@hunstadcenter.com (J.P. Hunstad).

0094-1298/06/$ – see front matter doi:10.1016/j.cps.2005.09.003
plasticsurgery.theclinics.com

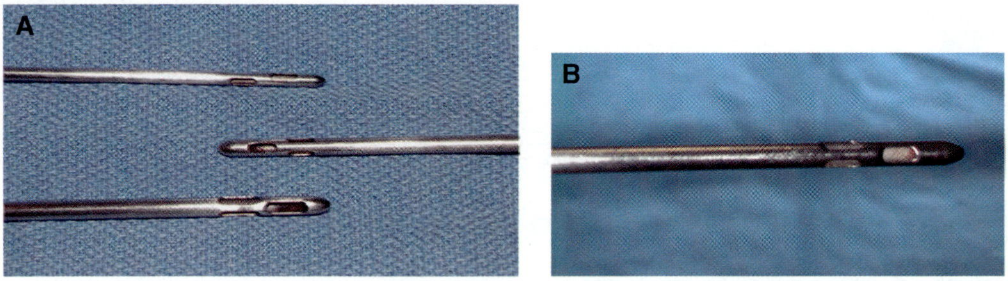

Fig. 1. (*A*) Multiple sizes of the pyramid tip cannula designed by Hetter. (*B*) Details of the pyramid tip.

weight. Many have tried multiple diets and exercise, unsuccessfully. Although this is not a procedure for weight loss, it can achieve improved body contour, overall size decrease, and act as a stimulus for further weight loss.

Cannulae

Illouz's first description used a large-diameter cannula, allowing a very aggressive removal of adipose tissue. Fat was pulled into the cannula openings, held there by vacuum pressure, and avulsed with cannula movement. As the technique began to be performed by other surgeons around the world, indications came to include patients who only needed body contouring for localized pockets of stubborn adiposity. This technique has evolved from essentially a "bump removal" procedure to a sophisticated body shaping and contouring method with cannula size reduction for more precise control of the fat removal and less risk of creating waviness commonly seen with a large-diameter cannula (personal communication with Mladick, 1996). This further allowed more gradual fat removal and decreased the risk of overresection and asymmetry.

Although the original single-port, blunt-tipped suction cannulae became popular, improvements for newer, more effective suction methods were subsequently introduced.

Today, cannula openings can be one sided or unidirectional, or they may be omni-directional and located circumferentially. The Pyramid or Las Vegas tip, designed by Hetter, has one distal and two proximal ports for suction in a unidirectional pattern and concentrated proximally, not adjacent to the skin [**Fig. 1**].

This is in comparison to the so-called Mercedes tip cannulae [**Fig. 2**], in which the ports are spaced evenly around the circumference of the cannulae and equidistant from the tip. When concerned with skin protection in areas such as over difficult bony prominences, more superficial suctioning, or in densely adherent areas, we prefer a directional blunt-tipped proximally concentrated cannula such as the Pyramid cannula. In areas such as the neck and face, Klein directional flattened cannulae [**Fig. 3**] glide easily through the relatively thin tissues, preserving the subdermal plexus of vessels. In the back and thicker areas, where dense adherent tissues exist, we employ basket cannulae [**Fig. 4**] a very aggressive *open cutting tipped* tool for fat aspiration in deeper tissues only.

Cannulae of ultrasound-assisted lipoplasty

In 7% to 10% of our patients, we find the ultrasound very helpful to liquefy fat before removal, particularly in the male back, chest, and for secondary procedures. Although bifunctional ultrasound cannulae that both liquefy and suction are available, we prefer to use a solid probe cannula. This maintains the liquid environment in

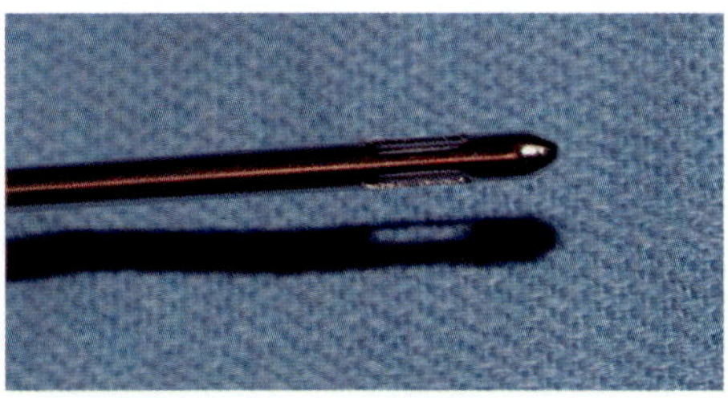

Fig. 2. Mercedes tip with evenly spaced ports equidistant from tip.

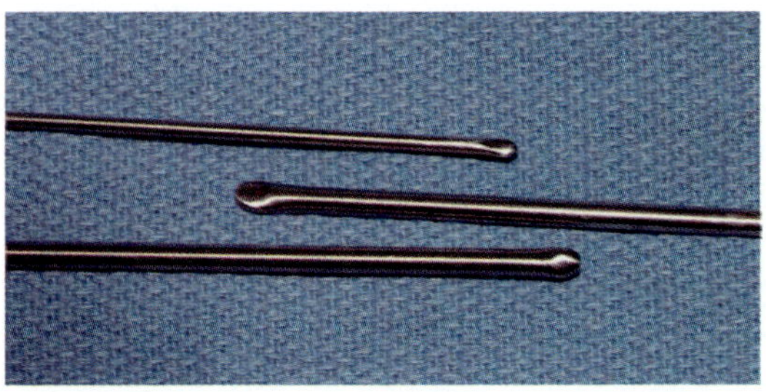

Fig. 3. Klein directional flattened cannulae for face and neck areas.

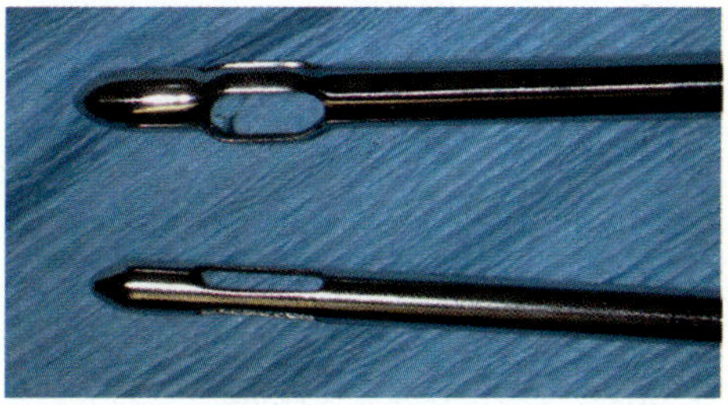

Fig. 4. Basket cannula compared with the Mercedes tip cannula.

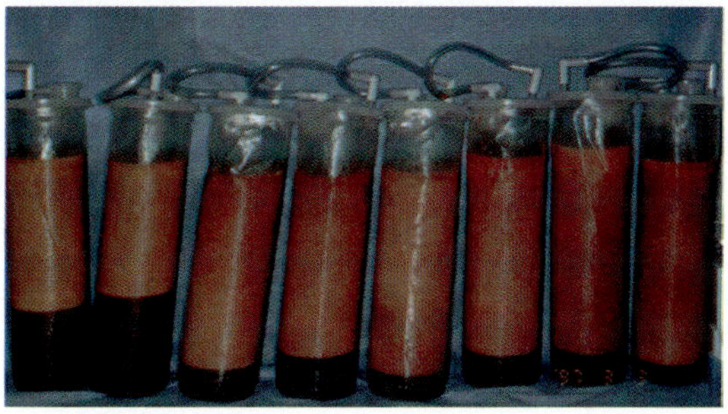

Fig. 5. Aspirated fat demonstrating the majority of the aspirate is yellow fat.

which ultrasound is most effective, dispersing the ultrasound energy more quickly and accelerating the procedure.

Safety guidelines

Our patients undergo liposuction procedures in our accredited facility. We also prefer general anesthesia provided by an experienced anesthesiologist for better control of the airway in all positions, for improved patient comfort, and for overall relaxation of the patient and surgeon. Those patients requiring or preferring to overnight in our facility, do so fully monitored, with a registered nurse at the bedside, and are released the following morning.

Recent recommendations made by the task force assembled by the American Society of Plastic Surgeons (ASPS) were prompted by reports of anesthetic complications, including deaths related to liposuction, and defined in the Practice Advisory on Liposuction, 2004 [5]. Anesthetic options should be selected by the anesthesia provider and plastic surgeon based on the overall health of the patient the estimated volume of the aspirate to be removed, and the postoperative dismissal plan. Although anesthesia may be delivered by either an anesthesiologist, a Certified Registered Nurse Anesthetist, or by another qualified health care provider, under physician supervision, the primary responsibility for the providing the anesthetic should be a physician [5]. Due to the risk of vasodilatation, hypotension, and fluid overload, it was not recommended by the task force that spinal or epidural anesthesia be used in the office setting. Combination anesthesia, such as intravenous, intramuscular, or oral analgesia with moderate sedation titrated to the patients comfort level can be an effective adjunct to infiltration anesthesia [5].

For treating obese patients, the ASPS Advisory group noted that there is an increased rate of complications associated with higher volumes of aspirates and number of regions treated [5]. It is their recommendation to treat those patients in whom total aspirates are expected to reach >5000 mL more cautiously by performing the procedure in an accredited facility or acute care hospital, and with the proper monitors and qualified overnight staff. In addition to these measures outlined for large-volume procedures, to avoid the need for transfusion, aspirates should contain mainly fat [Fig. 5].

Relative contraindications to liposuction include disease states such as diabetes, bowel, pulmonary, or bladder dysfunction, coronary artery disease, and immunodeficiency states, males with significant intraabdominal fat and huge girth, and patients with unrealistic expectations. They require a realistic explanation of results that may fall below their desire.

Current technique

The patient is marked standing in the photo suite preoperatively. Areas to be treated are drawn in a topographical manner, anticipating the feathering of the technique at the margins [Fig. 6]. Access sites

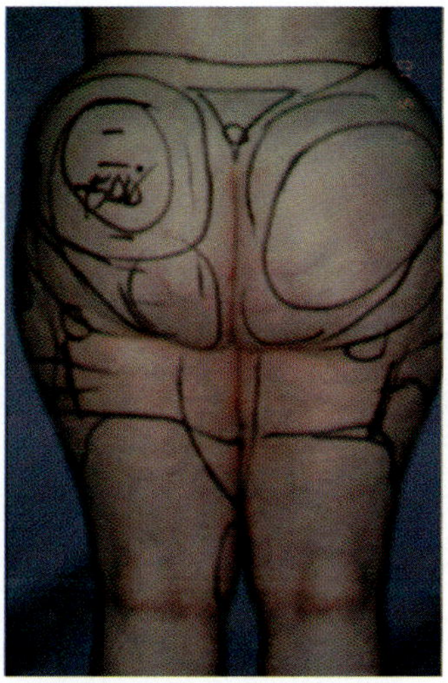

Fig. 6. Topographical diagram demonstrates feathering of the suction planned onto other body areas.

are discussed with the patient and agreed upon. The author has preferences for typical access sites; however, certain patient requests are common, and these are taken into consideration as long as it seems feasible with cannula length, patient size, and area to be treated.

The patient is placed supine on either the operating room (OR) gurney or table, depending on the areas to be treated. Sequential compression devices are placed on the patient and activated *prior* to the induction of general anesthesia. Intubation is via endotracheal tube due to the need unless the patient will remain supine in which a laryngeal mask airway could be appropriate. The patient is properly padded and warmed using a Bair hugger (Arizant Health Care, Eden Prairie, Minnesota), tumescent **fluid and IV fluids are warmed**, and general anesthesia induction is performed. The entry sites are prepped with betadine, and the tumescent fluid is infiltrated. The modified Hunstad tumescent fluid (warmed Lactated Ringers plus 25 mg Lidocaine and 1000 μg epinephrine) in the half strength is used, unless the estimated aspiration volume is considered large. If so, we further reduce the lidocaine to one quarter strength (12.5 mg/L).

The volume of fluid infiltrated depends on the tissue characteristics. Lighter, fluffier fat, such as the abdomen, takes up more tumescence as the tissues expand and fill. More dense tissues, such the back, are less distensible and fill more quickly with infiltration fluid. The endpoint is a firm, full, turgid, blanching tissue with a positive fountain sign [Fig. 7] [6].

Peau' de orange is undesirable due to the superficial nature of this fluid. Instead, infiltration should be into all layers, from the loose areolar plane above the deep muscle fascia to above the superficial fascia, tunneling the cannula throughout.

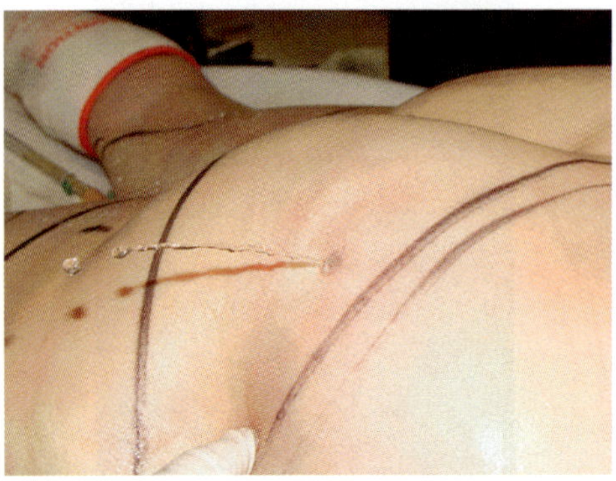

Fig. 7. Fountain sign demonstrating adequately infiltrated tissues.

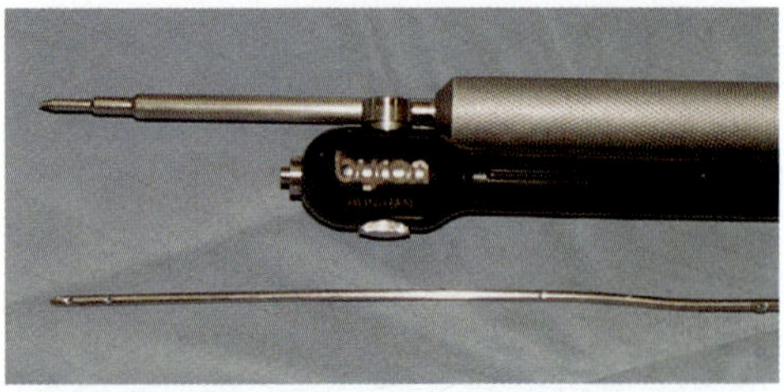

Fig. 8. Upper instrument is a stepped awl device for creating graded entry sites, lower instrument is a three-hole infiltration cannula.

Typically, a long 3-mm, multihole, blunt-tipped infiltration cannula (Byron, Tucson, Arizona) is used for this [Fig. 8]. Infiltration fluid is perfused through all areas to be suctioned and beyond.

Estimating the aspiration volume

For the plastic surgeon with limited experience, it can be helpful to preoperatively estimate the volume of anticipated fat removal to properly infiltrate the tissues, to have the warmed tumescent fluids readily available in the OR, and to anticipate postoperative care plans. The 60-cc Toomey syringe technique can be a helpful method of estimating these volumes. The aspirated volume using the proper tumescent technique is significantly larger than using the standard infiltration technique. Preoperatively, the surgeon should pinch the excess fat, imagining the size of a Toomey 60-cc syringe. Next, the number of syringes needed to equal the fat present should be counted and the volume to remove estimated through calculation [Fig. 9]. Intraoperatively, the surgeon should liposuction to within 10% of the estimated volume and measure the fat to verify adequacy of removal [7].

In the early 1980s, standard liposuction was taught with 10 passes of the cannula in a single tunnel followed by cannula repositioning, 10 more passes, and so on. This can leave skip areas and cause a washboard deformity. Now, we approach each area creating many tunnels, each with a single pass of the cannula, pulling it back completely in each pass. We perform all-layer liposuction in most regions, starting at the superficial plane and suctioning downward below the superficial fascia until reaching the deep fascia. The topographical markings made preoperatively are indicators of the treated areas and the point at which to begin feathering out the technique.

Asymmetries are addressed with careful attention to the volumes infused and aspirated. Clinical examination after the procedure endpoint is reached

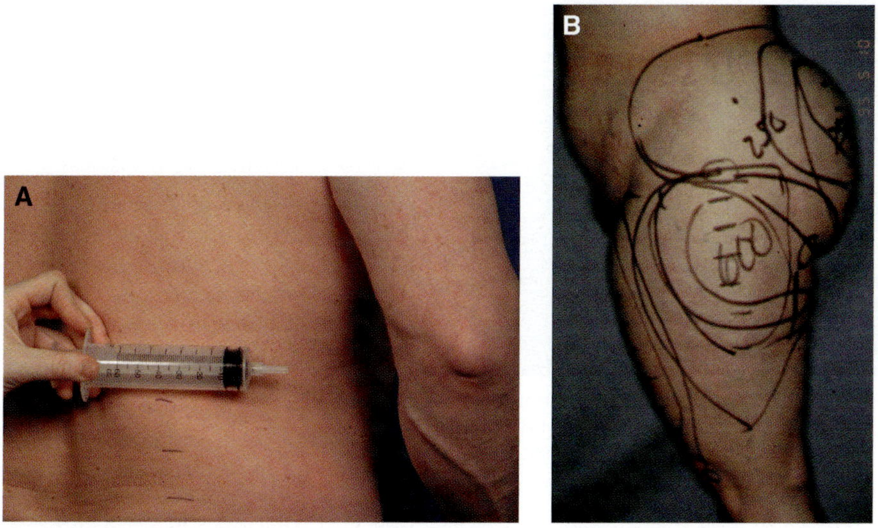

Fig. 9. Syringe (60 cc) technique to estimate the volume to be aspirated. (*A*) Diagram of the number of syringes to be filled with aspirated fat. (*B*) Estimate the total volume anticipated for removal, 600 cc.

should then be adequate to recognize and treat most asymmetries.

Syringe technique

The syringe technique popularized by Toledo [8] can be either an effective primary tool for all liposuction procedures or a useful inexpensive option for treatment of minor local areas. It has been reported before in the Clinics of Plastic Surgery [9], and continues to be, in this day of power-assisted liposuction, an excellent option for limited treatment areas in a manner identical to those treated with machine vacuum pumps. It is simply a combination of a Toomey tip syringe connected to the liposuction cannula with suction applied to the proximal end of the syringe. A locking ring holds the plunger back, creating the vacuum for suctioning. There is no tubing attached, which enables the operator to have more freedom, improved control, and enhanced precision. The other advantages of the syringe technique are (1) low cost, (2) silent OR, (3) accurate quantifiable volumes, and (4) ideal for harvest for fat injection. The disadvantages of this technique are that the suction can be lost at the access sites, particularly when using the short cannula or in small areas being treated. There is a definite need for an assistant in the OR, and it can be a relatively slow process compared with the motorized techniques. However, the gradual achievement of the final contour can be a benefit, as it decreases the chance of creating depressions and overresection. Difficult areas such as the face and neck are particularly well suited for syringe technique, especially for touchup liposuction or for use with fat injection. When treating large areas with significant volumes to be removed, larger, more aggressive cannulae will enable effective evacuation.

Suction-assisted lipoplasty

Suction-assisted lipoplasty, otherwise known as SAL, is the workhorse of liposuction. We use a remote liposuction pump to create a more inviting atmosphere in the OR (quieter) [**Fig. 10**]. Topographical lines made preoperatively assist the surgeon in identifying areas in need of treatment. A graded awl device creates the perfect hemostatic access site in the skin fitting the cannula to be used [**Fig. 11**]. The technique of suctioning inside of a pinch of tissue is not commonly used during the

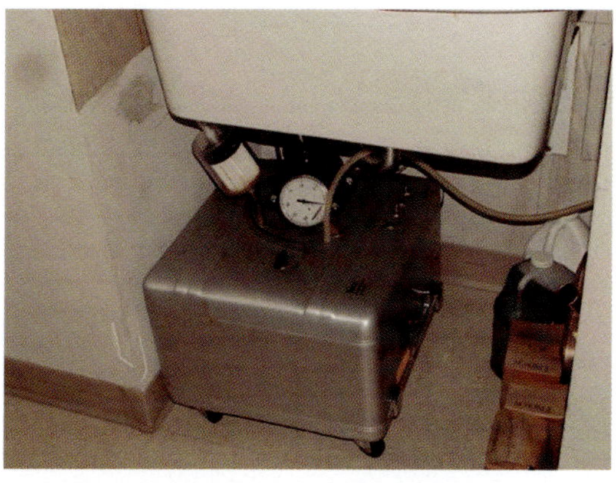

Fig. 10. Remote location for liposuction pump creates an inviting, quieter OR.

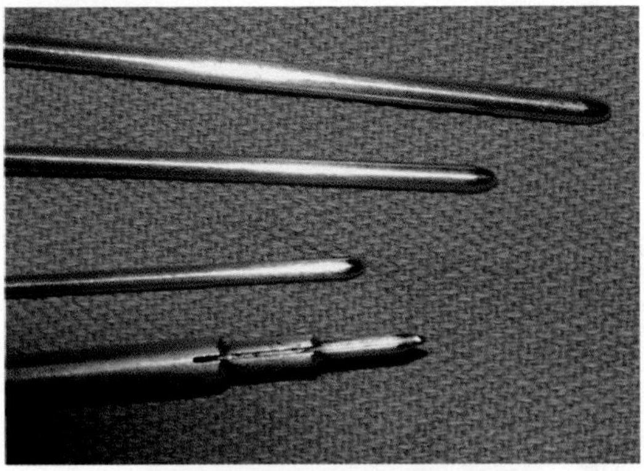

Fig. 11. Graded stepped awl shown with cannula of comparable diameter to level of the awl. Machined channel on side of awl opens puncture-resistant access sites.

process of liposuction, due to the possibility of inconsistent removal of fat from the overlying skin. We prefer the radial tunneling method of fanning out the cannula creating individual tunnels in multiple layers from which fat is removed sequentially at different levels. We begin the process in the upper level of fat and gradually descend below the superficial fascia as the tissues are reduced in thickness.

Superficial liposuction

Techniques of superficial liposuction, such as described by De Souza Pinto, Lewis, Gasparotti, and Toledo, and performed in the tissues above the superficial facial system, are applicable in any region of the body where significant skin retraction is desired [10]. Even in the most skilled surgical hands, however, it carries with it a higher risk of skin injury and must be differentiated from subdermal liposuction. Relying upon skin retraction, the technique is particularly valuable for the infragluteal fold when dermal sutures can result in buttock ptosis.

Subdermal lipo

Suctioning very superficially below the dermis can be very dangerous, and risk interruption of the delicate vascular plexus, carrying with it a high risk of subsequent waviness and irregularities. There are few indications for this technique. Some examples include the creation of a gluteal crease and for body etching.

Differential liposuction

Gilliland and Mentz used this term to describe the use of precise suction techniques to create a space devoid of fat outlining, for instance, the rectus muscles and their inscriptions, abdominal etching [11].

Ultrasound-assisted liposuction

Ultrasound energy applied to liposuction is useful when treating tissues that are extremely fibrous and for secondary procedures. Backs and male abdomens and breasts are all good examples of excellent times to use this technique. The procedure requires the surgeon to use caution with regard to the skin, as burning the skin can occur due to the friction and heat created with the cannula. Skin protectors are recommended. Originally, ultrasound used for industrial purposes was modified by Zocchi with solid cannulae, creating collapsing cavernous tissues [12]. This was a two-stage process, with emulsification followed by the use of skin rollers expelling the liquefied fat.

American surgeons requested the development of a hollow cannula that allowed both delivery of ultrasound waves and simultaneous fat aspiration. It was believed that this simultaneous application of energy and aspiration would to speed up the overall process. As delivery of the energy is most effective in a fluid environment, we prefer to deliver ultrasonic energy to achieve emulsification without aspiration. This is clinically determined by the loss of resistance to cannula passage. Post-emulsification evacuation is then performed using power-assisted liposuction (PAL)/SAL techniques. We perform about 10% of all liposuction procedures using the ultrasound machine, and we use a solid cannula. Suctioning out the fat is performed identically to standard suction, beginning at a superficial point and suctioning down toward the fascia. This technique appears to be efficient, using less time than without the ultrasound machine. Care should be taken to treat each side symmetrically and to avoid end-hits in the skin.

Power-assisted liposuction

PAL, developed initially by Microaire (MicroAire Surgical Instruments, Charlottesville, Virginia) has become important to liposuction. It functions similarly to SAL with a cannula that rapidly shifts back and forth in the tissues to more quickly and easily direct the fenestrations to fatty deposits in need of removal [**Fig. 12**]. The benefits are many, and include causing less physician fatigue, which probably allows for a more thorough complete liposuction result. Fat is more rapidly removed, decreasing OR time, we find less resistance to cannulae passage and an increase in accuracy overall, particularly

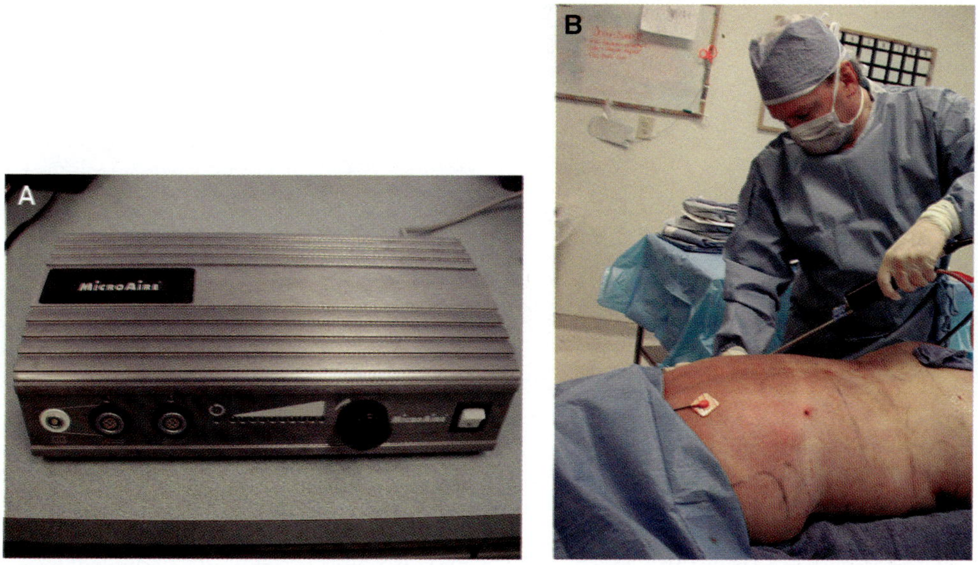

Fig. 12. (*A*) Microaire power-assisted liposuction machine and (*B*) its implementation in the OR.

in those areas near the entry sites, lessening the chance of leaving residual fatty deposits.

Liposuction of specific regions

Although patients will present with obvious localized areas of fat deposition, treatment should encompass the individual as a whole, and careful consideration of the entire body is recommended to assure proper contouring. For instance, treatment of the hips and waist, but failure to address neighboring regions of the body such the lateral thigh or the back, can result in an unbalanced appearance and patient dissatisfaction. Table 1 summarizes the approach that we use in our practice for the varying regions of the body presenting for liposuction.

Face/neck

Liposuction of the neck is a commonly performed adjuctive procedure to platysmoplasty and rhytidectomy procedures. It is useful for those patients with mild to significant thickness of the neck tissues, and often continues up onto the face. Occasionally, a patient suffering the ill effects of steroid use may be encountered requesting face and neck liposuction; however, more often it is the obese patient or one with a familial tendency who will present for this procedure. We inject the tumescent solution via a hand-held spring loaded injection system [**Fig. 13**A]. For either neck or face liposuction, a small directional cannula (1.5–3 mm) is recommended, keeping the ports directed away from the skin to avoid dermal trauma with dimpling and scarring caused by damage to the delicate

***Table 1:* The Hunstad approach to specific regions for treatment**

Location	Entry sites	Position	Range of infused volume	Drain
Abdomen	Groin, umbilicus, inframammary	Supine	3–6 L	Yes
Back	Bra-line (single or paired), buttocks, axilla	Prone	3–6 L	Yes
Hip rolls	Buttocks	Prone -> supine	1–3 L	No
Outer thigh	Gluteal crease, groin	Prone	1–3 L	No
Circumferential thigh	Groin, gluteal crease, knee	Prone -> supine	4–6 L	No
Neck	Postauricular submental	Supine	1/2 L	No
Arms	Anterior posterior axilla, elbow	Supine	1–2 L	No
Buttocks	Infragluteal, apical buttock	Prone	2–3 L	No
Inner thigh	Groin, infragluteal	Prone -> supine	1–2 L	No

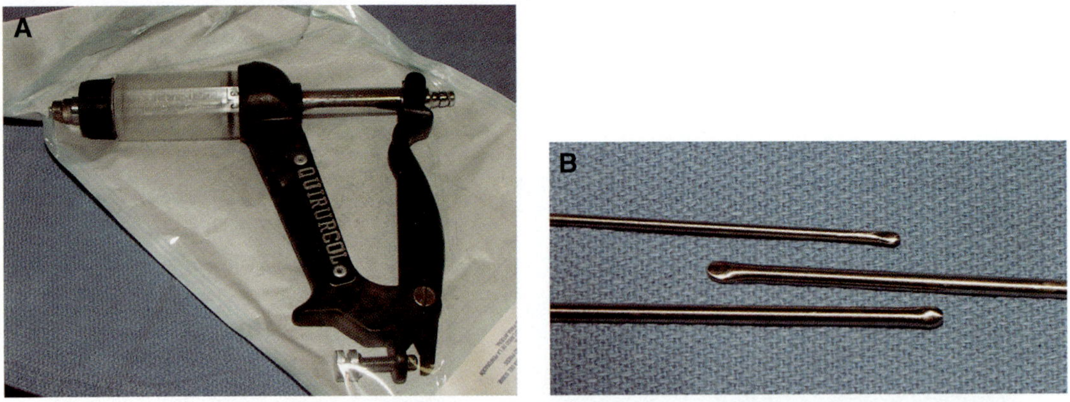

Fig. 13. (*A*) Hand-held infuser for tumescent fluid infiltration of the face. (*B*) Small Klein directional flat-tipped cannulae useful for the face and neck sculpting.

subdermal vascular plexus [Fig. 13B]. This is also an ideal time for use of the syringe technique to free the surgeon from the tethering of the tubing, to more accurately measure the volumes removed and more gradually reach the desired endpoint. A crisscross technique is important to treat the area without leaving residual waviness. This can be performed through a minute incision in the submental crease, behind the lobule in a postauricular position, or at the root of the helix. A slight undercorrection is strongly advised due to the improvement seen secondary to reabsorption of the tumescent solution and damaged fat cells [13]. The pinch technique can be used to assess adequacy of aspiration, symmetry, and resulting contour. Significant bruising and swelling can be uncomfortable, and the patient is encouraged to use a compressive neck garment postoperatively. Marginal mandibular nerve palsy is not unexpected with thorough or aggressive suctioning of the neck or over the mandible and jowls, and the patient should be warned in advance.

Abdomen

Indications for liposuction of the abdomen [Figs. 14 and 15] include those with minimal to moderate skin laxity and diastasis recti. Access sites preferred by these authors are in the bilateral bikini lines, which allow the entire lower abdomen to be adequately suctioned, in addition to the anterolateral hips. An intraumbilical access site is also used to suction the upper abdomen. The fat of the abdomen tends to be relatively soft and fluffy, absorbing the tumescence rapidly. One should be aware of the speed in which this fat can be suctioned, paying particular attention to the volumes being removed to avoid overresection defects. Although we prefer PAL, the syringe technique works well here to more gradually achieve the final contour. Care should be taken to thoroughly evaluate the abdomen for possible hernias or abdominal wall defects, which could lead to intraabominal perforation. The defects usually exist in the midline, and we believe a midline entry site should be avoided in the lower abdomen. Paired inguinal entry sites are preferred. Liposuction should gradually descend to a deeper level (below the superficial fascia) as more and more fat is removed. The potentially lethal sequelae of abdominal liposuction require a fully informed patient consent preoperatively and a knowledgeable practitioner.

Arms

The arms respond well with impressive retraction and redraping, and should be treated in a circumferential manner. Although the majority of complaints will be the inferior aspect of the arm, slenderizing the entire arm will produce a more optimal result. Care should be taken to avoid oversuctioning the medial arm area where the fat is thin, soft, and fluffy, and can be quite easily overdone. Patient selection again plays an important role for this area, as some patients will present with the "bat wing" deformity and nonretractable skin, unlikely to be improved with liposuction. We emphasize to all patients that liposuction thins, it does not tighten or lift!

The entry sites for this area are in the axilla and the elbow. The ulnar and volar forearms, too, can be improved with liposuction, creating a more complete result, and can be accessed via the antecubital fossa. Postoperatively, Ace-wraps, from the base of the fingers wrapped upwardly to the axilla with lessening pressure, can be safely removed the

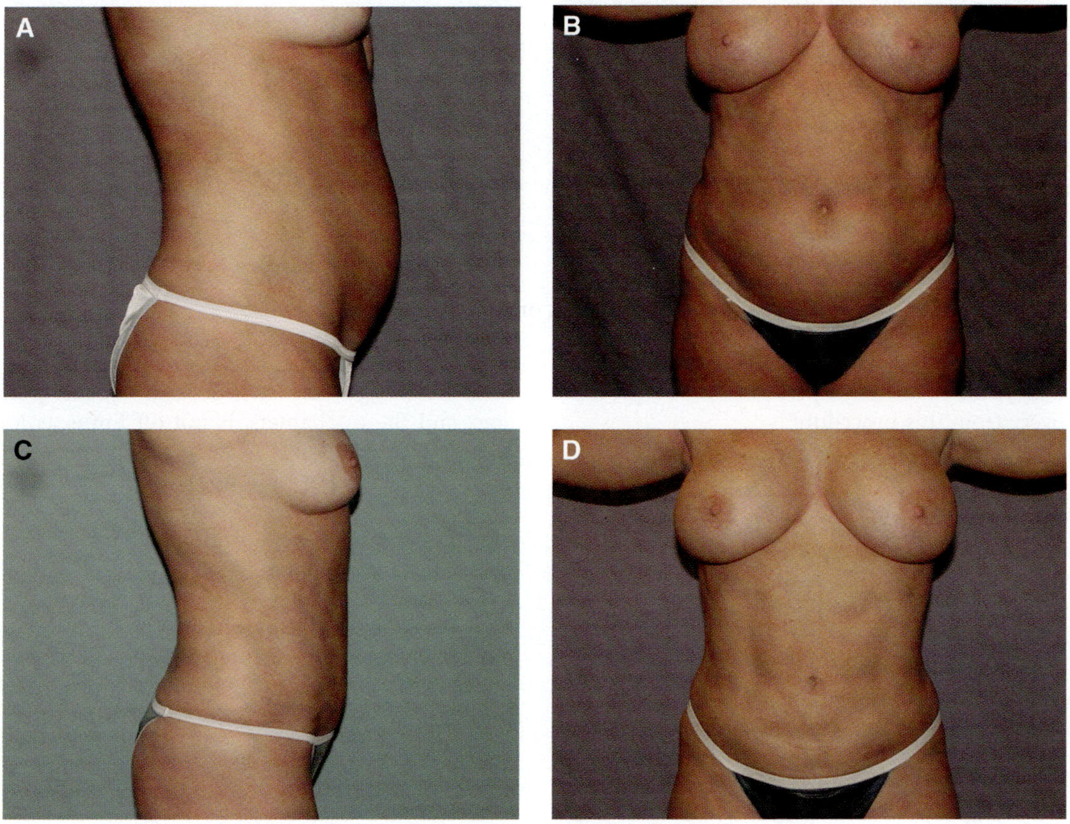

Fig. 14. (*A–D*) Preoperative and postoperative photos of abdominal liposuction.

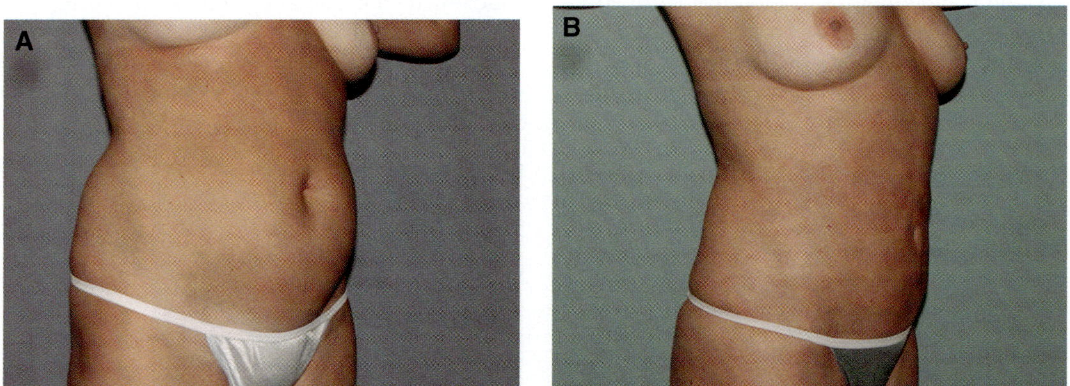

Fig. 15. (*A,B*) Preoperative and early postoperative photos of abdominal liposuction.

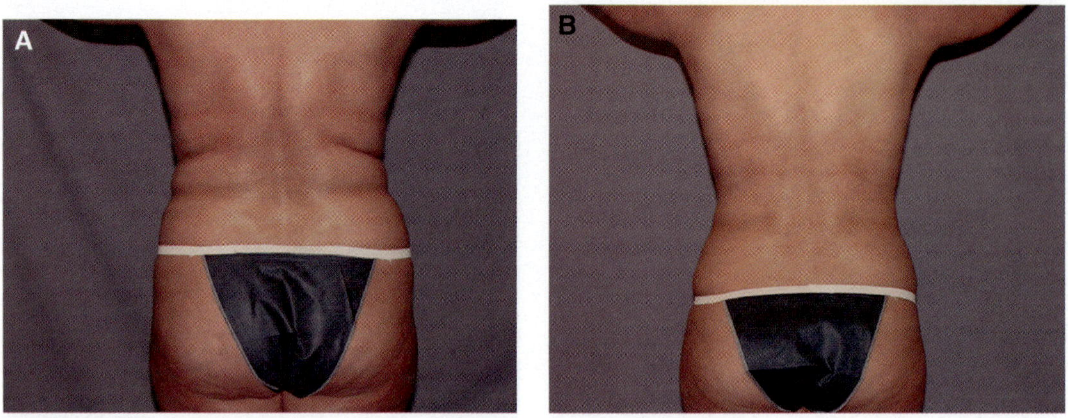

Fig. 16. (*A,B*) Preoperative and postoperative photos of back liposuction.

next day, and patients experience a very prompt recovery from this procedure.

Back

The back is a commonly treated area [Fig. 16], which is accessed by these authors through bilateral or unilateral bra-line and gluteal sites. It has more densely adherent, fibrous tissues, and we use the basket cannula for aggressive cutting-type resection and release of the tethered rolls beneath the scapula. A roll or bump may be used to gently flex the patient at the midline to more easily address the lumbar region.

Buttocks

Liposuction of the buttocks [Fig. 17] is often disputed as a safe procedure due to the risk of buttock ptosis following removal of supportive fat or structural tissues. The buttocks, previously thought to be off limits to liposuction for fear of the development of ptosis, are routinely treated. The so-called *Bermuda triangle*, the area defined by the gluteal apex and the trochanters, is not off limits as long as a uniform thickness of fat is maintained and a thorough tumescent infiltration is performed. This infiltration is critical to hydrate the tissues, allowing easy cannula passage, minimizing the chance of elastic fiber trauma, and promoting excellent skin retraction. Maintaining the supportive pillars originally described by Gasparotti [14] of the lower gluteal attachments will keep the position of the buttocks intact, while improving the contour, achieving an overall reduction in the size, and allowing the skin to redrape and retract properly. The access sites for this area are the gluteal apex and paired infragluteal entry sites.

Hip rolls

Significant improvement can be achieved with reduction in the size and contour of the hip rolls, primarily for the female patient. Commonly this is approached in combination with back liposuction or the lateral thigh. Entry sites are bilateral superior

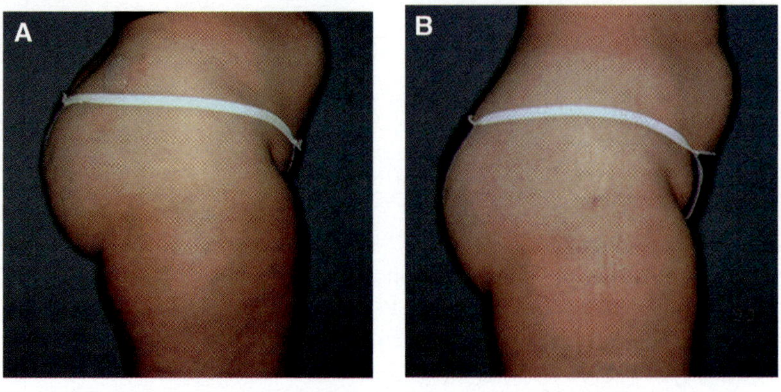

Fig. 17. (*A,B*) Preoperative and postoperative results of buttocks liposuction.

gluteal region, below the bikini line, and anteriorly in the inguinal crease.

Thighs

The thighs [Fig. 18] are a location that can be suctioned from many directions depending on the area being treated. Although in the past we used primarily the frog-leg position for circumferential thighs or saddlebag deformity, our approach has evolved into the use of sequential supine and prone positioning.

Particular attention must be paid to the effect of the buttock on the lateral thigh and infragluteal area. In relaxation, it may appear that the trochanteric deformity is quite severe, only to disappear with contraction of the buttocks. This change may suggest that the deformity of the lateral thigh is less severe, and the bulging seen on exam is actually due to the ptosis of the buttocks. Attention may then be turned to the buttock as the source of the problem [15].

Recovery after thigh liposuction is much more significant with circumferential thigh liposuction than with lateral or medial thigh due to the circumferential nature of the procedure. Despite this, patients who desire only medial or lateral thigh suctioning should be considered for circumferential thigh liposuction as it effectively diminishes the "heavy look" of the thigh and creates a longer, leaner appearance to the leg. Over 90% of our patients choose circumferential thigh liposuction. Entry sites for the thigh include the inguinal crease and the infragluteal crease and occasionally the peripatellar and posterior knees as indicated.

Calves/ankles

Requests for contouring of the lower leg are much less common. Because there is only a single layer of subcutaneous tissues between the skin and the deep fascia, this area is less forgiving in terms of resulting waviness and irregularities. Prolonged swelling is not unusual following treatment of this difficult area. Entry sites include paired popliteal fossa, paired peri-achilles tendon, and pretibial, although these are not ideal. Care must be taken to avoid injury to the underlying muscle, which can cause significant swelling and potentially a compartment syndrome. Postoperatively, compression

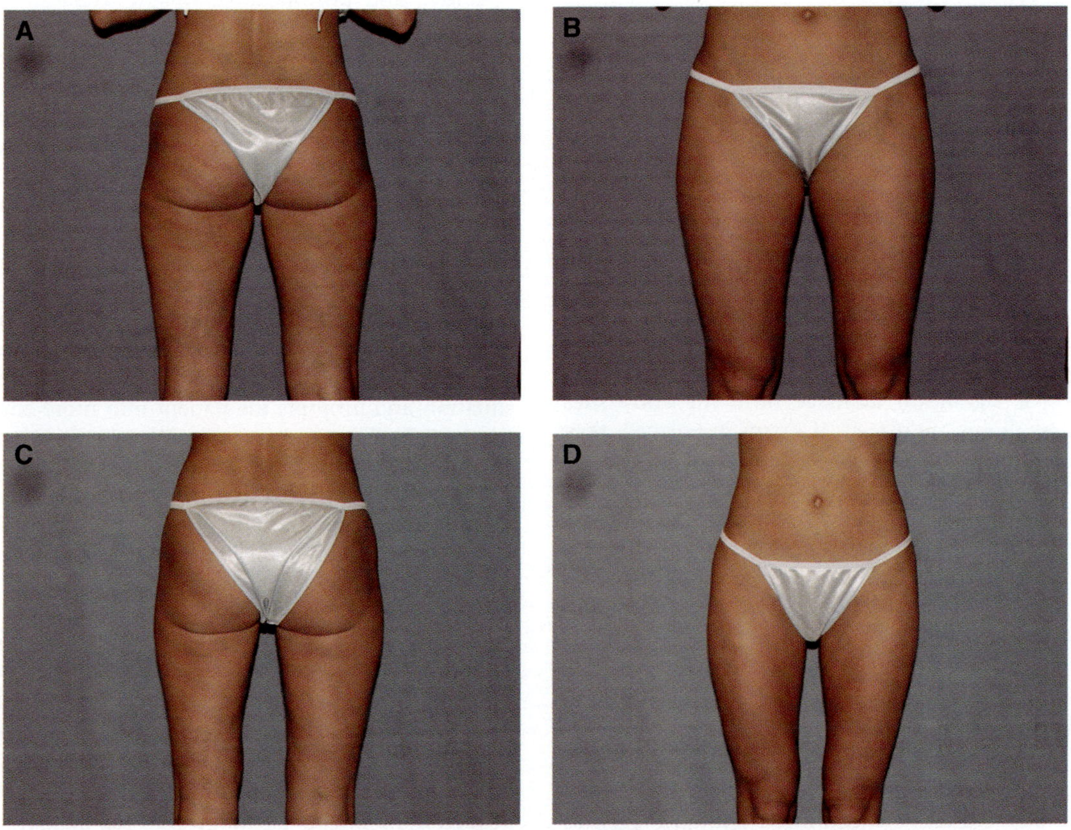

Fig. 18. (*A–D*) Preoperative and postoperative photos (1 year) following circumferential thigh liposuction.

hose, leg elevation, and sequential compressive garments can lessen the morbidity.

Touchup liposuction

Because anatomy and fat distribution vary by nature, liposuction is prone to require frequent touchups. When multiple bilateral areas are treated it is very possible to achieve a less than perfectly symmetric result. In these cases, however, a slight undercorrection is much more preferable to an overcorrection. Although touchup liposuction under local anesthesia is easily performed, fat grafting is a much more involved procedure and should be avoided if possible. The financial considerations for touchup procedures are individualized, yet should be spelled out ahead of time and agreed to by the patient.

Dressings

Evenly dispersed gentle postoperative compression is the goal. According to Illouz, this pressure should be between 17 and 21 mm of mercury to be both effective and harmless, as higher pressures may contribute to venous stasis [16]. This can be achieved through the use of compressive garments with the appropriate size chosen. Foam placed within the garments is used to more effectively distribute the pressure, especially at the flexion points and areas of possible creasing where it is helpful at minimizing bruising.

Postoperative care

Patients are routinely seen back in the office 1 to 2 days following surgery to assess their healing and answer any questions. Patients are sent home with a compressive garment over the area treated and expected to wear it for 3 to 8 weeks. Commonly, there is significant drainage from the entry sites unless drains are placed. If drains are placed, they are connected to a high-vacuum wall suction to facilitate more rapid fluid evacuation. For patients who overnight, they remain connected to suction until discharge. At the first postoperative visit, areas of skin that appear mottled are treated topically with a steroid cream to improve blood flow and diminish swelling.

Troubleshooting

It is important to remember that it is much easier to remove too much fat than to replace it. Cannula size and aggressive suctioning techniques such as PAL or ultrasound-assisted liposuction may lead to subtle asymmetries that should be addressed. Skin retraction can be quite impressive following a thorough liposuction. Subsequent skin retraction and fibrosis of the local tissues occurs for a number of weeks following surgery. An obvious defect at the time of surgery should be recognized and treated appropriately. Intraoperative lipo-filling is very effective in this regard, and fat injections can be performed in the same setting as the overresection to fill these areas to a certain extent. Appropriate methods of fat harvest must be used to achieve the best result. It should be remembered that more than one injection may be necessary, depending on the size of the defect.

Dissatisfied patients

It has been our experience that liposuction patients typically have a certain excess volume of fat overall. It is difficult for them to lose weight, and therefore they appeal to their plastic surgeon to assist them with this process. However, these same patients may have a tendency to fail to maintain their preoperative weight and instead gain weight postoperatively. To avoid the complaints typical at the 6-month postop visit, we have developed a system that includes a careful analysis of the patient's preoperative and postoperative weight. Without the patient's preoperative weight measurement, addressing weight gain after surgery becomes problematic. Furthermore, we always measure the true fat aspirate volume (omitting the fluid) and subtract this weight from the patient's preoperative weight, giving us the all-important GOAL WEIGHT. If a patient returns to the office and complains that the liposuction procedure was incompletely performed, that a certain treated area continues to be full, and insists upon a revision or redo operation, having these numbers is critical. When we share the preoperative weight, the weight of the remove fat, and their goal weight, it serves to diffuse a difficult situation and prompts the patient into more effective weight loss and exercise. If when patients return to the office they are over their goal weight, it can only be assumed that they have gained this weight since the time of surgery. If they subsequently desire additional liposuction surgery, they are much more willing to appropriately pay for it.

Undesirable outcomes

Preoperative evaluations and discussions of results the patient may expect from surgery are critical. There is only one chance for preoperative photos, weight measurement, and informed consent. Although normally liposuction results can be lifelong changes with proper weight management, patients

Table 2: **From ASPS practice advisory on liposuction, 2004**

Postoperative complications	
Minor	Small hematomas, seromas Minor contour irregularities
More severe	Fluid overload Infection Skin perforations Lidocaine toxicity Major contour defects Skin necrosis, thermal injury Adverse anesthetic reaction Pulmonary embolus/fat embolus
Severe	May require additional surgery Death

Abbreviation: ASPS, American Society of Plastic Surgeons.
Data from Iverson RE, et al. Practice advisory on liposuction. Plast Reconst Surg 2004;113(5):1478–90.

must be warned of the possibility of contour irregularities, asymmetries, or numbness. However rare, anesthetic and respiratory complications, transfusion requirements, and possible death complete the list of adverse events secondary to liposuction [see Table 2].

Summary

The apparent simplicity of liposuction and the ease with which it is performed, may lull the novice plastic surgeon into overlooking the evolutionary developments that have brought it to today's level of popularity in body contouring surgery. Patients who may benefit from liposuction range widely from the thin patient desiring contouring of localized areas of stubborn adiposity to the obese patient in whom diet has failed to control weight. One of the major drawbacks of liposuction is its ability to thin, but not tighten. Reliance upon skin retraction to affect a proper outcome will only lead to disappointment, and this patient may instead benefit from an excisional-type procedure. Careful patient selection, education, and proper administration of the technique as a primary or an adjunctive tool will help deliver the most desirable aesthetic result.

References

[1] Hait P, Schnur PL. History of the American Society of Plastic and Reconstructive Surgeons, 1931–1994. Plast Reconstr Surg 1994;94(4): 1A–105A.

[2] Kesselring UK. Regional fat aspiration for body contouring. Plast Reconst Surg 1983;72(5): 610–23.

[3] Illouz YG. Body contouring by lipolysis: a 5 year experience with over 3000 cases. Plast Reconst Surg 1983;72(5):591–7.

[4] Hunstad JP. Body contouring in the obese patient. Clin Plast Surg 1996;23(4):647–69.

[5] Iverson RE, Lynch DJ. Practice advisory on liposuction. Plast Reconstr Surg 2004;113:1478–90.

[6] Hunstad JP. The tumescent technique: an evolution. Presented at the 11th annual meeting of the Lipoplasty Society of North America. New Orleans; 1993.

[7] Hunstad JP. The tumescent technique: an evolution. Lipoplasty Newsletter 1994; Vol. 11, No. 29.

[8] Toledo L, Lewis CM. Why I use the syringe in superficial liposculpture. New York: Springer-Verlag; 1993.

[9] Hunstad JP. Addressing difficult areas in body contouring with emphasis on combined tumescent and syringe techniques. Clin Plast Surg 1996;23(1):57–80.

[10] De Souza Pinto EB. Superficial liposuction. In: Zaoli G, Zocchi ML, editors. Aesthetic plastic surgery. Zaoli (Italy): Piccin; 2003. p. 153.

[11] Mentz 3rd HA, Gilliland MD, Patronella CK. Abdominal etching: differential liposuction to detail abdominal musculature. Aesthetic Plast Surg 1993;17(4):287–90.

[12] Zocchi M. Ultrasonic liposculpturing. Aesthetic Plast Surg 1992;16(4):287–98.

[13] Lambros V. Fat contouring in the face and neck. Clin Plast Surg 1992;19(2):401–14.

[14] Gasparotti M. Superficial liposuction: a new application of the technique for aged and flaccid skin. Aesthetic Plast Surg 1992;16(2):141–53.

[15] Illouz YG. Body sculpturing by lipoplasty. Edinbrough: Churchill Livingstone; 1989. p. 81.

[16] Illouz YG. History and current concepts of lipoplasty. Clin Plast Surg 1996;23(4):721–30.

CLINICS IN PLASTIC SURGERY

Clin Plastic Surg 33 (2006) 27–37

Liposuction Anesthesia Techniques

Fábio Luís Ferrari Regatieri, MD*, Manuel Sanchez Mosquera, MD

We live in an era of incredible technologic advances. At the beginning of the last century, amputations were performed with rudimentary instruments using alcohol and opium to sedate the patient. Early in the last century, anesthesia was one of the most important medical discoveries, being used in procedures of various complexities, including plastic surgery and body contouring. Liposuction has evolved over the last 20 years with the help of new monitoring techniques and the discovery of safer drugs with little or no side effects.

Great advances have been made in the field of continuous venous anesthesia, with the use of pharmacokinetic model simulators allowing more detailed studies of the length and behavior of drugs. Microprocessed infusion pumps allow the choice of different dosage levels of specific drugs, a detail that improves the quality of the anesthetic act, allowing the anesthesiologist to reduce side effects and the recovery time from anesthesia, which also reduces the hospital costs to the patient.

The progress of venous anesthesia allows one to distinguish the fundamental components of anesthesia:

- Analgesia
- Amnesia
- Unconsciousness
- Patient immobility
- Elimination or reduction of autonomic responses (eg, tachycardia, hypertension)

One attempts to reach these stages by using specific drugs that achieve desired effects. Anesthetic options for liposuction are as follows:

- Local anesthesia
- Local anesthesia associated with sedation
- Regional anesthesia associated with or without sedation
- General anesthesia

The presence of an anesthesiologist during a surgical procedure performed under sedation or

Private practice, Rua Capote Valente, 640-82, São Paulo 05409-002, Brazil
* Corresponding author.
E-mail address: drfabio@anestesiologia.com.br (F.L.F. Regatieri).

0094-1298/06/$ – see front matter
doi:10.1016/j.cps.2005.08.003
plasticsurgery.theclinics.com

general or regional anesthesia is imperative for the safety of the patient, for maintenance, and for monitoring vital signs [1]. When described by Illouz [2] in 1980, liposuction in most cases was performed with epidural or general anesthesia. In 1987, Klein [3] introduced the tumescent technique, a new formula that allowed the surgeon to inject large amounts of local anesthetic solution in several areas of the body with small dosages of lidocaine, adrenaline, and saline at room temperature with or without sedation. In 1989, Toledo [4] altered Klein's formula, increasing the concentration of lidocaine and adrenaline and using Ringer's lactate instead of saline. Most of the authors' patients undergo liposuction with a combination of tumescent anesthesia as described by Klein and modified by Toledo associated with intravenous sedation.

This article discusses intravenous sedation, the authors' anesthesia of choice when performing most esthetic body contour refinement procedures. This technique is comfortable, safe, contemporary, and beneficial to the patient and medical crew. The preanesthesia evaluation is emphasized as a safety and high-quality action to any anesthesia procedure. Alternative anesthesia techniques are also discussed, including their possible advantages, disadvantages, indications, and counterindications.

Preanesthesia evaluation

An adequate preanesthesia evaluation is a quality and safety action that is extremely important to the anesthesia procedure. The preanesthesia evaluation involves a review of information from multiple sources that may include the patient's medical records, an interview, a physical examination, and the findings from medical tests and evaluations. Benefits may include, but are not limited to, safe perioperative care, optimal resource use, improved outcome, and patient satisfaction [5]. Any anesthesia technique should be chosen with the agreement of the surgeon, the anesthesiologist, and, of course, the patient during the preanesthesia evaluation.

The main intercurrent events during the perioperative period are a consequence of pre-existing clinical pathologies [6,7]; therefore, all efforts must be focused on the identification of disease and its treatment before surgery. That aspect is more important when dealing with esthetic and elective surgery for which, in theory, one has all the time needed to follow the procedure.

In 2001, the American Society of Anesthesiologists (ASA) Task Force published a Practice Advisory for Preanesthesia Evaluation that was amended in October of 2003. The advisory works as a good parameter in implementation of the preanesthesia evaluation in the surgeon's office. Most consultants and ASA members agree that for high surgical invasiveness, the initial assessment of pertinent medical records should be performed before the day of surgery by anesthesia staff. A majority of consultants and the ASA membership agree that the minimal preanesthetic physical examination should include an airway examination, a pulmonary examination including auscultation of the lungs, and a cardiovascular examination [8]. The authors' preanesthetic physical examination includes an assessment of the airway, lungs, and heart, with documentation of vital signs.

The authors recommend the application of patterned preanesthesia self-evaluation questionnaires to all probable surgery patients. This form should be written in a simple and objective way so anyone can understand the questions; patients may have major difficulties with technical words. One should address all of the pathologies relevant to the procedure, how they will be treated (medication names and doses), the past medical history, and possible habits and allergies. The questionnaire should be answered and signed by the patient and then thoroughly checked by the anesthesiologist. Remaining issues can be resolved through an interview with the patient. The physical examination should take into account the spine (if there is a possibility of spinal or epidural anesthesia) and the conditions of the airways to identify possible difficulties in intubation even if one does not intend to perform general anesthesia.

The ASA Task Force, consultants, and ASA members agree that preoperative tests should not be required routinely [8]. The Task Force recommends that preoperative tests be required or performed on a selective basis to guide or optimize perioperative management. The results of tests obtained from the medical record within 6 months of the surgery are generally acceptable if the patient's medical history has not changed substantially.

Required complementary preoperative tests involve a discussion. If it is known that a patient has some pathology, one should require tests to evaluate the status of the disease and the target organ [9,10]. Few anesthesiologists will attempt anesthesia in a hypertensive patient unless they have the patient's electrocardiogram (EKG) and a renal evaluation. The same care must be taken in a diabetic patient regarding the blood sugar test.

The major question is what to do with the healthy patient. Some physicians believe there is no need for any complementary tests in healthy patients who have no morbid or familiar history or habits that clearly lead to major risks. This posture must be respected under several points of view as economic or epidemiologic [10]; however, there is no guarantee of safety for the surgical team or patient and a possible risk of negligence. One must keep in mind not just the epidemiologic data but also the consequences that could arise from a subclinical pathology to the anesthesia or surgical procedures. An asymptomatic coagulopathy can cause serious damages in an epidural anesthesia or in a high-volume liposuction. A simple anemia, an almost ordinary condition, could compromise the result of certain surgeries if one has blood loss, unexpected or not.

Some procedures take place under local anesthesia plus analgesic sedation with the administration of high doses of local anesthetics and vasoconstrictors [11]. Even though several reports have shown that this is a safe procedure [12,13], one must consider the outcome in the "healthy" patient who has an intraventricular conduction disturbance that is asymptomatic. Is it wise not requiring a patient's EKG just because of economic or epidemiologic reasons?

As a routine, the authors request from all patients of any age a hemogram, a coagulogram, a blood sugar test, and an EKG. Extra tests are required based on the medical history (age, personal and family history, habits, pathologies, medication administered) and on the physical examination. A written clearance (about the patient's clinical condition) is recommended from the patient's personal physician. If there is any need to change the regular prescription for the patient, the authors talk to the physician.

The conditions responsible for most undesirable and critical events during the perioperative period are cardiac [10,14]. The authors also carefully evaluate patients with chronic lung disease, diabetics, and those with an increased risk of pulmonary thromboembolism [15].

Noncardiac surgical patients can be categorized as those who do not have a risk of coronary artery disease (CAD), those without known but at risk for CAD, and those with known CAD [10,14]. Recognized risks for CAD and perioperative ischemia include age over 70 years, diabetes, hypertension, hypercholesterolemia, tobacco use, and the presence of peripheral vascular disease. Of the routine preoperative tests, the EKG is one of the most important for patients, despite the fact that the EKG may be normal in 25% to 50% of patients who have CAD. The findings consistent with a prior heart attack, ongoing ischemia, or abnormal cardiac rhythm have all been shown to be associated with increased operative risk.

Hypertensive patients comprise 20% to 25% of surgical patients, and hypertension is known to be associated with a higher incidence of cardiovascular disease and diabetes. With approximately 65,000 deaths annually in the United States owing to perioperative cardiac complications, cardiac morbidity represents the leading cause of postoperative death. The incidence of perioperative hypertension and its attendant diseases in ambulatory surgery patients is likely to increase as the scope of surgery performed in ambulatory surgery centers broadens and as the general population ages [10]. All hypertensive patients must be compensate before elective procedures to prevent major complications (cardiac arrest, arrhythmias, hypertensive crises) and minor ones (edema, bleeding.

Patients with chronic lung disease may obtain benefits from respiratory physiotherapy before surgery, such as the prescription of bronchodilators and corticosteroids in the oncoming preoperative period [16]. Several studies have examined methods to minimize postoperative pulmonary complications in patients with chronic obstructive pulmonary disease (COPD). Gracey and coworkers [17] demonstrated that patients given a preoperative conditioning regimen of aerosol isoproterenol, oral theophylline, glyceryl guaiacolate, and chest physiotherapy had far fewer postoperative pulmonary complications (19%) than a historical cohort of clinically similar patients who did not receive a conditioning regimen (46%). They speculated that preoperative mobilization of secretions from the airways might have been the main benefit of the conditioning regimen, minimizing retention of secretions and consequent infection and atelectasis.

The best predictors of which patients will require extended (2–120 hours) ventilation following surgery are the preoperative arterial partial pressure of oxygen (PaO_2) and a dyspnea score (dyspnea at rest), not measurement of the pulmonary function, including FEV_1, FEV_1/FVC, peak flows, or measurement of the arterial partial pressure of carbon dioxide. Blood gas parameters and a dyspnea score have been shown to predict postoperative pulmonary morbidity in more recent studies as well.

Diabetes mellitus is one of the most common endocrine diseases affecting patients presenting for outpatient surgery. Appropriate perioperative management of diabetes is essential to reduce operative risks to diabetics, including metabolic derangement, impaired wound healing, and an increased risk of postoperative infection. Initial decisions regarding perioperative administration of glucose and insulin to diabetic patients are often made at the time of the preoperative visit, and the anesthesiologist can have a vital role in the initiation of safe diabetic management.

The most common causes of hypoglycemia in diabetic patients are related to the use of exogenous insulin or oral hypoglycemic agents. Goals of intraoperative glucose control in the diabetic patient

Table 1: **Mood-altering drugs and anesthetics**

Classes	Examples	Drug association problems	Serious reactions	Discontinuing
MAOIs	Phenelzine (Nardil), pargyline (Eutonyl), tranylcypromine (Parnate), deprenyl (selegiline Eldepryl)	Indirect-acting sympathomimetic substances (eg, ephedrine, tiramine–cheese) Narcotics	Convulsions Hyperpyrexic coma Hemodynamic instability Cardiac arrest	At least 2 to 3 weeks before any elective procedures
Tricyclic antidepressant drugs	Amitriptyline (Elavil, Endep, Limbitrol), imipramine (Imavate, Tofranil, Presamine), despiramine (Norpramin), doxepin (Adapin, Sinequan), nortriptyline (Aventyl, Pamelor)	MAOIs Vasoconstrictors Narcotics: phetidine Halothane Pancuronium	Hemodynamic instability Cardiac arrhythmias Cardiac arrest	At least 2 to 3 weeks before any elective procedures
SSRIs	Fluoxetine (Prozac), sertraline (Zoloft), paroxetine (Paxil), citalopram (Celexa), escitalopram (Lexapro)	Nonspecified general anesthetics Narcotics	Severe hypotension Cardiac arrhythmias Cardiac arrest Bleeding	No consensus: at least 3 to 7 days before elective procedures
Other antidepressants	Trazodone (Desyrel), bupropion (Wellbutrin), venlafaxine (Effexor), maprotiline (Ludiomil), mirtazapine (Remeron)			No consensus: at least 3 to 7 days before elective procedures
Phenothiazines	Chlorpromazine (Thorazine), promazine (Sparine), triflupromazine (Vesprin), fluphenazine (Prolixin), prochlorperazine (Compazine)	Nonspecified general anesthetics Spinal/epidural blocks	Severe hypotension Cardiac arrhythmias Potentiates hypnotics	No concensus
Butyrophenones	Droperidol and haloperidol (Haldol)	Nonspecified general anesthetics Spinal/epidural blocks	Hypotension Cardiac arrhythmias Potentiates hypnotics	No concensus
Lithium carbonate		Adespolarizant Neuromuscular blockers	Cardiac arrhythmias Prolongs neuromuscular block	No concensus
Cocaine		Local anesthetics Vasoconstrictors Narcotics	Seizures Hemodynamic instability Cardiac arrhythmias Cardiac arrest	

should be the prevention of hyperglycemia to avoid intraoperative diuresis and to minimize risks of postoperative wound infections, delayed healing, and central nervous system dysfunction. At the same time, control of blood glucose levels should not place the patient at significant risk for perioperative hypoglycemia. Most authorities agree that a blood glucose concentration between 120 and 200 mg/dL fulfills these goals [10].

Patients at risk for deep vein thrombosis (DVT) and its terrible consequence, pulmonary thromboembolism, must be identified mainly through their medical history data. One should document a prior history of DVT [18], cardiovascular disease, tabagism, prolonged sitting, bedrest or immobilization (eg, a long airplane or car trip) [19–21], recent surgery or trauma (especially hip, knee, or gynecologic surgery), fractures, childbirth within the last 6 months, and the use of medications such as estrogen and birth control pills. Risks also include a history of polycythemia vera, malignant tumor, and inherited or acquired hypercoagulability (changes in the levels of blood clotting factors making the blood more likely to clot).

Anesthesia and daily use medications

A complete discussion of the interaction of daily use medications and different types of anesthesia is beyond the scope of this article. Normally, the authors keep the use of drugs that the patient takes daily. Special attention is paid to antihypertensives, antiarrhythmics, and other drugs used to keep the respiratory and cardiovascular systems in good and controlled compensation. Actually, the authors recommend that patients take these drugs on the day of surgery. The oral ingestion of almost 20 mL of water with these drugs will not interfere with preoperative fasting. Drugs that interfere with blood coagulation, such as aspirin, which reduces the clumping or aggregation of blood platelets, and anticoagulants (eg, warfarin) could be an obstacle to surgery and to certain regional anesthesia techniques. Careful consideration is needed before telling patients to stop the intake of these drugs 10 to 15 days before surgery because their prescription may be related to the prevention and treatment of severe cardiovascular diseases.

One must consider the safety of the administration of drugs with an action over the central nervous system and their interaction with anesthetics and vasoactive drugs. Mood-altering drugs are the most frequently prescribed medications in the United States. They include monoamine oxidase inhibitors (MAOIs), selective serotonin reuptake inhibitors (SSRIs), phenothiazines, tricyclic antidepressant drugs, and drugs of abuse such as cocaine. Table 1 lists some interactions among mood-altering drugs and anesthetics, as well suggestions on how to deal with these clinical situations.

Despite the nonmedical belief that there is no risk associated with the use of herbal medications, the authors have noticed an increase in intraoperative bleeding owing to the use of ginkgo (*Ginkgo biloba*), the potentialization of the action of certain sedatives associated with St. John's Wort (*Hypericum perforatum*), and cardiac arrhythmias and arterial hypertension associated with the use of ephedra (*Ephedra sinica*).

Preoperative fasting

According to the ASA Task Force [22], "it's appropriate to fast from intake of clear liquids for 2 or more hours before procedures requiring general anesthesia, regional anesthesia or sedation/analgesia (monitored anesthesia care). Examples of clear liquids include, but are not limited to, water, fruit juices without pulp, carbonated beverages, clear tea, and black coffee. These liquids should not include alcohol. The volume of liquid ingested is less important than the type of liquid ingested."

The ASA Task Force also states, "it's appropriate to fast from intake of a light meal or non-human milk for 6 or more hours before elective procedures requiring general anesthesia, regional anesthesia, or sedation/analgesia (eg, monitored anesthesia care)." They also support a fasting period for a meal that includes fried or fatty foods or meat of 8 or more hours before elective procedures.

Preanesthetic medication

Preanesthetic medication has the function of diminishing the anxiety of the patient, collaborating with the acceptance of the new surrounding environment that is the surgical room, as well as diminishing hemodynamic changes such as tachycardia, increased blood pressure, and arrhythmia in the immediate period before the induction of anesthesia. It has a positive impact on the satisfaction of the patient, in addition to potentiating the effect of some sedatives. There are several possible medications that can be given for these purposes and several ways of administration. Examples that are part of the authors' daily practice are as follows:

The benzodiazepine midazolam has as its main advantage the promotion of a good anxiolytic effect and the induction of anterograde amnesia in a good percentage of patients [13]. It can be given intramuscularly (peak of action between 15 and 30 minutes) in a dosage ranging from 0.05 to 0.2 mg/kg or orally (peak of action between 30 and 60 minutes) in a dose ranging from 7.5 to 15 mg for adult patients.

The opioid meperidine (Demerol) is useful when the patient has some type of associated limitation pain (eg, surgical correction of broken bones). Beyond its sedative properties, it is a good analgesic; however, it is associated with an increased incidence of nausea and vomiting and, when used as epidural or spinal premedication, increases the incidence of arterial hypotension [23] in the period immediately after accomplishment of the blockade. It does not provide amnesia to the patient. The dose ranges from 1 to 2 mg/kg intramuscularly, limiting the dose to a maximum of 100 mg. The action occurs between 30 and 60 minutes.

Several studies have demonstrated the utility of clonidine as a preanesthetic drug. Its main advantages include sedative, anxiolytic, sympatholytic, and antisialogogue actions. It has the capacity to reduce the intraoperative doses of volatile anesthetics and opioids. Clonidine has been recommended as a preanesthetic drug in oral doses ranging from 2 to 5 μg/kg [24]. It intensifies the motor and sensitive blocks that result from the application of local anesthetics in epidural or peripheral nerve blocks [25]. Its main disadvantages are that it does not offer amnesia and requires a relatively long period (90 minutes) to take effect, frequently limiting its utility in ambulatory surgery.

Although one can associate medications with preanesthetic purposes, this is not a common practice, and there is not enough evidence in the medical literature to justify the eventual risk-benefit.

Safety conditions in the surgical room

Minimum conditions [26] of safety must exist to guarantee the integrity of the patient in any surgical or anesthetic procedure (if some unexpected adverse events happen). Resources that must be available in the anesthetic-surgical environment are as follows:

Disposable items

Nasal oxygen catheter
Suction catheter and aspiration device
Guedel airways (oropharyngeal airways)
Urethral catheter (Foley)
Intravenous catheter No. 22, 20, and 18 (Jelco or Insyte)
Laryngeal mask No. 3, 4, and 5
Endotracheal tubes 7, 7.5, 8, and 8.5
Electrodes for cardiac monitorization
Syringes and needles of different numbers

Equipment

Syringe infusion pump
Multiparametric monitor (EKG, pulse oxymeter, capnograph, and noninvasive automatic blood pressure)
Complete anesthesia machine
Laryngoscope
AMBU bag
Automatic defibrillator
Oxygen source, facial masks, and other devices for oxygen therapy

Drugs used in cardiopulmonary resuscitation and emergencies

Epinephrine
Lidocaine
Amiodarone
Atropine
Neostigmine
Magnesium sulfate 10%
β-blockers (intravenous)
β-2 agonists for parenteral use and inhalatory use
Hydrocortisone
Vasodilatators for intravenous use
Neuromuscular blockers
Antagonists: flumazenil, naloxone
Vasopressors: ephedrine, metaraminol

Aspects from the staff

The medical staff should be trained in an advanced life support protocol (eg, advanced cardiopulmonary life support or advanced trauma life support). The authors advise nonmedical staff to be trained in at least a basic life support protocol, especially if the surgery will be performed in an office-based structure.

Fluid replacement in lipoplasty

Fluid replacement is one of the most important aspects in the intraoperative handling of lipoplasty [26,27]. It intervenes with the hemodynamic stability of the patient and is an essential factor in postoperative recovery [28–30]. The adequate fluid balance is obtained considering the losses and the intake of fluids in the perioperative period. The anesthesiologist must give intravenous fluids to keep the intravascular volume. The goal is a normal cardiac output and a good tissue perfusion.

Estimating losses

Despite the fact that infiltration techniques decrease the blood loss, one must remember that lipoplasty provokes liquid losses in two ways: (1) volume is lost with the fat (intraoperative) and (2) volume is trapped with the edema fluid (intraoperative and mainly in the postoperative period). It is easy to estimate the first component of the losses, whereas one cannot say the same for the second one. Quantifying how much liquid is trapped under the form of posttraumatic edema is a sufficiently difficult exercise, not to mention that the fact that some determined areas trap more than others, and depends on the surgical technique and other factors related to the individual conditions of each patient.

Counting the intake

Apart from the fluids given intravenously, one must also consider the volume given through subcutaneous infusion of the anesthetic solution and the fact that it is not removed by lipoplasty. From a practical point of view, one can consider as losses the volume of removed fat and the volume of anesthetic solution removed. To restore the volume trapped in edema, we should consider clinical standards, such as hemodynamic stability (blood pressure, heart rate) and diuresis. In general, the authors give patients intravenously no more than 1 to 2 mL of saline solution or Ringer's lactate for each milliliter of removed fat. The volume of anesthetic solution that remains inside the patient after the liposuction of a certain area is considered.

An effort is made to maintain the parameter of blood pressure never inferior to 80% of the values at rest in healthful young patients. In patients with any cardiovascular pathology or the elderly, the drop does not have to be superior to 10% of the basal values. The volume of fluids given should be enough to produce diuresis of at least 0.5 to 1 mL/kg/h.

Anesthesia techniques

Several anesthesia techniques can be used for lipoplasty, each with its advantages and limitations. As mentioned previously [6,7,14], comorbidity is the primary predictor of anesthesia-related mortality and morbidity. Nevertheless, new studies [28] suggest that the maintenance of adequate levels of hypnosis (not so deep) to the anesthesia as well as hemodynamic stability during the procedure can have a greater importance in the full recovery of patients than previously imagined.

The following aspects must be taken into consideration when choosing the most appropriate technique for the type of procedure:

- Often, some surgeons prefer a certain type of anesthesia based on personal experiences or habit.
- As is true for surgeons, some anesthesiologists prefer a type of technique they are more acquainted to or familiar with.
- The technical complexity and length of the procedure is an important item in the choice of the anesthesia technique (eg, some types of regional anesthesia have a limited length of duration). Some basic conditions must be observed when determining which anesthesia technique will obtain the best result. This goal should always be a reference for the anesthesiologist.

The following items must be evaluated in the choice of the best anesthesia technique:

- Stable operative conditions ensure a safe surgical act (little bleeding, adequate muscle relaxation, hemodynamic stability). These conditions make the procedure much easier and decrease surgical time.
- Fast recovery of psychomotor and cognitive responses ensures that a precociously recovered cooperative patient will progress to hospital discharge.

Local plus sedation

Advantages

Infiltration of the solutions with local anesthetics and vasoconstrictors reduces bleeding and provides a good quality of intraoperative analgesia. The infiltrated solution should be warmed, minimizing perioperative hypothermia [31]. When it is well indicated, infiltration with anesthetic solutions allows lipoplasty to be performed under relatively light sedation, implying a short recovery time and acceptable costs.

Disadvantages

The infiltration is not always made in an adequate form; therefore, some areas will have a lack of analgesia that it is solved by going deeper in the sedation. This situation demands specific abilities of the anesthetist, who must be accustomed to dealing with control of the airways in deep levels of sedation. The deep sedation does not present clear advantages in relation to the general anesthesia in terms of complications, time of recovery, and cost.

Types of drugs

Currently, one can use drugs of fast onset and short action such as propofol and remifentanil for maintenance of hypnosis and analgesia during surgery. Propofol [32] acts by providing inhibition of supraspinal and spinal synapses, potentiating the effect of gamma-aminobutyric acid (GABA) receptors. It has no analgesic effect and has a fast onset (approximately 30 seconds). It causes dose-dependent respiratory depression, mainly when it is injected very fast. It diminishes the incidence of nausea and vomiting, an important aspect in the postoperative period and in the prevention of problems such as bleeding and the dehiscence of sutures. Because of its fast onset and short time of duration, the best way to administrate propofol is through an infusion pump, keeping an adequate therapeutic plasmatic level and preventing apnea, which optimizes the recovery time besides saving money.

The authors routinely use midazolam as a benzodiazepine for sleep induction and to obtain one of the most important and desirable effects of anesthesia, intraoperative amnesia, which is a useful effect to prevent the patient from experiencing surgical memories that can cause disturbances such as posttraumatic stress syndrome. The mechanism of action of the benzodiazepines occurs mainly in the cerebral cortex, with reinforcement of the inhibitory effects of several neurotransmitters such as GABA. Besides this property, midazolam has hypnotic, sedative, muscle relaxing, and anticonvulsive properties. It has no analgesic effect. Some authorities suggest that it presents a lesser incidence of nausea and vomiting in the postoperative period [33]. Owing to its pharmacokinetic characteristics, midazolam is the authors' choice among the benzodiazepines. The managed dose varies from procedure to procedure. Some factors influence the amount that must be given to keep the sedation level during the intraoperative period.

If other benzodiazepines are used as preanesthetic medication and their hypnotic effects are efficient, eventually only small doses of midazolam may be needed in the beginning of the surgery (from 1 to 3 mg intravenously) or may even be excluded. The authors use low doses if the patient is sensitive to these drugs (eg, elderly patients) or if the surgery will be short. Higher doses are used in patients who regularly use this medicine class or in extended duration surgeries.

Ketamine is another drug that can be used in sedation techniques. In low doses (from 0.25 to 0.5 mg/kg) associated with midazolam administration, it decreases significantly the consumption of opioids in the intraoperative period and of analgesics in the postoperative period [34,35]. Recently, excitatory neurotransmitters acting through N-methyl-D-aspartate (NMDA) receptors have been incriminated in the development and maintenance of hyperalgesia and allodynia and persistent postoperative pain. Apparently, these actions of ketamine are due to its properties as an antagonist of NMDA receivers. Mortero and coworkers [36] concluded that co-administration of small doses of ketamine with propofol attenuated propofol-induced hypoventilation, produced positive mood effects without perceptual changes after surgery, and may provide earlier recovery of cognition in patients under sedation (monitored anesthesia care).

The properties of clonidine have been described previously. In the recommended doses (from 2 to 5 μg/kg) given intravenously at the beginning of sedation in a small bolus of no more than 30 μg (to prevent bradycardia and brusque reductions of the arterial pressure), clonidine is useful as an adjuvant in sedation techniques.

The authors use some opioids for analgesia, such as meperidine or fentanyl. The right dose is adjusted by giving these drugs in a small bolus (20 mg of meperidine, 25 μg of fentanyl) until the desired effect is achieved. Because one should keep the patient breathing spontaneously, it is necessary to individualize the dose from patient to patient to produce appropriate analgesia without causing respiratory arrest. Because it is important to respect the onset of each drug, appropriate attention to time is needed to raise the proper level of sedation.

A new opioid, remifentanil [37], which is metabolized by plasmatic enzymes and has a very fast onset and short time of action, can be used in sedation techniques; however, as is true for propofol, the best way to use this drug is through an infusion pump to optimize its use and safety.

Epidural anesthesia

Epidural anesthesia is another technique that is widely used to provide analgesia in lipoplasty. The quality of its analgesia is superior to that provided by infiltration with solutions. Patients tend to tolerate the surgery very well with a relatively light sedation. It presents the advantage of working with a total mass of local anesthetic inferior to that needed in the technique described in the previous section. Despite being a consummative fact, the incidence of toxicity for local anesthetics must be superior when the epidural technique is used, as related in some articles in the medical literature.

This apparent contradiction is sufficiently justified by the fact that the epidural space is highly vascularized, and, usually, great amounts of local anesthetics are injected in a few seconds. Consequently, possible inadvertent intravascular administration may occur, quickly increasing the plasmatic level of these substances with consequent intoxication. The absorption of local anesthetics from subcutaneous tissue [3] is slow (plasmatic peak between 12 and 24 hours after the administration), allowing their removal together with the fat before being absorbed. Moreover, the slow absorption makes possible the metabolization of these drugs by the organism before reaching dangerous plasmatic levels.

Epidural anesthesia used to be indicated in procedures limited to a few segments to preserve the hemodynamic stability of the patient. Too extensive epidural blockades are frequently associated with hypotension and must be avoided or limited to patients with good cardiac reserve. Lipoplasty with aspiration of great volumes under extensive epidural anesthesia is often followed by hemodynamic instability.

Even when using epidural anesthesia, the authors recommend the infiltration of warmed solution at 37°C [31] with vasoconstrictors (eg, normal saline 0.9% with epinephrine 1:500,000) in the liposuction area to minimize bleeding [38]. This technique is the main choice of many surgical teams because of other advantages such as excellent analgesia [23] (intraoperative and postoperative), good control of anesthetic time (the continuous technique), and low cost. Because one does not enter the subarachnoid space, the puncture can be done through the thoracic or lumbar level depending on where the procedure will be carried through. Lipoplasty of thoracic, abdominal, or dorsal high segments can be performed with a thoracic epidural (puncture between T8 and T10). Surgeries at inferior segments that involve the abdomen, gluteus, or inferior members can be performed through the lumbar technique (punctures between L2 and L4).

The formal counterindications to epidural anesthesia are refusal of the patient, previous alterations of the vertebral column, coagulopathy, hemodynamic instability, some cardiac diseases, and infections at the puncture site.

Spinal anesthesia

Spinal anesthesia is associated with decreased epinephrine secretion during the surgery and the postoperative period, whereas epidural anesthesia is associated with decreased cortisol secretion. Neither epidural nor spinal anesthesia inhibits insulin secretion when sensory levels are below T7. Spinal and epidural anesthesia may have some advantages for diabetic patients regarding the anesthetic effects on glucose metabolism. Spinal anesthesia is a useful technique for lipoplasty below the umbilical area with a surgical time inferior to 3 hours. In these conditions, this technique is safe with few side effects and is inexpensive. As is true for epidural anesthesia, extensive spinal blockades are associated with hemodynamic instability. The quality of the anesthesia and the muscular relaxation in the blocked area are excellent, and the administration of opioids for spinal anesthesia provides good analgesia in the first 24 hours of the postoperative period.

The use of spinal microcatheters for continuous spinal anesthesia has fell into disfavor owing to the high number of complications, making long procedures impractical with this type of anesthesia. As is true for the epidural technique, the authors suggest the infiltration of warmed solution at 37°C [31] with a vasoconstrictor (eg, normal saline 0.9% with epinephrine 1:500,000) in the liposuction area to minimize bleeding. The counterindications are the same as for the epidural technique.

General anesthesia

General anesthesia is always an option for the accomplishment of any surgical procedure. Besides providing adequate control of ventilation and hemodynamic parameters, it is a good choice for extensive lipoplasties or those associated with other surgical procedures. A new generation of drugs gives great flexibility in the technique and short recovery periods. Beyond propofol, introduced more than a decade ago, other anesthetics such as remifentanil (opioid) [37], cisatracurium (neuromuscular blocker), and sevoflurane and desflurane (inhalant anesthetics) are examples of drugs with minimum residual effect, fast elimination, and few side effects.

The relative disadvantage of general anesthesia is the cost of the procedure. The authors believe that improvement in security and reduction of complications and hospital time that occur by using these drugs, compensate for their higher price. If prices get lower, these drugs can become more popular. The infrastructure monitorization must be improved. The administration of venous anesthetics with this profile usually demands the use of infusion pumps, and the use of inhalant anesthetics implies having specific and adequate vaporizers.

Summary

Liposuction is a common and safe procedure that can be performed under several anesthesia techniques. The preanesthesia evaluation is a security and quality factor for the procedure. The use of new medications contributes to safer anesthesia, improves the satisfaction of the patient, and reduces the discharge time and the side effects associated with anesthesia. Selection of the best technique should take into account the characteristics of the patient, the extent and length of the surgery, the surgeon's preferences, and the anesthesiologist's skills.

References

[1] ASA's standards for basic anesthetic monitoring (approved by the ASA House of Delegates on October 21, last amended on October 27, 2004). Available at: http://www.asahq.org/publicationsAndServices/standards/02.pdf. Accessed June 2005.

[2] Illouz YG. A new method for localized lipodystrophies. Rev Chir Esthet 1980;19(6):3–10.

[3] Klein JA. The tumescent technique for liposuction surgery. Am J Cosmetic Surg 1987;4:263–7.

[4] Toledo LS. Superficial syringe liposculpture. Annals of the International Symposium-Recent Advances in Plastic Surgery, March 3–5, 1990, São Paulo, Brazil. p. 446.

[5] Mendes FF, Mathias LAST, Durval Neto GF, et al. Impact of preoperative outpatient evaluation clinic on performance indicators. Rev Bras Anestesiol 2005;55(2):175–87.

[6] Kawashima Y. Annual study of anesthesia-related mortality and morbidity in the year 2001 in Japan: the outlines report of Japanese Society of Anesthesiologists Committee on Operating Room Safety. Masui 2003;52(6):666–82.

[7] Fleisher LA. Risk of anesthesia. In: Miller RD, editor. Anesthesia. 6th edition. San Francisco: Churchill Livingstone Elsevier; 2005. Chapter 24, p. 893–920.

[8] Arens JF. Practice advisory for preanesthesia evaluation (approved by the House of Delegates on October 17, 2001, and last amended on October 15, 2003). A report by the American Society of Anesthesiologists Task Force on Preanesthesia Evaluation, supported by the American Society of Anesthesiologists. Available at: http://www.asahq.org/publicationsAndServices/preeval.pdf. Accessed June 2005.

[9] Fischer SP. Cost-effective preoperative evaluation and testing. Chest 1999;115(5):96–100.

[10] Van Norman GA. Preoperative assessment of common diseases in the outpatient setting. Anesthesiol Clin North Am 1996;14(4):631–54.

[11] Fulda GJ, Khan SU, Zabel DD. Special issues in plastic and reconstructive surgery. Crit Care Clin 2003;19(1):91–108.

[12] Klein JA. Anesthetic formulation of tumescent solutions. Dermatol Clin 1999;17(4):751–9.

[13] Burk RW, Guzman-Stein G, Vasconez LO. Lidocaine and epinephrine levels in tumescent technique liposuction. Plast Reconstr Surg 1996; 97(7):1379–84.

[14] Hollenberg SM. Preoperative cardiac risk assessment. Chest 1999;115(5):51–7.

[15] Davison SP, Venturi ML, Attinger CE, et al. Prevention of venous thromboembolism in the plastic surgery patient. Plast Reconstr Surg 2004; 114(3):43E–51E.

[16] Kheradmand F, Wiener-Kronish JP, Corry DB. Assessment of operative risk for patients with advanced lung disease. Clin Chest Med 1997; 18(3):483–94.

[17] Gracey DR, Divertie MB, Didier EP. Preoperative pulmonary preparation of patients with chronic obstructive pulmonary disease: a prospective study. Chest 1979;76:123–9.

[18] Murin S. Comparison of outcomes after hospitalization for deep venous thrombosis or pulmonary embolism. Thromb Haemost 2002; 88(3):407–14.

[19] Gajic O, Sprung J, Hall BA, et al. Fatal acute pulmonary embolism in a patient with pelvic lipomatosis after surgery performed after transatlantic airplane travel. Anesth Analg 2004;99: 1032–4.

[20] Schwarz T. Venous thrombosis after long-haul flights. Arch Intern Med 2003;163(22):2759–64.

[21] Shields GP. Validation of the Canadian clinical probability model for acute venous thrombosis. Acad Emerg Med 2002;9(6):561–6.

[22] Warner MA. Practice guidelines for preoperative fasting and the use of pharmacologic agents to reduce pulmonary aspiration: application to healthy patients undergoing elective procedures. A report by American Society of Anesthesiologists. Available at: http://www.asahq.org/publicationsAndServices/NPO.pdf. Accessed July 2005.

[23] Block BM, Liu SS, Rowlingson AJ, et al. Efficacy of postoperative epidural analgesia: a meta-analysis. JAMA 2003;290(18):2455–63.

[24] Eisennach JC, Marc DE, Klimscha W. α2-Adrenergic agonists for regional anesthesia. Anesthesiology 1996;85:655–74.

[25] Gaumann DM, Brunet PC, Jirounck P. Clonidine enhances the effects of lidocaine on C-fiber action potential. Anesth Analg 1992;74:719–25.

[26] Grocott MPW, Mythen MG, Gan TJ. Perioperative fluid management and clinical outcomes in adults. Anesth Analg 2005;100(4):1093–106.

[27] Trott SA, Beran SJ, Rohrich RJ, et al. Safety considerations and fluid resuscitation in liposuction: an analysis of 53 consecutive patients. Plast Reconstr Surg 1998;102(6):2220–9.

[28] Monk TG, Saini V, Weldon BC, et al. Anesthetic management and one-year mortality after noncardiac surgery. Anesth Analg 2005;100:4–10.

[29] Rao RB, Ely SF, Hoffman RS. Deaths related to liposuction. N Engl J Med 1999;340(19):1471–5.

[30] Gilliland MD, Coates N. Tumescent liposuction complicated by pulmonary edema. Plast Reconstr Surg 1997;99(1):215–9.

[31] Toledo LS, Regatieri FLF, Carneiro JDA. The effect of hypothermia on coagulation and its implications for infiltration in lipoplasty: a review. Aesthetic Surgery Journal 2001;21(1):40–4.

[32] Mackenzie N, Grant IS. Propofol for intravenous sedation. Anaesthesia 1987;42:3–6.

[33] Bauer KP, Dom PM, Ramirez AM, et al. Preoperative intravenous midazolam: benefits beyond anxiolysis. J Clin Anesth 2004;16(3):177–83.

[34] Joshi GP. Multimodal analgesia techniques and postoperative rehabilitation. Anesthesiology Clin North Am 2005;23:185–202.

[35] Kapfer B, Alfonsi P, Guignard B, et al. Nefopam

and ketamine comparably enhance postoperative analgesia. Anesth Analg 2005;100:169–74.
[36] Mortero RF, Clark LD, Tolan MM, et al. The effects of small-dose ketamine on propofol sedation: respiration, postoperative mood, perception, cognition, and pain. Anesth Analg 2001; 92(6):1465–9.
[37] Evron S, Glezerman M, Sadan O, et al. Remifentanil: a novel systemic analgesic for labor pain. Anesth Analg 2005;100(1):233–8.
[38] Knize DM. Use of preoperative subcutaneous "wetting solution" and epidural block anesthesia for liposuction in the office-based surgical suite. Plast Reconstr Surg 1997;100(7):1867–74.

ELSEVIER
SAUNDERS

CLINICS IN PLASTIC SURGERY

Clin Plastic Surg 33 (2006) 39–46

Liposuction and Tumescent Surgery

Joseph P. Hunstad, MD, FACS[a,*], Marguerite E. Aitken, MD, MFA[b]

- Tumescent technique
- Content of fluid
- Quantity of fluid
- Lidocaine toxicity
- Estimating infiltration volumes
- Current techniques
- Complications
- Summary
- References

The first accounts of fat removal via closed techniques can be attributed to the European community. Joseph Schrudde presented a fat-removal procedure utilizing the sharp uterine curette at the international congress in Cologne, Germany, in 1972 [1], while in 1977, Yves-Gerard Illouz began using blunt-suction techniques for fat removal in France. He describes his first case being performed as "a procedure of love" on a close friend who desired resection of a lipoma from her back [2]. As an actress, she expressed concern regarding scarring, and he considered his options for shorter scar techniques. Having seen the obstetrician's using suction for uterine evacuations, he felt this would be a safe and effective option meeting his needs for both resection and the shortest possible scar [2]. With the success of this procedure over other closed techniques, blunt suction-assisted lipectomy or "liposuction" has become the primary means of body contouring.

Illouz improved his technique, reporting in 1983 on greater than 3000 cases where he injected a hypotonic hyaluronidase solution to emulsify the adipose tissues and enable aspiration via fat suctioning, essentially describing a "wet" technique [3].

This blunt tunneling under the skin rather than sharp undermining limits local tissue injury to structures such as lymphatics and nerves [3]. Fournier, also working in Paris at the time, preferred to omit the hypotonic solution, describing instead, a "dry" technique. This was claimed to be faster, had less tissue distortion, provided a better understanding of the volume of fat aspirated, and lessened the risk of adverse reactions to the hyaluronidase. As with Illouz' cases, the suction cannulae were blunt round/tipped instruments #5 to #10 (5–10 mm) in size. For patients in whom 1 to 2 liters of fat was aspirated, however, they required transfusion to prevent shock [4].

Illouz' wet technique grew in popularity based on advantages including hydrodissection of the tissue planes, transformation of the fat into a fluffier state, making the procedure less physically demanding, and most importantly, reduced bleeding due to vasoconstriction and to the pressure gradient caused by the large volume of fluid and the epinephrine in the wetting solution [5]. This technique was then popularized in the Untied States by surgeons, most notably Hetter, Grazer, and Teimourian. In 1984, Hetter [6] introduced low-dose epinephrine into the solution, which had previously been prohibited due to interactions with the general anesthetic fluothane [5,7]. This technique was performed similarly to Illouz' wet technique of injecting limited volumes of normal saline, distilled water with epinephrine, and hyaluronidase into the subcutaneous tissues by needle-stick injection. Hetter outlined, on the basis of 10 pa-

[a] The Hunstad Center, 8605 Cliff Cameron Drive, Suite 100, Charlotte, NC 28269, USA
[b] Plastic Surgery Associates, P.C., Grand Plaza Place, 220 Lyon Street NW, Suite 700, Grand Rapids, MI 49503, USA
* Corresponding author.
E-mail address: jpg1@hunstadcenter.com (J.P. Hunstad).

0094-1298/06/$ – see front matter doi:10.1016/j.cps.2005.09.002
plasticsurgery.theclinics.com

tients studied pre- and postoperatively, that the addition of low-dose epinephrine could be safely used with the newer anesthetic agents and allowed a greater volume of fat to be aspirated for the same change in hematocrit [6]. However, despite the use of this wet technique, blood losses were still significant, and transfusions typically correlated with the volumes of fat aspirated. Aspirated fat (1.5 liters) would require 1 unit of autologous or donated blood transfusion, 2 liters of fat to 2 units of blood, and 3 liters of fat to 3 units of blood, with this being the endpoint. The average appeared, at that time, to be 3 cc of fat removed associated with 3 cc of blood transfusion.

Originally, guidelines recommended supplemental intravenous fluid that was three times the volume of the aspirate to treat NPO status, third spacing, and fluid shifts. In 1992, Hunstad found that the introduction of tumescent fluid and its subsequent absorption balanced the anticipated volume shifts caused by aspiration and fat removal [8]. Difficulties with pulmonary edema and fluid overload caused surgeons to rethink intravenous fluid requirements after the addition of subcutaneous solutions, and recently, the American Society of Plastic Surgeons made recommendations in a Practice Advisory on Liposuction [9]. In the fluid management section of these practice guidelines it is emphasized to monitor all fluid intake and output accurately, to consider maintenance requirements, preexisting deficits such as overnight fasting, and intraoperative losses of aspirated tissue and third-space deficits. We also recommend these guidelines.

Tumescent technique

The profound vasoconstrictive effects caused by the tumescent solution can also be advantageous for procedures other than liposuction [**Fig. 1**]. The donor site of a skin graft can be tumesced to reduce the bleeding to nearly nothing, making not only the dressing application simpler, but the site virtually pain free at the end of the case. In burn surgery, the infiltration of warm tumescent fluids offers further advantages of decreasing core body temperature loss, minimizing bleeding and the need for transfusion, and lessening the overall operative time.

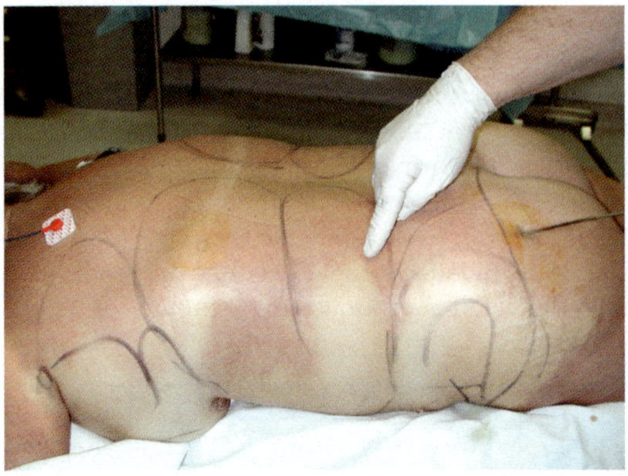

Fig. 1. Infiltration with tumescent solution leads to profound vasoconstriction of the vessels of the skin, readily apparent after 10 to 20 minutes.

Breast reduction surgery, by any method, once required transfusion due the high volume of blood loss. Now, with the addition of tumescent solution placed into either the retromammary space or the subcutaneous tissues or both, blood loss is nearly zero. Other breast surgeries, which can be improved with the use of tumescent solution, include augmentation mammoplasty, capsulectomy, and mastectomy with reconstruction. Both rhytidectomies and abdominoplasties benefit from the use of tumescence to hydrodissect the tissue planes, simplifying the sharp dissection, facilitating flap elevation, and removing the obscuring effects of blood. Hair restoration procedures are greatly improved and pain free with tumescence solution [10]. Its use is also expanded into other specialties, such as urology. Once, prostatectomies were invariably a bloody procedure carrying a high risk of nerve injury. Now, early cases are being performed with excellent results due to the hemostatic effects of tumescent solutions [11]. We continue to anticipate the expanding use of this technique into other specialties.

Safety is of utmost concern when it comes to aesthetic surgery, particularly when using the tumescent technique. Relative contraindications to the technique for use in liposuction, include those patients who fall below an ASA class of I or II (as defined by the American Society of Anesthesiologists), and those taking anticoagulation who require continual treatment, that is, artificial heart valves, history of deep vein thrombosis/pulmonary embolism, atrial fibrillation, or any condition that merits ongoing anticoagulation.

Content of fluid

The wet technique evolved, with increasing infiltration volumes, into the tumescent technique. In 1987, Klein [12] coined this phrase describing the injection of large volumes of saline, dilute epinephrine, and lidocaine to expand the tissues to the point of being swollen, firm, and turgid. Klein made other important contributions to the technique of tumescence for liposuction including analyzing its safety in large volume infiltrations, maximum lidocaine dosages, and its method of delivery [13–15].

Table 1: **Modified Hunstad tumescent fluid solutions**

	Normal (half) strength solution (<5000 mL aspirate)	Large volume (quarter) strength solution (>5000 mL aspirate)
Lactated Ringers	1000 cc	1000 cc
1% Lidocaine plain	25 cc	12.5 cc
Epinephrine 1:1000	1 cc	1 cc
Final concentrations	Lidocaine — 0.05% Epinephrine — 1:1,000,000 Temp 38–40 degrees Celsius	Lidocaine — 0.0125% Epinephrine — 1:1,000,000 Temp 38–40 degrees Celsius

In 1992, we simplified the Klein formula to utilize Lactated Ringers (or Hartmann's solution) versus saline for a reduced load of sodium as well as a more neutral pH of 6.5 [8,16]. Importantly, this fluid is warmed from 38°C to 40°C to reduce core body temperature loss and postoperative morbidity. Currently, we have reduced the lidocaine dosage even further to between 12.5 and 25 mL of 1% lidocaine depending on the volume of anticipated aspirates [Table 1]. This maintains our lidocaine dosage at or below 35 mg/kg, which has been repeatedly shown to be extremely safe. Regardless of the lidocaine content, the epinephrine dosage is the same (1 mg, 1:1000), and remains the most important ingredient in this recipe.

Quantity of fluid

The tumescent technique has been defined by the ratio of fluid infiltrated versus fluid aspirated, and is typically described as 3 to 4:1 versus the wet technique 1:1. Undue emphasis, however, is placed on these ratios.

The surgeon's best guide for proper infiltration is to achieve the tumesced state, the final endpoint of strong tissue turgor. Ratios offer a difficult and meaningless guide to assist the anesthesiologist in fluid delivery during the case. When the overall anticipated suction volume is small, such as in a 3 to 5 liters case, it is much more feasible to use an expected tumescent ratio. However, when the volumes rise to greater levels of aspirate removed, the ratios approach 1:1, regardless of the number of regions being treated. When the patient is obese or when the number of sites being treated is high, it is also more likely that the ratio will approach 1:1, even with associated large volume infiltration. Ratios may seem helpful, but in general, the best approach is ongoing communication with the anesthesiologist and limitation of intravenous fluid delivery due to absorption of tumescent fluid both during and after the case. Continuous clinical evaluation remains the most important guideline for safe fluid administration.

At our institution, the aspirates of the tumescent technique have a much reduced hematocrit and are virtually bloodless due to the effects of the epinephrine and pressure of the fluid on the local tissues [16–18]. Where the wet technique would produce a blood loss of approximately 150 to 300 mL/L of aspirate, the effects of the tumesced state produce blood loss of only 6 to 7 mL/L of aspirates! Because the volumes infused to reach the tumescent state can be quite large, concern may exist regarding the absorption of lidocaine systemically and the time required for infusion of these large volumes.

Using a hand-pressurized bag or a gas-pressurized infuser to provide rapid infusion of fluids, time for infiltration can be much reduced. In our hands, 5 to 6 liters of fluid can be infused over a period of 10 to 15 minutes [16].

Lidocaine toxicity

Lidocaine toxicity is always a concern, and is due to the sodium channel blocking effects normally exerted upon nerves, also affecting the membranes of the brain, heart, and arteriolar smooth muscle. Typically the manifestation of this toxicity occurs first in the brain with symptoms of central nervous system excitation such as light headedness, dizziness, auditory and visual disturbances, and eventually convulsions. Evidence of higher blood levels are brain depression, impaired impulse conduction in the heart, decreased myocardial contractility, and dilatation of arteriolar smooth muscle [18]. Diazepam will raise the threshold for such events to occur, while addition of epinephrine reduces the availability of the lidocaine beyond the infiltration sites [18]. Although it remains reasonable that a slower rate of subcutaneous infiltration would raise blood levels of lidocaine at a slower rate, enabling observation of the symptoms of toxicity, studies performed at our institution show otherwise. A prospective analysis of 220 consecutive patients undergoing increasing rates of standard tumescent infiltration found no significant change in blood levels after infiltration compared to those during infiltration (average 0.8 μg/mL) [17].

Another important study of lidocaine levels analyzed two patients infiltrated with tumescent fluid,

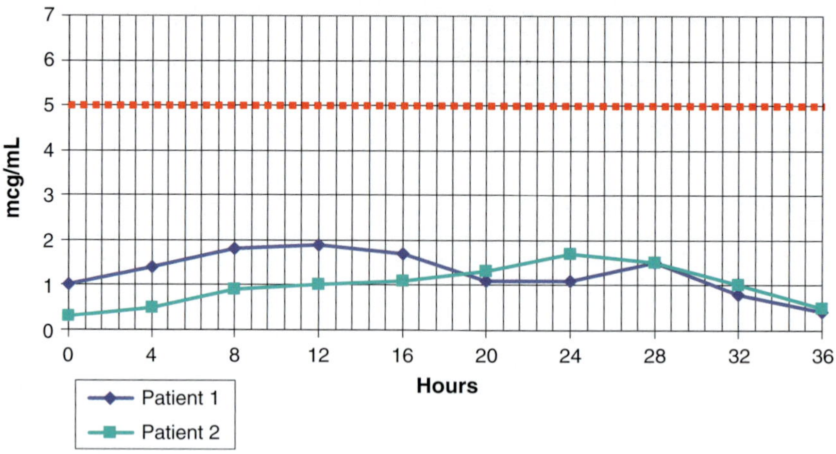

Fig. 2. Levels of lidocaine measured every 4 hours postoperatively, not exceeding 2 μg/mL and well below maximum lidocaine levels.

but not suctioned. The levels of lidocaine were evaluated at 4-hour intervals for 36 hours, and found never to exceed 2 μg/mL, well below the 5 μg/mL level where concern for toxicity arises [Fig. 2].

Rubin also found while studying the levels of lidocaine absorption postinfiltration, that although local pressures in the tumesced tissues can be raised to 300 mmHg, the absorption of lidocaine is not significantly affected by these high pressures but is delayed in those fluids containing low dose epinephrine [19,20].

Although many investigators have shown that it is safe to administer higher doses of lidocaine, we believe caution should be taken to avoid the delivery of doses greater than 35 mg/kg [13]. We feel there is no reason to significantly exceed this recommendation (35 mg/kg), as this level has repeatedly been shown to be very safe. If greater volumes of infiltrated fluid are expected for treatment of multiple sites or high-volume aspirations, the dosage of lidocaine should be reduced in the tumescent solution. In the obese patient with an anticipated fat removal of 10 to 12 liters, it is not unusual to infuse 10 to 15 liters of tumescent fluid or more. Realistically, the ratio of fluid to aspirate in these cases ranges from 1.5:1 to 1:1, but intravenous fluids should again be minimized to prevent fluid overload or pulmonary edema postoperatively [16].

Estimating infiltration volumes

The plastic surgeon experienced in liposuction needs no assistance in the estimation of fluid to be infiltrated. However, for purposes of verification, for those surgeons new to the concepts of tumescent liposuction or for those who desire some direction in choosing volumes to infuse, we suggest a simple tool. In our practice, an estimate of the anticipated fat aspirate is not a straight line estimation of the volume to be infused. However, it is possible to estimate the volume of fluid to be infused based simply on observational techniques.

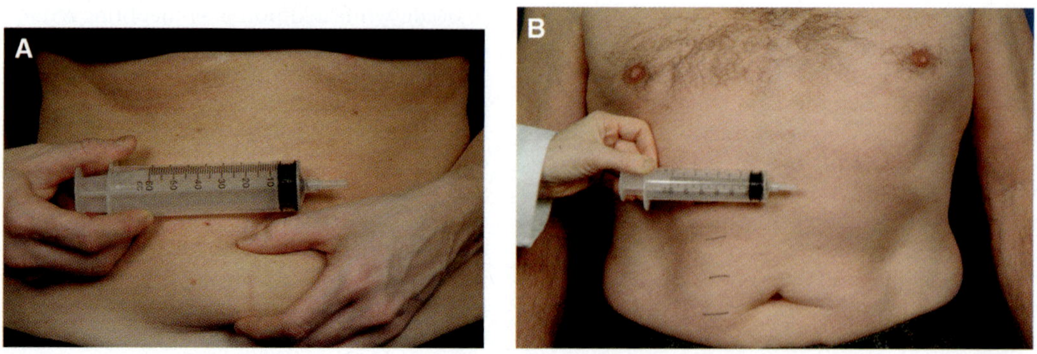

Fig. 3. Technique for estimating the volume of fat to be aspired. (*A*) Pinching the skin to minic the syringe size. (*B*) Count the number of syringes anticipated and calculate the estimated aspiration.

The physician should study in the preoperative examination the tissues to be treated via the pinch technique, comparing them with the volume of a standard 60-cc syringe. With the patient standing, enough muscle contraction exists to properly evaluate the excess subcutaneous fat in most body areas as a pinch between the index finger and the thumb, mimicking the diameter of a 60-cc syringe [Fig. 3]. For a certain region, each "60-cc syringe" volume to be suctioned should be counted and multiplied by 60 to estimate the fat aspirate. The infiltration volume can then be determined, depending on the total volume to be suctioned, the type of fat present, and the desired level of tumescence. In our practice, at least 100 mL to 200 mL of tumescent fluid is administered for each "60-cc syringe" volume, for a ratio of greater than 2:1. Intraoperative adjustments must be as needed to achieve an endpoint of tumescence as described above. The total of estimated fat for removal is used as a guideline. A good rule of thumb is to aspirate to within 10% of this value and use clinical judgment at this point to determine the endpoint.

Current techniques

All preoperative markings are performed in the photo suite prior to surgery. The patient is actively involved in the location of entry sites as well as areas to be treated. Topographical markings help to delineate those regions to be significantly reduced, those in which only light suctioning will be adequate, and for areas to be avoided or treated with lipoinjection.

Although tumescent solution provides a certain level of anesthesia and pain control, the majority of our patients undergo general anesthesia simply for comfort and control of the airway in all positions, particularly for prone cases or those that require extended periods of time. After sequential compression devices are placed, induction is performed in the supine position on the operating room (OR) gurney and the patient is subsequently rolled, following anterior tumescent infiltration, into a prone position on the table and padded for protection of nerves and pressure points.

Infiltration via entry sites shown [Fig. 4] is performed using a CO_2 pressurized tumescent delivery system [Fig. 5] (Circon Corporation, BC, Canada) allowing for a constant maintenance of pressure and using a flow-control handle of a 3-mm blunt tipped, multiple-hole infiltration cannula and a flow control handle (Byron) facilitating fluid delivery.

The entry site is prepped with betadine and the cannula wiped with betadine prior to creation of each new access site. The solution is delivered to

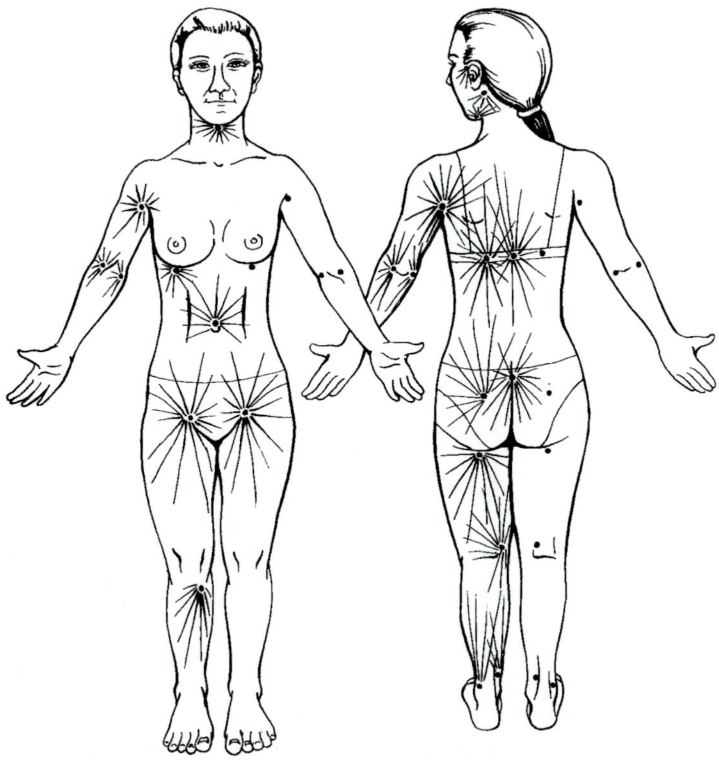

Fig. 4. Location of preferred entry sites for infiltration and suction.

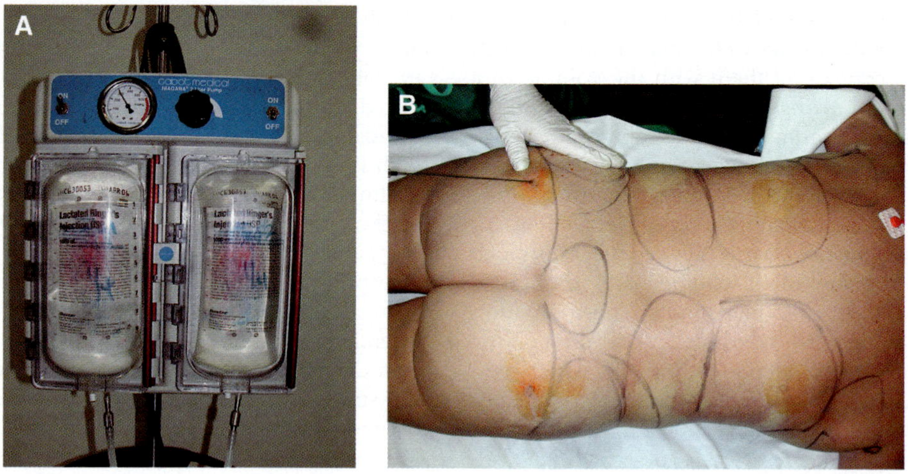

Fig. 5. (*A*) Gas pressurized tumescence infiltration system. (*B*) Utilizing tumescent infiltration.

the prefascial, intermediate and superficial levels—all levels to be subsequently suctioned. The endpoint for infiltration is evaluated by both inspection of blanching due to the effects of epinephrine and by a palpable level of turgidity and a firm, tight, fullness of the entire area being treated. A positive *fountain sign* is an excellent indicator that the tissues are adequately hydrated.

On the OR wall hangs a linear graph depicting the liters of standard tumescence solution versus patient weight in kilograms to confirm at a glance the limitations in volume based on lidocaine levels that can be infused safely [**Fig. 6**]. As the effects of epinephrine are the key to bloodless surgery, it is imperative to wait at least 20 minutes after infiltration to take effect. This is another reason to complete the anterior tumescent infiltration and turn the patient to a prone position for infiltration of the posterior areas, to waste little precious and expensive OR time. The effectiveness lidocaine within the tissues is almost immediate.

We recommend the use of our intraoperative graph to track, in real time, the volumes of fluid and supernatant fat aspirated per site and per side to better establish the fluid balance on a site by site basis [**Fig. 7**]. This enables both the surgical and anesthesia personnel to continuously monitor aspirates.

Complications

Complications due to tumescent surgery and liposuction include skin devascularization, permanent or temporary nerve damage, contour irregularities, skin laxity, asymmetries and death due to excessive aspiration, fluid imbalance, and lidocaine toxicity. Proper patient selection and the administration of the appropriate technique are critical to ensure a

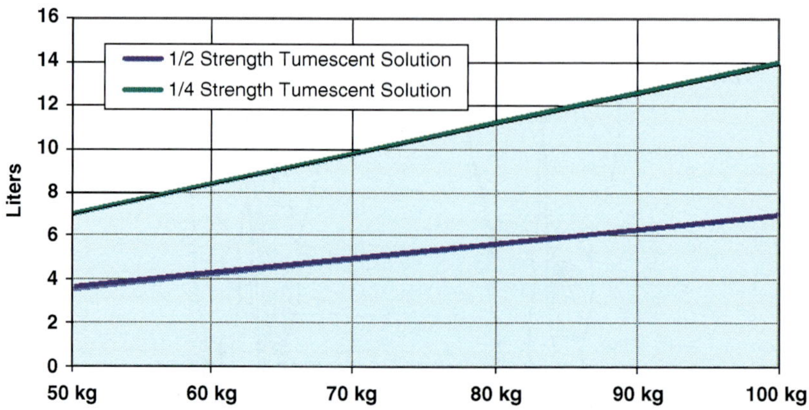

Fig. 6. Quick reference graph depicting number of liters that can be infused based upon desired lidocaine maximum dosage and patient weight.

A

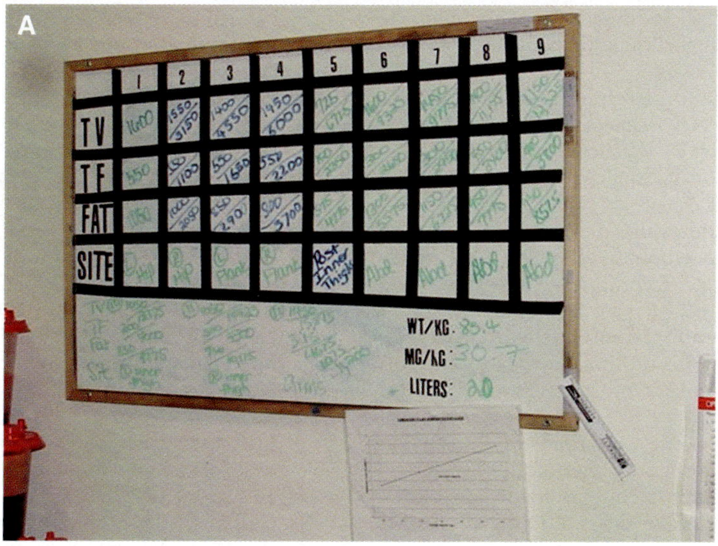

B

	1	2	3	4	5	6	7	8	9	10
TV (mL)										
TF (mL)										
FAT (mL)										
UAL										
SITE										

Fig. 7. (*A*) Chart depicting information on aspirates. (*B*) Chart for aspirate recording. All volumes are recorded after aspirate has settled, approximately 20 minutes. FAT, supernatant fat (calculated); SITE, location of procedure; TF, total infranatant fluid; TV, total aspirate volume; UAL, ultrasonic on time (seconds).

good aesthetic result. The major concern with tumescent surgery is the overuse of the solution and possible respiratory complications, that is, pulmonary edema, the mechanism of which is both fluid overload and potentially high doses of lidocaine leading to depressed cardiac myocontractility [21,22]. The most effective solution for safe aesthetic surgery is to abide by the recommendations put forth by the ASPS task force. Constant communication with anesthesia personnel experienced in the care of liposuction patients is critical to safe surgery, and we have recommended methods here to enable this exchange.

Summary

When guidelines for tumescent surgery are followed, treatment of patients with a broad range of concerns can be extremely effective. Whether its use is as a primary technique as in liposuction, or as an adjunct to another procedure such as reduction mammoplasty, the effects of reduced blood loss, pain control, and fluid management make it a powerful tool for the surgeon. Constant awareness of volumes infiltrated and aspirated, as well as the patient's clinical status, are critical in the safe delivery of tumescent surgery.

References

[1] Hait P, Schnur PL. History of the American Society of Plastic and Reconstructive Surgeons, 1931–1994. Plast Reconstr Surg 1994;94(4): 1A–105A.

[2] Illouz YG. Personal discussion with Hunstad JP during a meeting in Puerto Vallarta, Mexico, October 2004.

[3] Illouz YG. Body contouring by lipolysis: a 5-year experience with over 3000 cases. Plast Reconstr Surg 1983;72(5):591–7.

[4] Fournier PF, Otteni FM. Lipodissection in body sculpting: the dry procedure. Plast Reconstr Surg 1983;72(5):598–601.

[5] Illouz YG. History and current concepts of lipoplasty. Clin Plast Surg 1996;23(4):721–30.

[6] Hetter GP. The effect of low-dose epinephrine on the hematocrit drop following lipolysis. Aesthetic Plast Surg 1984;8(1):19–21.

[7] Weigt HU, Kwok WM, Rehmert GC, et al. Modu-

lation of cardiac sodium current by alpha1-stimulation and volatile anesthetics. Anesthesiology 1997;87(6):1507–16.
[8] Hunstad JP. The tumescent technique: an evolution. Lipoplasty Newsletter, 1994; Vol. 11, No. 29.
[9] Iverson RE, Lynch DJ. Practice advisory on liposuction. Plast Reconstr Surg 2004;113(5):1478–90; discussion 1491–5.
[10] Hunstad JP. Addressing difficult areas in body contouring with emphasis on combined tumescent and syringe techniques. Clin Plast Surg 1996;23(1):57–80.
[11] May J, McGovern F. Hemostatic hydrodissection: a new technique to promote nerve-sparing during radical retropubic prostatectomy. Curr Urol Rep 2005;6(1):1.
[12] Klein JA. Tumescent technique for liposuction surgery. Am J Cosm Surg 1987;4:263.
[13] Klein JA. Tumescent technique for regional anesthesia permits lidocaine doses of 35 mg/kg for liposuction. J Dermatol Surg Oncol 1990;16:248–63.
[14] Klein JA. Tumescent technique for local anesthesia improves safety in large volume liposuction. Plast Reconstr Surg 1993;92(6):1085–101.
[15] Burk 3rd RW, Guzman-Stein G, Vasconez LO. Lidocaine and epinephrine levels in tumescent technique liposuction. Plast Reconstr Surg 1996; 97(7):1379–84.
[16] Hunstad JP. Body contouring in the obese patient. Clin Plast Surg 1996;23(4):647–69.
[17] Hunstad JP. The tumescent technique: an evolution. Presented at the 11th annual meeting of the Lipoplasty Society of North America. New Orleans; 1993.
[18] Hunstad JP. Liposuction of the hips and thighs. In: Evans G, editor. Operative plastic surgery. New York: McGraw Hill; 2000. p. 93–125.
[19] Hetter GP. Lipoplasty: the theory and practice of blunt suction lipectomy. 2nd edition. Boston: Little, Brown and Co.; 1990. p. 138–9.
[20] Rubin JP. The tumescent technique: the effect of high tissue pressure and dilute epinephrine on absorption of lidocaine. Plast Reconst Surg 1999;103(3):990–6.
[21] Gilliland MD, Commons GW, Halperin B. Safety issues in ultrasound-assisted large-volume lipoplasty. Clin Plast Surg 1999;26(2):317–35.
[22] Gilliland MD, Coates N. Tumescent liposuction complicated by pulmonary edema. Plast Reconstr Surg 1997;99(1):215–9.

ELSEVIER
SAUNDERS

CLINICS IN PLASTIC SURGERY

Clin Plastic Surg 33 (2006) 47–53

Fat Injection: A 20-Year Revision

Luiz S. Toledo, MD[a,*], Raul Mauad, MD[b]

The search for an ideal method to correct soft-tissue defects by autologous means has always been a concern in plastic surgery. Fat injection has been a controversial subject for many years. The first decades of the twentieth century were filled with reports of progress made in the field of fat grafting, but interest waned only to reawaken in the 1970s.

The first communication about fat transplantation was presented by Neuber [1] in 1893, followed by reports by Czerny [2], Lexer [3], and Rehn [4]. In 1911, Bruning [5] was the first to inject autologous fat into the subcutaneous tissue for the purpose of soft-tissue augmentation. In 1956, Peer [6] showed that the survival rate for fat grafts could be as high as 50%.

In the last 20 years, several different techniques of lipoinjection have been developed, but a standard procedure has not been adopted by all practitioners. There is no agreement as to the best way of processing the fat to ensure maximal take and viability of the graft. Other controversial issues include the ideal cannula for harvesting and reinjection, the presence of blood in the transplanted fat, trauma, air exposure, contamination of the graft, durability, and fat cell survival. Newly emerging approaches to fat tissue engineering with the use of cultured autologous preadipocytes may improve the technique of fat injection and transplant.

The 1980s: the first liposuction studies

With the development of liposuction, the process of harvesting fat became an outpatient procedure. In the 1980s, Illouz [7–10] and Fournier [11,12] developed an easy approach to fat transfer by syringe harvesting, called "microlipoinjection" by Fournier [11]. This process became possible after the advent of liposuction. Fat grafting became the simplest and easiest method among the different techniques used to correct the soft tissues for facial contour [13–16] and, if needed, to replace soft tissue in areas such as augmentation and reshaping the buttocks, thighs, calves, and ankles [17,18], trochanteric depressions [19], scar depressions, small wrinkles, depressions of the face and Romberg's disease [20,21], the nasolabial fold, liposuction sequelae, and the fingers and hands [22].

Toledo [23] showed improvement of superficial irregularities, depressions, "cellulite," and liposuction sequelae to varying degrees depending on the problem, with high patient satisfaction when the reality of the improvement was explained preoperatively. Chajchir and Benzaquen [24] showed that autogenous graft tissue was more successful than homologous and heterologous tissue in eliminating deep defects in the skin surface. Lipoinjection began to be used as a graft by innumer-

[a] Private practice, Av. Brg. Luiz Antonio, 4442, São Paulo 01402-002, Brazil
[b] Private practice, R. Manoel Cebrian Ferrer, 60, São Paulo 04023-070, Brazil
* Corresponding author.
E-mail address: lstoledo@netpoint.com.br (L.S. Toledo).

0094-1298/06/$ – see front matter doi:10.1016/j.cps.2005.08.002
plasticsurgery.theclinics.com

ous surgeons for the modification of facial and body contour, including in the chin, cheekbones, nasolabial folds, lips, labiomandibular folds, glabella, foreheads, nose, buttocks, and legs [14,17, 25–57].

Autologous fat grafting has been a controversial subject for a long time. It has strong advocates as well as strong critics, such as Ersek [58] (who later changed his mind about the procedure, incorporating it into his armamentarium), Fredericks [59], Goldwyn [60], Samdal and coworkers [61], and Smahel [62]. The main disadvantage is the high absorption rate of the injected fat, which can reach up to 70% of its volume [20,63]. Fredericks wrote in 1988 that "The converse of that argument is that the emotional and financial investments by the patient are not justified for a short-lived improvement that tantalizes and ultimately disappears." In 1988, Illouz [9] published long-term results for 167 cases in which the fat injection technique was performed, including his disappointment with the use of fat to fill wrinkles in the face (later, Illouz used the technique when necessary). Guerrerosantos and coworkers [47] found that fat transplanted into subcutaneous tissue was impossible to identify or separate from the already existent fat but when infiltrated into the muscle seemed to be permanent.

Reports by Guerrerosantos [47] and Eppley [64] and their coworkers suggest that there is a better take of the fat cells when they are injected into the muscle. Toledo injects fat into the subcutaneous tissue or muscle, depending on the area and the problem to be corrected. Nevertheless, in some areas (face, ankles), there is no available muscle to inject fat where it is needed.

A review of the use of free autologous fat grafts was published by Billings and May [65] in 1989, and a histologic review was conducted by Smahel [62] in 1986. The cell survival theory proposes that some of the graft adipose tissue survives after the host reaction subsides. Some fat really integrates as a graft, whereas the rest is probably involved in an inflammatory reaction.

Fat grafts have become an important and reliable procedure in plastic surgery. As Chajchir and Benzaquen [32] wrote in 1989, "...the early results obtained, the increasing number of patients asking for the fat injection, and their high level of satisfaction makes us recommend this method as effective."

Deburge and coworkers [66] reported the experimental use of fat grafts thicker than 5 mm applied to prevent postoperative peridural fibrosis after surgery on the lumbar spine. Van Akkerveeken and coworkers [67] observed the fate of the fat graft in spinal surgery using CT scanning, and Weisz and Gal [68] reported a 40-month survival of a free fat graft in the spinal canal postlaminectomy.

Many articles have been written on experiments in animals [69–72] showing results in agreement with those of Peer and consistent with his cell survival theory. Experimental studies in rats performed by Eppley and coworkers [73,74] suggested that, for the fat cells to survive, they should be mixed previously with basic fibroblast growth factor (bFGF) alone or dextran beads pretreated with bFGF. These findings suggest that the addition of cell-specific bioactive peptides that affect the preadipocyte cell line or the fibroblastic components of the recipient site will improve postoperative fat graft weight maintenance. Insulin has also been mixed with fat cells by Bircoll [75] and Silkiss and Baylis [76] in an attempt to improve cell take, but this process has been abandoned, and the efficacy of insulin treatment remains unproved. Research performed by Boyce and coworkers [77], including the development of preadipocyte transplants and the hormonal manipulation of fat grafts, may improve the long-term results of fat transplantation.

Asaadi and Haramis [78] have reported successful follow-ups after 5 years and advocate the technique. Severe complications are rare and are usually caused by the use of inappropriate instrumentation. Egido and coworkers [79] have published cases of middle cerebral artery embolism and visual loss after fat injection in the glabellar area, probably owing to intravascular injection by using a sharp needle instead of a blunt one. Trockman and coworkers [80] reported complications of penile injection of autologous fat owing to bad technique.

Hunter and Baker [81] have used fat grafting successfully in ophthalmology to treat enophthalmos by orbital injection of a fat autograft, and Santarosa and Blaivas [82] have used the technique in urology, performing periurethral injection of autologous fat for the treatment of sphincteric incontinence.

Contrary to the theory that 3-mm threads of fat are best for reinjection, McFarland [83] suggests that "pearl" grafts have a better take. Schorr and coworkers [84] reported greater long-term soft-tissue augmentation and graft survival with insulin-treated free fat pearl grafts. The pearl or almond-shaped fat graft was initially performed by Loeb [85] to treat the nasal-jugal groove.

Based on the experience of Carpaneda and Ribeiro [86], the viability of the fat graft decreases if the graft diameter is greater than 3 mm. These researchers showed that the fat's ability to obtain nutrition through plasmatic imbibition occurs approximately 1.5 mm from the vascularized edge. Their studies originated the technique of injecting 3-mm thick threads of fat, leaving space for neovascularization.

Review of autologous fat transfer during the last 10 years: techniques, survival, and longevity

In 1994, Niechajev and Sevcuk [87] reported on nine cases of idiopathic constitutional subcutaneous fat atrophy in the cheek area treated by the autologous transplantation of fat for purely esthetic reasons. The fat graft suspension was obtained by the low-power aspiration technique with the use of a vacuum pump. The contour defects were initially overcorrected by approximately 50% more volume than required. Delicate tissue handling and the small total amount of fat transplanted by careful distribution in the recipient tissues are probably the factors responsible for the long-lasting improvement in these patients.

Also in 1994, Carpaneda and Ribeiro [86] concluded that the percentage of graft viability depends on the thickness and geometrical shape and is inversely proportional to the graft diameter if grafts with a diameter greater than 3 mm are considered.

In 1995, Coleman [88] documented the amount and rate of reabsorption of fatty tissue transplanted using his technique. A selected crease was infiltrated with autologous fatty tissue using a nearby crease as a control. Photographs were taken in the first week and at least yearly over 6 years. This experiment demonstrated the potential lasting nature of corrections performed with the transplantation of fatty tissue and is supported by over 400 infiltrations into the nasolabial folds in the authors' practice.

In 1995, Hunstad [89] evaluated the combined tumescent and syringe techniques for liposuction. Liposuction aspirates using the modified tumescent technique were compared and contrasted with liposuction aspirates obtained using the "dry" and "wet" technique. A critical analysis of the limitations of this combined technique was also described, noting added time requirements and difficulties with undercorrection of deformities, the need for reoperation, and methods for determining the endpoint of the procedure, as well as addressing large-volume liposuction problems. Advantages included eliminating the need for general anesthesia, lessening blood loss and postoperative bruising, greater accuracy and precision, and overall high patient satisfaction.

In 1996, Chajchir [34] reported the results of long-term follow-up (from 1984 to 1994) of fat injection to correct soft-tissue defects using the patient's own fatty tissue obtained by liposuction. The main goal was to find a successful procedure to obtain a good specimen graft and long-term results. This task was not easy because of the high reabsorption of fatty tissue.

In 1996, Toledo [56] reported 8-year results with syringe liposculpture, a technique for the treatment of localized fat deposits, to remodel the body and the face using disposable syringes and fine-tip cannulas. He started working on a combination of syringe liposculpture and superficial liposuction to treat the superficial layer of fat, resulting in "superficial liposculpture." Syringe liposculpture of the face can be offered as an alternative to rhytidoplasty and a complement to other techniques to improve the appearance with minimal morbidity.

Also in 1996, Pereira and Radwanski [55] presented their experience with fat grafting for the treatment of contour deformities of the buttocks and lower limbs. This method has been termed *liposculpture* and consists of removing adipose tissue by a cannula and syringe and cleaning the aspirated material with saline. All external contact is carefully avoided, preventing contamination. Fat grafting is performed in multiple tunnels in a deep plane. Fat absorption was estimated by clinical evaluation to be less than 20% of volume. A low rate of complications (less than 3%) supports the opinion that this method is an efficient and safe procedure to correct or enhance contour deformities of the lower limbs.

In 1996, Guerrerosantos [48] described that the combination of liposuction and lipoinjection was rapidly becoming the procedure of choice for achieving symmetry and better contour of the back torso and middle third of the body. Its versatility makes it suitable for most body contour deformities. Fat graft long-term survival was presented. This procedure has been used by the authors during the past 12 years.

In 1997, Schuller-Petrovic [90] reported his experience performing microlipotransplantation of autologous fat to correct contour defects, mainly of the face, since 1987. He treated a total of 176 patients with different tissue defects. With a follow-up as long as 8 years, the best results were with scars and atrophies.

In 1997, Coleman [37] described the placement of small amounts of fatty tissue in multiple tunnels, of utmost importance in the quest for survival of fatty tissue and an esthetically appropriate correction. Successful three-dimensional sculpting requires attention to patient preparation, meticulous planning, and fastidious photographic evaluation. The potential applications of this new tool in esthetic and reconstructive surgeries are profound. Lipostructure represents a safe, long-lasting method of recontouring the face with autologous tissue.

In 1998, Guerrerosantos [49] reported a 10-year experience combining rhytidoplasty (including systematizing superficial musculoaponeurotic system and platysma plication) with lipoinjection, placing thin rolls of autologous fat into the facial and cervical muscles or at least under the fascia. The results revealed a high success rate with few minor complications.

In 1999, Amar [91] presented his experience with autologous fatty tissue transplantation. He called his method "microinfiltration of adipocytes." Fat was harvested with the technique of syringe liposuction without trauma and was refined and placed in an intricate layering of autologous fatty tissue with anatomic patented microcannulas. This procedure, named lipostructure by Coleman, is not a lipofilling or "liposculpture" as described by Fournier in 1989. By focusing on the procedure as an autotransplantation fat grafting technique and fully respecting the delicate nature of the fat cell, Amar has been able to document a high rate of success with 3 years of follow-up.

In 2000, De Pedroza [92] reported the results for 1350 liposculptures performed over a period of 6.5 years. A total of 879 patients had buttock augmentation. The hypothesis that applied fat grafts are real grafts was demonstrated. The grafts were not only real but were also able to live and persist with the patient, growing if the patient gained weight over the gluteus area and not losing circumference when the patient reduced weight. In 2000, Peren [93] presented the authors' experience with gluteus augmentation with autologous fat grafts and liposuction methods, having recorded the evolution of gluteus reshaping with autologous intramuscular fat graft injections. Long-term results were emphasized.

Also in 2000, Guerrerosantos [49] presented his experience with two types of patients: (1) older persons with thin facial soft tissues, in whom the combination of lifting and lipoinjection gives good results; and (2) patients with progressive hemifacial atrophy caused by Parry-Romberg's syndrome, in whom normal or almost normal facial contour can be achieved. The long-term survival of fat grafts was presented.

In 2000, Sommer and Sattler [94] studied the controversy surrounding the longevity of correction in autologous fat grafts and its relation to adipocyte survival. The reported long-term fat graft survival rates differed widely depending on the harvesting method, means of reinjection, injection site, and evaluation methods. They demonstrated histologic findings of aspirated adipose tissue and compared the findings with reports in the literature. The clinical longevity of correction after autologous fat transfer is determined by the degree of augmentation resulting from the amount of fibrosis induced and the number of viable fat cells. Survival of aspirated fat cell grafts depends mainly on the anatomic site, the mobility and vascularity of the recipient tissue, and underlying causes and diseases, and less on harvesting and reinjection methods.

In 2001, Shoshani and coworkers [95] examined the role of frozen storage as a means of preserving the fat obtained by suction-assisted lipectomy for repeated procedures. Human adipose tissue obtained by suction-assisted lipectomy was stored in a domestic refrigerator at −18°C for 2 weeks. After thawing, the fat was injected into nude mice. Grafts were dissected out and compared 15 weeks postinjection. The injected fat survived in the study and control groups. There were no significant differences between fat graft weight and volume or in any of the histologic parameters examined; therefore, it was concluded that fat obtained by suction-assisted lipectomy could be preserved for future use by freezing.

In 2002, Coleman [39] presented a reliable technique of autologous fat grafting for long-lasting rejuvenation of the dorsum of the hand. Small intact parcels of fatty tissue are harvested with a syringe and a blunt 3-mm cannula. Most of the nonviable components are removed from the harvested subcutaneous material by centrifugation, decanting, and wicking. A 17-gauge blunt cannula is used to place the fat in minuscule parcels of tissue with many passes through five or six tiny incisions in the hand. Separation of the tiny parcels of fat maximizes contact between the surfaces of the transplanted fat and surrounding recipient tissues to encourage integration, anchoring, and long-term survival.

In 2003, Butterwick and Lack [96] presented their experience with 100 patients who underwent a new technique known as fat autograft muscle injection in which fat was injected within the muscles of facial expression. The fat was harvested in an atraumatic and sterile manner. Centrifuged fat was then injected with specific blunt-tipped cannulas for different muscle groups. The majority of patients underwent a partial versus full-face procedure. Facial volume restoration with the fat autograft muscle technique is a systematic approach for facial volume restoration. It offers the potential for symmetric, long-term results.

In 2004, Aygit and coworkers [97] designed an experimental study to assess the viability and revascularization of intramuscularly injected fat autografts. Fat autografts were performed on the right side of a rabbit, and the left side was used as control. Scintilographic imaging and histopathologic examination of the limbs were performed after injection of adipose tissue on days 15, 30, 45, 60, 90, and 120. The technetium-99m increased uptake indicated that there was viable fat tissue in this region. Histopathologic evaluation revealed that adipose tissue survived in more than 50% of the graft area in all of the animals. These findings show that fat autografts can survive in muscle tissue with less than 50% fibrotic change.

In 2004, Guerrerosantos [50,51] reported a new simple method for preparing fat for injection and published an article in which a fat graft was used for the treatment of palatopharyngeal and velopharyngeal incompetence. Some authorities [98–102] advocate using newly emerging approaches when fat tissue engineering principles are applied. These approaches are sophisticated, complex, and expensive procedures. The use of culture autologous preadipocytes may be a way to improve the techniques of lipoinjection and transplant.

Even using available technology, fat grafting has become in the last 20 years the treatment of choice of many plastic surgeons for facial and body contour soft-tissue augmentation in reconstructive and esthetic surgery.

References

[1] Neuber GA. Fettransplantation. Verh Dtsch Ges Chir 1893;22:66.
[2] Czerny A. Plastischer Ersatz der Brustdrose durch ein Lipoma. Chir Kongr Verhandl 1895; 216:2.
[3] Lexer E. Freire fettgewebstranplantation. Dtsch Med Wochenschr 1910;36:46.
[4] Rehn E. Die fettransplantation. Arch Klin Chir 1912;98:1.
[5] Bruning P [cited by Broeckaert TJ]. Contribution a l'étude des greffes adipeuses. Buli Acad R Med Belgique 1919;28:440.
[6] Peer LA. The neglected "free fat graft": its behavior and clinical use. Am J Surg 1956;92:40.
[7] Illouz YG. De l'utilization de la graisse aspiré pour combler les defects cutanés. Rev Chir Esthet Lang Franc 1985;10:13.
[8] Illouz YG. The fat cell graft: a new technique to fill depressions. Plast Reconstr Surg 1986;78:122.
[9] Illouz YG. Present results of fat injection. Aesthetic Plast Surg 1988;12(3):175–81.
[10] Illouz YG. Fat injection: hope or reality? In: Illouz YG, De Villers YT, editors. Body sculpturing by lipoplasty. Edinburgh: Churchill Livingstone; 1989. p. 389–95.
[11] Fournier PF. Microlipoextration et microlipoinjection. Rev Chir Esthet Lang Franc 1985;10: 36–40.
[12] Fournier PF. Facial recontouring with fat grafting. Dermatol Clin 1990;8:523–37.
[13] Toledo LS. Liposculpture of the face and body. In: Toledo LS, editor. Annals of the International Symposium Recent Advances in Plastic Surgery. São Paulo, March 3–5, 1989. p.177–92.
[14] de la Fuente A, Tavora T. Fat injections for the correction of facial lipodystrophies: a preliminary report. Aesthetic Plast Surg 1988; 12(1):39–43.
[15] Levy S, Pitombo V. Facial graft. In: Toledo LS, editor. Annals of the International Symposium Recent Advances in Plastic Surgery. São Paulo, March 3–5, 1989. p.163–9.
[16] Pitombo V, Levy S. Fat graft in the face (evolution). In: Toledo LS, Pinto ES, editors. Annals of the International Symposium Recent Advances in Plastic Surgery. São Paulo, March 28–30, 1990. RAPS International Corporation; 1990. p. 204–11.
[17] Matsudo PK, Toledo LS. Experience of injected fat grafting. Aesthetic Plast Surg 1988;12(1): 35–8.
[18] Gonzalez R. Buttocks contouring: prosthesis and fat grafting. In: Toledo LS, Pinto ES, editors. Annals of the International Symposium Recent Advances in Plastic Surgery. São Paulo, March 28–30, 1990. RAPS International Corporation; 1990. p. 263–72.
[19] Lewis CM. Correction of deep gluteal depression by autologous fat grafting. Aesthetic Plast Surg 1992;16(3):247–50.
[20] Moscona R, Ullman Y, Har-Shai Y, et al. Free-fat injections for the correction of hemifacial atrophy. Plast Reconstr Surg 1989;84(3):501–7 [discussion, 508–9].
[21] Chajchir A, Benzaquen I. Liposuction fat grafts in face wrinkles and hemifacial atrophy. Aesthetic Plast Surg 1986;10(2):115–7.
[22] Aboudib Jr JH, Castro CC, Gradel J. Beautifying the hands. In: Toledo LS, Pinto ES, editors. Annals of the International Symposium Recent Advances in Plastic Surgery. São Paulo, March 28–30, 1990. RAPS International Corporation; 1990. p. 197–203.
[23] Toledo LS. Syringe liposculpture: a two-year experience. Aesthetic Plast Surg 1991;15(4):321–6.
[24] Chajchir A, Benzaquen I. Fat-grafting injection for soft-tissue augmentation. Plast Reconstr Surg 1989;84(6):921–4 [discussion, 935].
[25] Aboudib Jr JHC, Cardoso de Castro C, Gradel J. Hand rejuvenescence by fat filling. Ann Plast Surg 1992;28:559.
[26] Baroudi R. Personal approach in fat transplantation. Presented at the16th Annual Symposium on Aesthetic Plastic Surgery, University of Guadalajara, 1998.
[27] Bolivar de Souza Pinto E, Erazo IPJ, Prado Filho FSA, et al. Superficial liposuction. Aesthetic Plast Surg 1996;20:111.
[28] Cardenas-Camarena L, Lacouture AM, Tobar-Losada A. Combined gluteoplasty: liposuction and lipoinjection. Plast Reconstr Surg 1999; 104(5):1524–31.
[29] Carraway JH, Mellow CG. Syringe aspiration and fat concentration: a simple technique for autologous fat injection. Ann Plast Surg 1990; 24(3):293–6.

[30] Carraway JH. Discussion: enhancing the take of injected adipose tissue by a simple method for concentrating fat cells. Plast Reconstr Surg 2005;115(1):202–3.
[31] Chajchir A, Benzaquen I. Liposuction fat grafts in face wrinkles and hemifacial atrophy. Aesthetic Plast Surg 1986;10(2):115–7.
[32] Chajchir A, Benzaquen I. Fat-grafting injection for soft-tissue augmentation. Plast Reconstr Surg 1989;84(6):921–34.
[33] Chajchir A, Benzaquen I, Wexler E, et al. Fat injection. Aesthetic Plast Surg 1990;14(2):127–36.
[34] Chajchir A. Fat injection: long-term follow-up. Aesthetic Plast Surg 1996;20(4):291–6.
[35] Coiffman F. Lipoinjection complications. In: Hinderer U, editor. Plastic surgery, vol. 2. Amsterdam: Excerpta Medica; 1992. p. 759–60.
[36] Coleman SR. Long-term survival of fat transplants: controlled demonstrations. Aesthetic Plast Surg 1995;19(5):421–5.
[37] Coleman SR. Facial recontouring with lipostructure. Clin Plast Surg 1997;24(2):347–67.
[38] Coleman SR. Structural fat grafts: the ideal filler? Clin Plast Surg 2000;28(1):111–9.
[39] Coleman SR. Hand rejuvenation with structural fat grafting. Plast Reconstr Surg 2002;110(7): 1731–44.
[40] Colic MM. Lip and perioral enhancement by direct intramuscular fat autografting. Aesthetic Plast Surg 1999;23(1):36–40.
[41] Ellenbogen R. Free autologous pearl fat grafts in the face: a preliminary report of a rediscovered technique. Ann Plast Surg 1996;16:179.
[42] Ellenbogen R. Autologous fat injection [invited comment]. Ann Plast Surg 1990;24:297.
[43] Ellenbogen R. Autologous fat injection [letter]. Plast Reconstr Surg 1991;88:543.
[44] Ellenbogen R. Fat transfer: current use in practice. Clin Plast Surg 2000;27(4):545–56.
[45] Gatti JE. Permanent lip augmentation with serial fat grafting. Ann Plast Surg 1999;42(4): 376–80.
[46] Gonzalez-Ulloa M. Gluteoplasty: a ten-year report. Aesthetic Plast Surg 1991;15(1):85–91.
[47] Guerrerosantos J, Gonzalez-Mendoza A, Masmela Y, et al. Long-term survival of free fat grafts in muscle: an experimental study in rats. Aesthetic Plast Surg 1996;20(5):403–8.
[48] Guerrerosantos J. Autologous fat grafting for body contouring. Clin Plast Surg 1996;23(4): 619–31.
[49] Guerrerosantos J. Simultaneous rhytidoplasty and lipoinjection: a comprehensive aesthetic surgical strategy. Plast Reconstr Surg 1998; 102(1):191–9.
[50] Guerrerosantos J. Long-term outcome of autologous fat transplantation in aesthetic facial recontouring: sixteen years of experience with 1936 cases. Clin Plast Surg 2000;27(4):515–43.
[51] Guerrerosantos J. A new simple method used to prepare fat for injection. Aesthetic Plast Surg 2004;29(1):23.
[52] Guerrerosantos J, Chicas M, Rivera H. Palatopharyngeal lipoinjection: an advantageous method in velopharyngeal incompetence. Plast Reconstr Surg 2004;113(2):776–7.
[53] Lambros V. Fat injections for aesthetic facial rejuvenation. Aesthetic Surg J 1997;17:190.
[54] Levy S, Pitombo V. Rhytidoplasty: the use of microliposuction and microlipoinjection. Rev Bras Cir 1988;78:311.
[55] Pereira LH, Radwanski HN. Fat grafting of the buttocks and lower limbs. Aesthetic Plast Surg 1996;20(5):409–16.
[56] Toledo LS. Syringe liposculpture. Clin Plast Surg 1996;23(4):683–93.
[57] Wilkinson T. Lip enhancement techniques: short-and long-term results. In: Toledo I, editor. Annals of the International Symposium Recent Advances in Plastic Surgery. São Paulo, 1992. p. 75–6.
[58] Ersek RA. Transplantation of purified autologous fat: a 3-year follow-up is disappointing. Plast Reconstr Surg 1991;87(2):219–27.
[59] Fredericks S. Transplantation of purified autologous fat: a 3-year follow-up is disappointing [discussion]. Plast Reconstr Surg 1991;87:228.
[60] Goldwyn RM. Unproven treatment: whose benefit, whose responsibility [editorial]. Plast Reconstr Surg 1988;81:946.
[61] Samdal F, Skolleborg KC, Berthelsen B. The effect of preoperative needle abrasion of the recipient site on survival of autologous free fat grafts in rats. Scand J Plast Reconstr Surg Hand Surg 1992;26(1):33–6.
[62] Smahel J. Adipose tissue in plastic surgery. Ann Plast Surg 1986;16(5):444–53.
[63] Horl HW, Feller AM, Biemer E. Technique for liposuction fat reimplantation and long-term volume evaluation by magnetic resonance imaging. Ann Plast Surg 1991;26(3): 248–58.
[64] Eppley BL, Smith PG, Sadove AM, et al. Experimental effects of graft revascularization and consistency on cervicofacial fat transplant survival. J Oral Maxillofac Surg 1990;48(1): 54–62.
[65] Billings Jr E, May Jr JW. Historical review and present status of free fat graft autotransplantation in plastic and reconstructive surgery. Plast Reconstr Surg 1989;83(2):368–81.
[66] Deburge A, Benoist M, Lassale B, et al. The fate of fat grafts used in surgery of the lumbar spine. Rev Chir Orthop 1988;74(3):238–42.
[67] Van Akkerveeken PF, Van de Kraan W, Muller JW. The fate of the free fat graft: a prospective clinical study using CT scanning. Spine 1986; 11(5):501–4.
[68] Weisz GM, Gal A. Long-term survival of a free fat graft in the spinal canal: a 40-month postlaminectomy case report. Clin Orthop 1986; 205:204–6.
[69] Wetmore SJ. Injection of fat for soft tissue augmentation. Laryngoscope 1989;99(1):50–7.

[70] Matthews RD, Christensen JP, Canning DA. Persistence of autologous free fat transplant in bladder submucosa of rats. J Urol 1994; 152(2 Pt 2):819–21.
[71] Kononas TC, Bucky LP, Hurley CBS, et al. The fate of suctioned and surgically removed fat after reimplantation: a volumetric and histologic study in the rabbit. Plast Reconstr Surg 1993;91:763.
[72] Curi MM, Singer MJM, Iaconelli LM, et al. Autologous fat graft: experimental study. In: Toledo LS, Pinto ES, editors. Annals of the International Symposium Recent Advances in Plastic Surgery. São Paulo, March 28–30, 1990. RAPS International Corporation; 1990. p. 213–92.
[73] Eppley BL, Snyders Jr RV, Winkelmann T, et al. Autologous facial fat transplantation: improved graft maintenance by microbead bioactivation. J Oral Maxillofac Surg 1992;50(5):477–82 [discussion, 482–3].
[74] Eppley BL, Sidner RA, Platis JM, et al. Bioactivation of free-fat transfers: a potential new approach to improving graft survival. Plast Reconstr Surg 1992;90(6):1022–30.
[75] Bircoll M. Autologous fat transplantation. Plast Reconstr Surg 1987;79(3):492–3.
[76] Silkiss RZ, Baylis HI. Autogenous fat grafting by injection. Ophthal Plast Reconstr Surg 1987; 3(2):71–5.
[77] Boyce RG, Nuss DW, Kluka EA. The use of autogenous fat, fascia, and nonvascularized muscle grafts in the head and neck. Otolaryngol Clin North Am 1994;27(1):39–68.
[78] Asaadi M, Haramis HT. Successful autologous fat injection at 5-year follow-up. Plast Reconstr Surg 1993;91:755.
[79] Egido JA, Arroyo R, Marcos A, et al. Middle cerebral artery embolism and unilateral visual loss after autologous fat injection into the glabellar area [letter]. Stroke 1993;24(4):615–6.
[80] Trockman BA, Berman CJ, Sendelbach K, et al. Complication of penile injection of autologous fat. J Urol 1994;151(2):429–30.
[81] Hunter PD, Baker SS. The treatment of enophthalmos by orbital injection of fat autograft. Arch Otolaryngol Head Neck Surg 1994; 120(8):835–9.
[82] Santarosa RP, Blaivas JG. Periurethral injection of autologous fat for the treatment of sphincteric incontinence. J Urol 1994;151(3):607–11.
[83] McFarland JE. The free autogenous fat graft: a comparison of the fat "pearl" and fat "cell" graft in an animal model. Ophthal Plast Reconstr Surg 1988;4(1):41–7.
[84] Shorr N, Christenbury JD, Goldberg RA. Free autogenous "pearl fat" grafts to the eyelids. Ophthal Plast Reconstr Surg 1988;4(1):37–40.
[85] Loeb R. Naso-jugal groove leveling with fat tissue. Clin Plast Surg 1993;20(2):393–400 [discussion, 401].
[86] Carpaneda CA, Ribeiro MT. Percentage of graft viability versus injected volume in adipose autotransplants. Aesthetic Plast Surg 1994;18(1):17–9.
[87] Niechajev I, Sevcuk O. Long-term results of fat transplantation: clinical and histologic studies. Plast Reconstr Surg 1994;94(3):496–506.
[88] Coleman SR. Long-term survival of fat transplants: controlled demonstrations. Aesthetic Plast Surg 1995;19(5):421–5.
[89] Hunstad JP. Tumescent and syringe liposculpture: a logical partnership. Aesthetic Plast Surg 1995;19(4):321–33.
[90] Schuller-Petrovic S. Improving the aesthetic aspect of 50ft tissue defects on the face using autologous fat transplantation. Facial Plast Surg 1997;13(2):119–24.
[91] Amar RE. Adipocyte microinfiltration in the face or tissue restructuration with fat tissue graft. Ann Chir Plast Esthet 1999;44(6):593–608.
[92] De Pedroza LV. Fat transplantation to the buttocks and legs for aesthetic enhancement or correction of deformities: long-term results of large volumes of fat transplant. Dermatol Surg 2000;26(12):1145–9.
[93] Peren PA, Gómez JB, Guerrerosantos J, et al. Gluteus augmentation with fat grafting. Aesthetic Plast Surg 2000;24(6):412–7.
[94] Sommer S, Sattler G. Current concepts of fat graft survival: histology of aspirated adipose tissue and review of the literature. Dermatol Surg 2000;26(12):1159–66.
[95] Shoshani O, Ullmann Y, Shupak A, et al. The role of frozen storage in preserving adipose tissue obtained by suction-assisted lipectomy for repeated fat injection procedures. Dermatol Surg 2001;27(7):645–7.
[96] Butterwick KJ, Lack EA. Facial volume restoration with the fat autograft muscle injection technique. Dermatol Surg 2003;29(10):1019–26.
[97] Aygit AC, Sarikaya A, Doganay L, et al. The fate of intramuscularly injected fat autografts: an experimental study in rabbits. Aesthetic Plast Surg 2004;28(5):334–9.
[98] Har-Shai Y, Lindenbaum ES, Gamliel-Lazarovich A, et al. An integrated approach for increasing the survival of autologous fat grafts in the treatment of contour defects. Plast Reconstr Surg 1999;104(4):945–54.
[99] Katz AJ, Llull R, Hedrick MH, et al. Emerging approaches to the tissue engineering of al. Clin Plast Surg 1999;26(4):587–603.
[100] Moore Jr JH, Kolaczynski JW, Morales LM, et al. Viability of fat obtained by syringe suction lipectomy: effects of local anesthesia with lidocaine. Aesthetic Plast Surg 1995;19(4):335–9.
[101] Huss FR, Kratz G. Adipose tissue processed for lipoinjection shows increased cellular survival in vitro when tissue engineering principles are applied. Scand J Plast Reconstr Surg Hand Surg 2002;36(3):166–71.
[102] Viterbo F, Marques M, Valente M. Fat-tissue injection versus graft: experimental study in rabbits. Ann Plast Surg 1994;33(2):184–92.

ELSEVIER
SAUNDERS

CLINICS IN
PLASTIC
SURGERY

Clin Plastic Surg 33 (2006) 55–62

Adipose Tissue: Stem Cells and Beyond

Sunil S. Tholpady, MS, MD, PhD[a,*], Ramon Llull, MD, PhD[b], Roy C. Ogle, PhD[a], J. Peter Rubin, MD[c], J. William Futrell, MD[c,d], Adam J. Katz, MD[a]

Until recently, the biology of adipose tissue has been primarily the purview of biochemists and endocrinologists. The reasons for this are apparent from the traditional functions that fat and mature adipocytes were thought to perform. For many years it was assumed that fat was primarily and simply a dormant reservoir of energy for storage and production. Energy stored as free glucose can only sustain the human body for a few minutes, whereas that in glycogen is sufficient for support after an overnight fast. By contrast, large amounts of energy can be stored in relatively small amounts of fat. When given enough water, an average human can sustain a 30- to 40-day fast based on the energy from small amounts of fat.

In the late 1980s, it became apparent that adipose tissue was a dynamic organ that participated in the metabolism of sex steroids [1]. Soon thereafter came the discovery of other adipose-specific bioactive factors, such as leptin [2], which again demonstrated the functionality of adipose tissue signaling on local and systemic levels. This knowledge has changed the understanding of adipose tissue as a passive entity to one that is intimately involved in homeostasis, energy metabolism, neuroendocrine function, immune regulation, and structural support and protection of vital organs.

Because its normal function is tied so closely to the maintenance of cell function and normal health, aberrations in body fat depots can have devastating consequences. All too familiar examples are the health penalties paid by the overweight and obese, that is, hypertension, heart disease, diabetes, musculoskeletal degeneration, and a host of prothrombotic and proinflammatory states. Lipodystrophies in which fat depots can be normal in amount but inappropriately distributed can pose additional challenges, including a propensity toward a specific metabolic syndrome.

[a] Departments of Plastic and Reconstructive Surgery, Cell Biology, and Neurosurgery, University of Virginia Health Sciences Center, Charlottesville, VA 22908, USA
[b] Department of Cell Biology, University of Barcelona Medical School, Barcelona, Spain
[c] Division of Plastic Surgery, University of Pittsburgh Medical Center, University of Pittsburgh, Pittsburgh, PA, USA
[d] Bioengineering, Carnegie-Mellon University, Pittsburgh, PA, USA
* Corresponding author. Department of Plastic and Reconstructive Surgery, University of Virginia Health Sciences Center, Charlottesville, VA 22908.
E-mail address: sst8a@virginia.edu (S.S. Tholpady).

doi:10.1016/j.cps.2005.08.004
plasticsurgery.theclinics.com

Despite the knowledge that fat and individual adipocytes perform important functions, historically and in the hands of surgeons, such substances are often considered little more than a soft tissue that is regularly traversed in surgical procedures. A primary intended goal in many plastic surgery procedures is to remove fat if it exists in excess, or if lacking, to augment the area with fat grafts. Plastic surgeons are now in the unique position of being able to harvest and conduct basic and clinical research on the inter- and intraperson differences between fat deposits, as well as the components of fat beyond just the stem cells. This article highlights potential uses for harvested fat and describes the current state of the art regarding adipose stem cells (ASCs).

Components of adipose tissue

Adipose tissue extracellular matrix

The extracellular matrix of every tissue should be thought of as a biologically multifunctional substrate that cells require for their survival. The extracellular matrix sequesters and releases growth factors, attracts and repels appropriate cell types, and is intimately and reciprocally involved in the growth, proliferation, and differentiation of resident cells.

The extracellular matrix of adipose tissue is poorly characterized. Only collagens type I to VI have been studied out of more than 25 collagens known to exist. All of these collagens are present except for type II, which is a predominantly cartilaginous collagen [3–6]. Studies in the authors' laboratory indicate that types VII, XIV, XV, XVIII, and XXVII collagen are also produced by cells present in freshly isolated liposuction tissue. Laminin and fibronectin are present in moderate quantities [5–7]. Growth factors are present wherever extracellular matrix exists, and adipose tissue is no exception. In addition to its endocrine function, cells within fat secrete transforming growth factor-beta, platelet-derived growth factor, and fibroblast growth factor, among other substances, as shown from microarray data.

Neither extracellular matrix proteins nor growth factors have been studied adequately in adipose tissue. A better understanding of these components will enhance the understanding, design, and practice of various procedures and techniques, such as free fat grafting. Because successful and predictable fat grafting involves the removal of tissue from its blood supply, and subsequently requires expedient and optimal revascularization, a better appreciation of the factors that impact the adipogenic process and its links to angiogenesis will help transition fat grafting from an "art" to a "science." Studies of the nature of the extracellular matrix are also important so that individual factors can be isolated and defined. Fat tissue can be obtained in voluminary amounts, facilitating large-scale purification of proteins from the extracellular matrix. An example of this isolation is the purification of laminin, which has been shown to have remarkable neural regenerative properties. Although mouse laminin can be purified, it is unsuitable for human use because of the possibility of immune attack/rejection with subsequent cross-reaction and autoimmunity against endogenous human laminin. Future isolation and use of purified autologous laminin from human fat would conceivably remove such risk.

Cellular components of adipose tissue

Fat contains multiple resident cell types besides adipocytes. These cells include preadipocytes, endothelial cells, smooth muscle cells, pericytes, fibroblasts, and ASCs. Additionally, liposuction aspirates can potentially contain any cell type that normally circulates, including classic immune cells (B and T cells, natural killer cells, mast cells, macrophages, monocytes), hematopoietic stem cells, or endothelial progenitor cells. Any preparation derived from liposuction aspirate or excised abdominoplasty tissue most likely contains some relative permutation of this dynamic microenvironment in which multiple cell types coexist.

Studies involve separating populations of cells based on the expression of cell surface markers. In one such experiment, cells derived from the stromal fraction of fat were sorted based on their expression of CD31, a cell surface marker indicative of the endothelium. CD31+ cells highly expressed other markers of endothelial origin, whereas CD31− cells were able to differentiate into fat, bone, cartilage, and nerve [8]. Other studies have shown the presence of CD11b and CD11c surface markers on a subpopulation of cells extracted from the stromal fraction of liposuction aspirates [9]. These markers are present on macrophages and osteoclasts among other cells. Indeed, preliminary work at the University of Virginia suggests that at least a subpopulation of adipose-derived stem cells is capable of differentiating into osteoclastlike phenotypes under appropriate conditions.

The identification, purification, and characterization of the diverse cell populations within fat tissue serves a purpose greater than merely expanding the knowledge base of its basic biology. The ability to distinguish and isolate purified ASC populations from other morphologically similar cell types within fat will likely expedite their therapeutic application. Even "contaminating" cells (ie, non-ASCs) have potential value. For example, endothelial cells might be used to create new blood vessels or to augment the growth of existing vessels. Hematopoietic precursor cells obtained from fat and its matrix could be used to supplement bone marrow reconstitution procedures. All of these uses and many others would be associated with little morbidity using tissue that would otherwise be discarded following commonly performed procedures.

Adipose stem cells

Although fat contains individual cells and constituent matrix components of value, recent interest and excitement in fat biology has arisen from the description of a heterogenous mix of cells present within the stromal vascular fraction of liposuction aspirate. These cells, termed *adipose stem cells* as suggested by an international panel of investigators working in this field (International Fat Applied Technology Society 2nd International Meeting held in October 2004 at Pittsburgh, Pennsylvania), are capable of differentiating into fat, bone, cartilage, muscle, nerve, and other yet to be defined tissues [**Fig. 1**] [10,11]. Because of their origin, these cells do not carry the ethical overhead present in the heated debates regarding embryonic stem cells. They are one of the several cell types garnered from several differing sources collectively known as adult stem cells. Although adult stem cells may not have the flexibility and extended differentiation capacity seen in embryonic stem cells, their human application is more likely in the near future.

With emerging evidence suggesting that human subcutaneous adipose tissue contains cells with extensive and even unrecognized developmental plasticity, interest has rapidly grown in their therapeutic potential. As the field matures, it is becoming increasingly difficult to ignore the fact that there are obvious and profound similarities between ASCs and marrow mesenchymal stem cells (MSCs). In fact, much of the research performed on ASCs has been based on previous work with stromal cells derived from bone marrow, or bone marrow–derived stem cells (BMSCs). Both cell populations represent the stromal cell fraction isolated from an adipose depot (subcutaneous tissue for ASCs, bone marrow for MSCs) based on their adherence to tissue culture plastic. Even more explicit, these two cell types are remarkably similar with respect to morphology, growth, and transcriptional and cell surface profiles [9,12]. The two cell types display remarkably similar developmental behavior in vitro and in vivo. Indeed, ASCs may simply represent an MSC fraction resident within the subcutaneous space. From a translational perspective, ASCs provide the relative advantages of abundance, expendability, and ease of harvest.

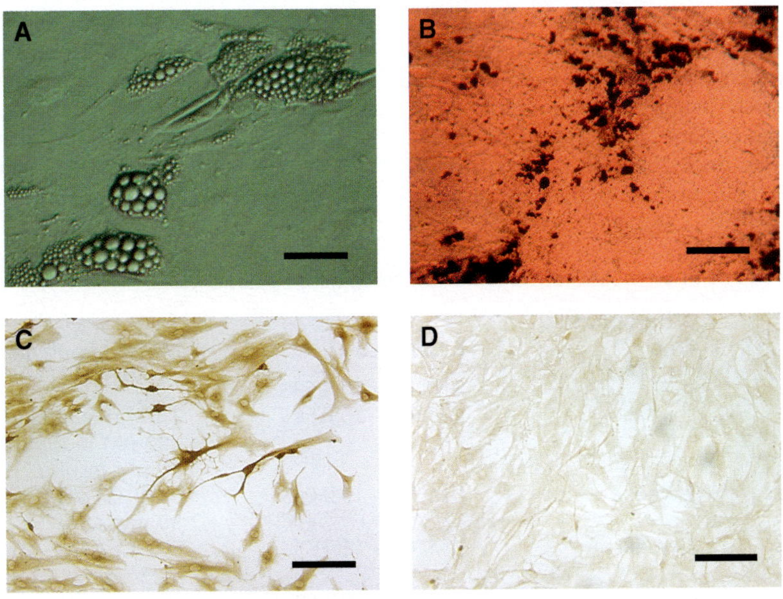

Fig. 1. Differentiation of ASCs to (*A*) fat, (*B*) bone, and (*C*) nerve. (*A*) Note the lipid droplets present within the adipocytes after 3 weeks in adipogenic media. (*B*) ASCs that differentiated to bone secrete mineralized matrix as detected by Von Kossa staining. (*C*) Neural cells created in 6 hours stain heavily for TUJ1, a neural marker. (*D*) TUJ1 staining is much less apparent in undifferentiated ASCs. (*From* Tholpady SS, Katz AJ, Ogle RC. Mesenchymal stem cells from rat visceral fat exhibit multipotential differentiation in vitro. Anat Rec A Discov Mol Cell Evol Biol 2003;272(1):398–402; with permission.)

In vitro and in vivo differentiation

Differentiation of ASCs into fat is perhaps the most expected developmental possibility and most likely reflects a shared or overlapping identity with historically described preadipocytes. Complete differentiation is accomplished using a specific differentiation protocol [Table 1] and requires 3 weeks. Lipid can be seen within cells after 1 week, and these depots enlarge and coalesce with time. Molecular markers for fatty differentiation are also upregulated within the 3-week time frame [11,13]. Fat grafting as a technique may rely not only on transplantation of mature adipocytes with the development of new vascularization for survival of the cells but also on the ASC fraction that can differentiate into adipocytes and also support new blood vessel growth.

Chondrogenic differentiation often uses a technique known as "micromass culture." ASCs are cultured at high density to encourage the formation of a sphere of cells. When given exposure to the correct differentiative media within this sphere, the cells differentiate to chondrocytes and secrete a cartilaginous matrix [14,15]. The completed process again requires 3 weeks.

The differentiation of ASCs into myocytes occurs with the lowest yield and reproducibility of all the differentiated cell types reported in the literature. Successful myogenesis is reflected in the formation of multinucleated fibers that express myogenic markers such as myoD, myogenin, and myosin heavy chains [10,16]. The morphologic and genotypic changes associated with this developmental cascade take approximately 4 to 6 weeks. In addition to the relatively lengthy developmental time course and low conversion rate, a growing number of laboratories, including the authors', have found it difficult to reproduce published findings consistently when attempting the myogenic induction of human ASCs (S.S. Thopaldy, unpublished data, 2003).

Bony differentiation also requires a lengthy time frame, at the end of which cells secrete mineralized matrix. Transformed cells also express mature osteoblast-specific markers such as osteopontin, osteocalcin, and CBFA-1 [11,17,18]. In vivo experimental studies have been performed in which ASCs have demonstrated the capacity to heal bony defects [19]. In that study, ASCs were implanted into a mouse critical size calvarial defect. Such a model does not heal over the lifetime of the animal; therefore, it is an ideal method to study any regenerative or reparative effect a given treatment may have. ASCs were shown to cause regeneration of such defects, but not as well as isolated osteoblasts [19].

At least one case report involving ASCs in the clinical setting has been published. A traumatic calvarial defect complicated by chronic infection in a 7-year-old girl was treated with autologous ASCs. Cells were implanted with bone fragments and fibrin glue placed between resorbable polymeric sheets [20]. Treatment in this manner yielded complete bony coverage of the defect. Two important points arise from this study. First, evidence supports (but does not entirely prove owing to limited long-term follow-up) the notion that ASC implantation is not harmful and, second, that it does not have a deleterious effect on bone healing. It is impossible to determine the relative effect, if any, of the undifferentiated ASCs on bone regeneration in this case report because the osteoconductive and osteoinductive properties of fibrin and bone fragments contributed to the final healed result [21].

The case report used ASCs that were removed and reimplanted in one operative session, demon-

Table 1: Methods of in vitro ASC differentiation to selected phenotypes

Differentiated phenotype	Differentiative time	Basal media	Media supplements
Control		DMEM + 10%FBS	
Adipocytes	3 weeks	DMEM + 10%FBS	1 μM dex, 500 μM IBMX, 200 μM indomethacin, 10 μM insulin
Osteoblasts	3 weeks	DMEM + 10%FBS	0.01 μM VD3, 10 mM β-GP, 50 μM ASAP
Chondrocytes	3 weeks	DMEM + 1%FBS	50 nM ASAP, 10 ng/mL TGF-β1, 6.25 μg/mL insulin
Myocytes	6 weeks	DMEM + 10%FBS + 5% HS	50 μM hydrocortisone
Neurons	6 hours	DMEM	1–10 mM β-ME

Abbreviations: ASAP, ascorbate-2-phosphate; β-GP, beta-glycerophosphate; β-ME, beta-mercaptoethanol; dex, dexamethasone; DMEM, Dulbecco's Modified Eagle's Medium; FBS, fetal bovine serum; HS, horse serum; IBMX, 3-Isobutyl-1-methylxanthine; VD3, vitamin D3.

strating the feasibility of autologous, cell-based therapy within the surgical setting. Although this approach may prove to be the preferred model for ASC-based therapies, several important questions remain. Regulatory concerns may require that devices or solutions that are used to isolate cells at the bedside or in the operating room setting yield a population of cells that is consistent, reproducible, and predictable with regard to phenotype, quality, yield, and therapeutic potential and efficacy. Ironically, it is unclear and unproven whether "freshly" isolated ASCs are similar in form or function to those that have been processed in culture. Most, if not all, in vitro and in vivo studies published to date have used either culture-enriched ASCs or flow cytometry–enriched subpopulations isolated based on specific cell surface markers [22]. It remains unclear whether the developmental plasticity observed in ASCs (and other adult stem cell populations for that matter) is the result of epigenetic changes related to culture conditions, or part of the innate or inherent potential of such cells within their native in situ setting. This important issue certainly deserves further study.

Differentiation of ASCs to neural cells is perhaps the least anticipated possibility among all cell types. Because fat is of mesodermal origin, its transmutation to a tissue of ectodermal origin was not thought to be possible. Neural differentiation was first described in BMSCs [23], and these observations were extended to ASCs by several other groups [13,24–26]. Conversion of ASCs to neural-like cells takes less than 6 hours and can be induced by reducing agents and drugs that increase cAMP [24–26]. One animal study has been conducted to elucidate the capacity of ASCs to improve function following middle cerebral artery occlusion. ASCs were implanted into the ventricles of animals with demonstrated functional deficits. The ASCs migrated along white matter tracts and became resident in damaged areas of the brain. In addition to ASC expression of neural-specific genes, functional recovery of the animals was observed [27].

ASCs are also capable of reconstituting bone marrow. Injection of extracted ASCs into lethally irradiated mice can rescue the hematopoietic forming elements of the animal [28]. ASCs were found not only in the bone marrow of the injected animals but also in the blood and spleens of the animals. This finding indicates that ASCs either contain a population of cells that have hematopoietic progenitors, or that they are capable of initiating and sustaining the endogenous recovery of bone marrow components.

ASCs also secrete angiogenic and survival factors that may support the growth of existing tissue [9,29]. Reperfusion injury and cell damage associated with extremity replants or flap reconstructions can be ameliorated with autologous ASC treatments. In a mouse model of an ischemic hind limb, treatment with ASCs resulted in an increased hind limb survival rate [22]. ASCs were shown to engraft into the host tissue with concomitant increases in capillary density and blood flow. Two possibilities can explain this result. ASCs may be differentiating and engrafting into host tissues, resulting in recovery of function previously lost by damaged cells, or ASCs may be secreting factors that support the tissue while it becomes revascularized.

Limitations of adipose stem cell technology

Several problems and limitations exist concerning the basic biology and clinical applications of ASCs. At a fundamental level, do ASCs fulfill criteria to be considered stem cells? Originally, stem cells were defined as cells capable of unlimited self-renewal and having the capacity to differentiate into any given cell type. ASCs are not immortal and reach a state of senescence as they are passaged. Additionally, it is generally accepted that, although ASCs have multipotential differentiating capacity, embryonic stem cells are thought to differentiate into more cell types than can adult stem cells. Further research is required to verify the validity of this assumption.

When implanted in vivo, do differentiated ASCs function as well as the cells they putatively replace? Differentiation during development follows a pattern of gene expression that is not replicated when ASCs differentiate in vitro [30,31]. Subtle differences in the expression of proteins may modify the behavior of differentiated ASCs when compared with normal differentiated cell types. It is also possible that, instead of replacing a damaged cell in vivo, ASCs are merely fusing with them and supporting their survival. This possibility, suggested in a few studies, has not been replicated in others [32,33].

Perhaps the greatest confusion in the study of ASCs relates to the variability among various cells referred to as ASCs. In addition to the fact that ASCs represent a heterogeneous population of cells, other differences exist, including intra- and inter-person variation, extraction method differences, and culture condition differences. Intraperson differences relate to differences in fatty tissue derived from different anatomic sites (eg, abdomen, thighs, infrapatellar, visceral, subcutaneous). It is well known that disparities exist in metabolism and fat storage among adipocytes from these sources [34–37]. Although not yet reported in the literature, indirect evidence suggests depot-specific differences among other cell types in fat. ASCs derived from separate patients also display proliferative and differentiative variations. Age and sex can greatly influence ASC behavior [34,38,39]. Increasing age can lead to a decrease in the general proliferative activity of ASCs [34]. ASCs differentiated into fat show a greater expression of fat-related genes in female mice versus male mice [39]. Whether these differences are true for other differentiated cell types remains to be seen. Gene expression profiling of ASC populations gathered from patients will also generate data relating to interperson differences. One such study demonstrated only a 66% concordance in the genes expressed between three patients [9].

ASC populations may also differ owing to the method of fat harvest. Although liposuction aspirate was first used to extract ASCs, abdominoplasty specimens can also yield ASCs that differentiate into all known cell types. Studies profiling the relative levels of cells expressing surface markers in liposuction versus abdominoplasty specimens do not completely agree and are sometimes in conflict. A possible explanation may be differences in the cell types that are gathered during the two procedures. Liposuction causes a sustained and concentrated tissue insult in the presence of intact perfusion, resulting in systemic release of proinflammatory mediators [40,41]. These mediators cause cells throughout the body to be mobilized and recruited. Abdominoplasty, on the other hand, results in the removal of fat from its blood supply, potentially limiting the influx and migration of circulating and distant cells. It is possible that cells obtained from liposuction-harvested tissue may vary in the relative quantity, quality, or type as compared with those isolated from an excised abdominoplasty specimen. Cells obtained from ultrasonic liposuction specimens may have additional variation.

Culturing cells in vitro causes a significant change in the genes expressed. The shift from a three-dimensional in vivo environment to a two-dimensional in vitro culture dish is accompanied by upregulation in cytoskeletal components, cell cycle proteins, and tissue-specific genes [8]. Differences may exist between the in vitro behavior of differentiated cells and the in vivo behavior of implanted cells. These same differences may also exist when considering and comparing freshly isolated versus cultured ASCs.

Dangers of adipose stem cell technology

Liposuction and abdominoplasty are frequently performed surgical procedures with relatively low complication rates. Likewise, autologous fat grafting is commonly performed, and these procedures pose little unknown danger to patients. Because ASCs were described in the literature only 4 years ago [11], more research must be done to determine the safety of their implantation in humans. Encouraging results have been gathered from the one study of ASCs implanted into a young girl with no obvious deleterious effects [20]. Nevertheless, ASC implantation poses two potential dangers as determined from the BMSC literature. BMSCs have unique immunomodulatory properties and can downregulate T-cell proliferation and activation [42,43]. Additionally, in many cases, they are able to evade an immune response [44–46]. ASCs apparently share this property with BMSCs [47]. Although this property might obviate the development of autoimmune, graft versus host reactions, or transplant rejection, it may also allow occult cancers to evade immune surveillance. A study performed in mice demonstrates this point. Mice were injected with B16 melanoma cells concurrently with BMSCs (subcutaneously or intravenously). B16 melanomas did not form tumors but when combined with BMSCs were a nidus for tumor growth [48]. Further long-term studies and vigilance are required to further elucidate the extent of this concern.

Homing to sites of injury or chronic inflammation is another property that BMSCs (and most likely ASCs) possess [49–54]. BMSCs home to damaged gastric mucosa as seen in an animal model of *Helicobacter pylori* infection. In that study, mice were lethally irradiated to kill all endogenous bone marrow cells and were then implanted with marrow labeled with β-galactosidase, a histologically traceable marker. Within 1 year, labeled cells were seen in the glands of the gastric mucosa. Surprisingly, the bone marrow cells were found to have undergone transformation to high-grade gastrointestinal intraepithelial neoplasia, a precursor of gastric adenocarcinoma [55]. The relevance of this finding to the clinical use of ASCs has not yet been determined, but repeated infusions of ASCs may prove to provide building blocks for cancerous conditions resulting from chronic inflammatory conditions. Clearly, ASC biology remains a young field that is primed for extensive growth in the future.

Summary

Adipose tissue contains many cells and proteins that are of value not only because of their possible therapeutic applications but also because of the low cost of harvest and delivery. Plastic surgeons, with an operative domain that covers almost every major fat depot, have a unique opportunity and a vested interest in expanding basic and clinical research into the various facets of adipose biology. The harvest and manipulation of ASCs, a plastic surgery innovation, promises to affect every major field of medicine. Although regeneration of tissue is the most obvious application, their immunomodulatory and tissue support properties may change treatments for heart disease, stroke, renal failure, autoimmune disorders, transplants, and many other disparate afflictions. The ability to access quickly and easily and to administer large numbers of autologous (and possibly allogeneic) cells has the potential to make ASCs a practical, appealing, and valuable clinical therapy.

References

[1] Siiteri PK. Adipose tissue as a source of hormones. Am J Clin Nutr 1987;45:277–82.

[2] Zhang Y, Proenca R, Maffei M, et al. Positional cloning of the mouse obese gene and its human homologue. Nature 1994;372:425–32.

[3] Carpaneda CA. Collagen alterations in adipose autografts. Aesthetic Plast Surg 1994;18(1):11–5.

[4] Cryer A, Van RL. Characterization of the collagen types synthesized by human and rat adipocyte precursors in vitro. Eur J Clin Invest 1982;12(3): 235–8.

[5] Nakajima I, Yamaguchi T, Ozutsumi K, et al. Adipose tissue extracellular matrix: newly organized by adipocytes during differentiation. Differentiation 1998;63(4):193–200.

[6] Nakajima I, Muroya S, Tanabe R, et al. Extracellular matrix development during differentiation into adipocytes with a unique increase in type V and VI collagen. Biol Cell 2002;94(3): 197–203.

[7] Ono M, Aratani Y, Kitagawa I, et al. Ascorbic acid phosphate stimulates type IV collagen synthesis and accelerates adipose conversion of 3T3–L1 cells. Exp Cell Res 1990;187(2):309–14.

[8] Boquest AC, Shahdadfar A, Fronsdal K, et al. Isolation and transcription profiling of purified uncultured human stromal stem cells: alteration of gene expression after in vitro cell culture. Mol Biol Cell 2005;16(3):1131–41.

[9] Katz AJ, Tholpady A, Tholpady SS, et al. Cell surface and transcriptional characterization of human adipose-derived adherent stromal (hADAS) cells. Stem Cells 2005;23(3):412–23.

[10] Zuk PA, Zhu M, Ashjian P, et al. Human adipose tissue is a source of multipotent stem cells. Mol Biol Cell 2002;13(12):4279–95.

[11] Zuk PA, Zhu M, Mizuno H, et al. Multilineage cells from human adipose tissue: implications for cell-based therapies. Tissue Eng 2001;7(2): 211–28.

[12] Pittenger MF, Martin BJ. Mesenchymal stem cells and their potential as cardiac therapeutics. Circ Res 2004;95(1):9–20.

[13] Tholpady SS, Katz AJ, Ogle RC. Mesenchymal stem cells from rat visceral fat exhibit multipotential differentiation in vitro. Anat Rec 2003; 272(1):398–402.

[14] Huang JI, Zuk PA, Jones NF, et al. Chondrogenic potential of multipotential cells from human adipose tissue. Plast Reconstr Surg 2004;113(2): 585–94.

[15] Erickson GR, Gimble JM, Franklin DM, et al. Chondrogenic potential of adipose tissue-derived stromal cells in vitro and in vivo. Biochem Biophys Res Commun 2002;290(2):763–9.

[16] Mizuno H, Zuk PA, Zhu M, et al. Myogenic differentiation by human processed lipoaspirate cells. Plast Reconstr Surg 2002;109(1):199–209.

[17] Halvorsen YC, Wilkison WO, Gimble JM. Adipose-derived stromal cells—their utility and potential in bone formation. Int J Obes Relat Metab Disord 2000;24(Suppl 4):S41–4.

[18] Halvorsen YD, Franklin D, Bond AL, et al. Extracellular matrix mineralization and osteoblast gene expression by human adipose tissue-derived stromal cells. Tissue Eng 2001;7(6):729–41.

[19] Cowan CM, Shi YY, Aalami OO, et al. Adipose-derived adult stromal cells heal critical-size mouse calvarial defects. Nat Biotechnol 2004;22(5):560–7.

[20] Lendeckel S, Jodicke A, Christophis P, et al. Autologous stem cells (adipose) and fibrin glue used to treat widespread traumatic calvarial defects: case report. J Craniomaxillofac Surg 2004;32(6):370–3.

[21] Urist MR. Bone: formation by autoinduction. Science 1965;150:839–99.

[22] Miranville A, Heeschen C, Sengenes C, et al. Improvement of postnatal neovascularization by human adipose tissue-derived stem cells. Circulation 2004;110(3):349–55.

[23] Woodbury D, Schwarz EJ, Prockop DJ, et al. Adult rat and human bone marrow stromal cells differentiate into neurons. J Neurosci Res 2000; 61(4):364–70.

[24] Safford KM, Safford SD, Gimble JM, et al. Characterization of neuronal/glial differentiation of murine adipose-derived adult stromal cells. Exp Neurol 2004;187(2):319–28.

[25] Safford KM, Hicok KC, Safford SD, et al. Neurogenic differentiation of murine and human adipose-derived stromal cells. Biochem Biophys Res Commun 2002;294(2):371–9.

[26] Ashjian PH, Elbarbary AS, Edmonds B, et al. In vitro differentiation of human processed lipoaspirate cells into early neural progenitors. Plast Reconstr Surg 2003;111(6):1922–31.

[27] Kang SK, Lee DH, Bae YC, et al. Improvement of neurological deficits by intracerebral transplantation of human adipose tissue-derived stromal cells after cerebral ischemia in rats. Exp Neurol 2003;183(2):355–66.

[28] Cousin B, Andre M, Arnaud E, et al. Reconstitution of lethally irradiated mice by cells isolated from adipose tissue. Biochem Biophys Res Commun 2003;301(4):1016–22.

[29] Rehman J, Traktuev D, Li J, et al. Secretion of angiogenic and antiapoptotic factors by human adipose stromal cells. Circulation 2004;109(10): 1292–8.

[30] Neuhuber B, Gallo G, Howard L, et al. Reevalua-

tion of in vitro differentiation protocols for bone marrow stromal cells: disruption of actin cytoskeleton induces rapid morphological changes and mimics neuronal phenotype. J Neurosci Res 2004;77(2):192–204.
[31] Lu P, Blesch A, Tuszynski MH. Induction of bone marrow stromal cells to neurons: differentiation, transdifferentiation, or artifact? J Neurosci Res 2004;77(2):174–91.
[32] Terada N, Hamazaki T, Oka M, et al. Bone marrow cells adopt the phenotype of other cells by spontaneous cell fusion. Nature 2002;416(6880): 542–5.
[33] Ying QL, Nichols J, Evans EP, et al. Changing potency by spontaneous fusion. Nature 2002; 416(6880):545–8.
[34] Van Harmelen V, Rohrig K, Hauner H. Comparison of proliferation and differentiation capacity of human adipocyte precursor cells from the omental and subcutaneous adipose tissue depot of obese subjects. Metabolism 2004;53(5): 632–7.
[35] Bruun JM, Lihn AS, Madan AK, et al. Higher production of IL-8 in visceral vs. subcutaneous adipose tissue: implication of nonadipose cells in adipose tissue. Am J Physiol Endocrinol Metab 2004;286(1):E8–13.
[36] Bakker AH, Van Dielen FM, Greve JW, et al. Preadipocyte number in omental and subcutaneous adipose tissue of obese individuals. Obes Res 2004;12(3):488–98.
[37] Tchkonia T, Giorgadze N, Pirtskhalava T, et al. Fat depot origin affects adipogenesis in primary cultured and cloned human preadipocytes. Am J Physiol Regul Integr Comp Physiol 2002;282(5): R1286–96.
[38] Sen A, Lea-Currie YR, Sujkowska D, et al. Adipogenic potential of human adipose derived stromal cells from multiple donors is heterogeneous. J Cell Biochem 2001;81(2):312–9.
[39] Ogawa R, Mizuno H, Watanabe A, et al. Adipogenic differentiation by adipose-derived stem cells harvested from GFP transgenic mice including relationship of sex differences. Biochem Biophys Res Commun 2004;319(2):511–7.
[40] Kenkel JM, Brown SA, Love EJ, et al. Hemodynamics, electrolytes, and organ histology of larger-volume liposuction in a porcine model. Plast Reconstr Surg 2004;113(5):1391–9.
[41] Lipschitz AH, Kenkel JM, Luby M, et al. Electrolyte and plasma enzyme analyses during large-volume liposuction. Plast Reconstr Surg 2004; 114(3):766–75.
[42] Gotherstrom C, Ringden O, Tammik C, et al. Immunologic properties of human fetal mesenchymal stem cells. Am J Obstet Gynecol 2004; 190(1):239–45.
[43] Krampera M, Glennie S, Dyson J, et al. Bone marrow mesenchymal stem cells inhibit the response of naive and memory antigen-specific T cells to their cognate peptide. Blood 2003; 101(9):3722–9.
[44] Maitra B, Szekely E, Gjini K, et al. Human mesenchymal stem cells support unrelated donor hematopoietic stem cells and suppress T-cell activation. Bone Marrow Transplant 2004;33(6): 597–604.
[45] Le Blanc K. Immunomodulatory effects of fetal and adult mesenchymal stem cells. Cytotherapy 2003;5(6):485–9.
[46] Tse WT, Pendleton JD, Beyer WM, et al. Suppression of allogeneic T-cell proliferation by human marrow stromal cells: implications in transplantation. Transplantation 2003;75(3):389–97.
[47] Puissant B, Barreau C, Bourin P, et al. Immunomodulatory effect of human adipose tissue-derived adult stem cells: comparison with bone marrow mesenchymal stem cells. Br J Haematol 2005;129(1):118–29.
[48] Djouad F, Plence P, Bony C, et al. Immunosuppressive effect of mesenchymal stem cells favors tumor growth in allogeneic animals. Blood 2003; 102(10):3837–44.
[49] Borue X, Lee S, Grove J, et al. Bone marrow-derived cells contribute to epithelial engraftment during wound healing. Am J Pathol 2004;165(5): 1767–72.
[50] Badiavas EV, Abedi M, Butmarc J, et al. Participation of bone marrow derived cells in cutaneous wound healing. J Cell Physiol 2003;196(2): 245–50.
[51] Gupta S, Verfaillie C, Chmielewski D, et al. A role for extrarenal cells in the regeneration following acute renal failure. Kidney Int 2002;62(4): 1285–90.
[52] Poulsom R, Forbes SJ, Hodivala-Dilke K, et al. Bone marrow contributes to renal parenchymal turnover and regeneration. J Pathol 2001;195(2): 229–35.
[53] Theise ND, Henegariu O, Grove J, et al. Radiation pneumonitis in mice: a severe injury model for pneumocyte engraftment from bone marrow. Exp Hematol 2002;30(11):1333–8.
[54] Kotton DN, Ma BY, Cardoso WV, et al. Bone marrow-derived cells as progenitors of lung alveolar epithelium. Development 2001;128(24): 5181–8.
[55] Houghton J, Stoicov C, Nomura S, et al. Gastric cancer originating from bone marrow-derived cells. Science 2004;306(5701):1568–71.

ELSEVIER
SAUNDERS

CLINICS IN PLASTIC SURGERY

Clin Plastic Surg 33 (2006) 63–73

Subdermal Liposuction: Long-Term Experience

Carlo Gasperoni, MD*, Paolo Gasperoni, MD

Suction lipectomy has become popular because an effective body reshaping is achievable with inconspicuous scars. The need for better results led the authors to focus their attention on the pitfalls of the classic liposuction technique, their causes, and possible ways of solution. The subdermal liposuction was introduced [1] to enhance the results obtainable with the widepread technique originally proposed by Illouz.

From an historic point of view, Illouz [2] improved the technique of suction used by Fisher, who was considered the father of liposuction, having described it for the first time in 1976 [3]. Fischer used a vacuum system and a special blunt cannula with a window on one side, named the cellusuctiotome. It had an electric device that cut the fat that penetrated inside its lumen. In 1978, Kesselring [4] proposed the aspiradeps, another instrument consisting of a sharp cannula that permitted cutting and aspirating at the same time. All of these cutting instruments caused significant injuries to blood and lymphatic vessels and, as a consequence, blood and lymphatic collections. Illouz introduced a blunt cannula derived from the Karman uterine cannula with no cutting device that allowed one to preserve blood and lymphatic vessels and the fibrous connections between skin and muscle. That technique was associated with much less complications and was reliable enough to become widely accepted [2]. Blood and lymphatic collections, the major complications of the Fisher technique, were significantly reduced. The skin connections with the muscles were no longer severed, permitting a more physiologic healing with less skin depressions caused by scarring in the subcutaneous layer.

One of the main concerns of Illouz was to treat only the deep layer of fat to avoid skin irregularities. In fact, use of the large gauge cannulas at that time (from 6 mm upward) close to the skin surface could lead to irregularities. Illouz recommended going deep into the adipose tissue, 1 to 2 cm below the dermis, to respect the integrity of the superficial fat and to avoid adhesions that might cause unesthetic dimples or furrows. It was considered mandatory not to suction the superficial fat. In 1989, the authors presented the method of subdermal liposuction [1], introducing a new way of thinking. In the authors' experience, many unsatisfactory results were caused by the lack of attention to the role of the superficial layer of fat and the inability to treat it properly [5,6]. In the following

Clinica Quisisana, Via Gian Giacomo Porro 5, 00197 Roma, Italy
* Corresponding author.
E-mail address: cgasperoni@hotmail.com (C. Gasperoni).

0094-1298/06/$ – see front matter
doi:10.1016/j.cps.2005.08.006
plasticsurgery.theclinics.com

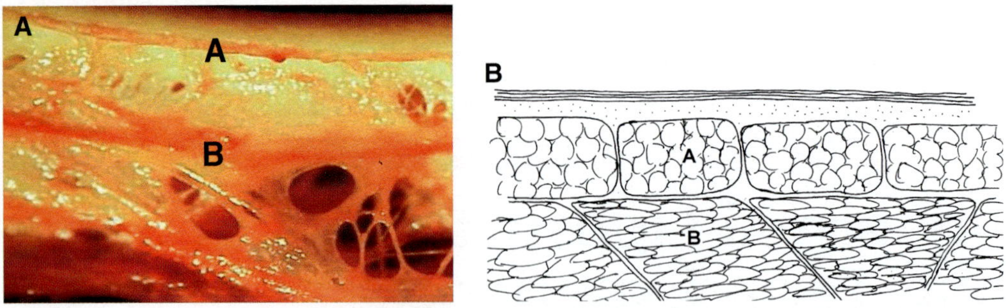

Fig. 1. SFS in the abdominal region. Photograph shows (*A*) skin and (*B*) fascia superficialis. The areolar fat layer is above the fascia superficialis. The lamellar layer is under the fascia superficialis. Schematic representation shows the subcutaneous fat encased in the SFS. (*A*) Areolar fat with fibrous septae of the SFS perpendicular to the skin surface. (*B*) Lamellar fat with oblique septae containing loose fat.

years, several groups published articles on this new subject, representing a revolution of the liposuction technique [7–11].

When examining the subcutaneous layer, great structural differences can be observed in a comparison of the superficial layer with the deep one. These two layers are anatomically [12] and functionally [13] distinct. The superficial fascial system (SFS) divides the fat in areolar (more superficial) and lamellar (deeper) layers [Fig. 1A,B]. The areolar layer consists of fat lobules located between the dermis and the fascia superficialis encased in a structure of fibrous septae typically perpendicular to the skin surface and connecting it to the fascia superficialis [Fig. 2]. This layer is stiffer than the deeper lamellar one mostly owing to the fact that it is encased in a fibrous structure, and apparently also because the fat lobules have a more elastic consistency. When the fat lobules of the areolar layer increase their volume, they stretch the vertical septae that pull down the skin surface, causing visible dimples, so-called "cellulitis" [Fig. 3]. Skin dimples and hollows may also be caused by significant irregularities of the subcutaneous fat layer or may be iatrogenic.

The deeper lamellar layer is softer and is encased in the deeper part of the SFS, the one that connects the fascia superficialis to the deeper muscles and fascias. The areolar layer is considered a structural fat, meaning that it wraps up all the external parts of the body, except those where no fat is present. This fat cannot enhance its volume much with fattening, nor can it reduce it with thinning. Its main function is to be a pad, serving as a protection and shock absorber. The superficial areolar layer is esthetically important because it hides the deeper structure anatomy. This pad is significantly reduced in body builders, because they find it esthetically pleasant to show the details of the deeper yet normally hidden structures.

The lamellar layer is deeper and greatly changes its volume during fattening or thinning. It is considered the real energy storage place of the body and is evidently present in areas where the body fattens the most [13]. These areas are different in males and females. The reasons why they are different are obviously genetic and hormonal related, but the authors did not find specific studies in the literature to clarify this topic. These considerations are important when planning a successful liposuction. Liposuction performed in the superficial layer only does not reduce the deep lamellar layer, which is the layer that may thicken even ten times when fattening occurs [12]. If one desires to obtain a stable result, the liposuction must be carried into this deep part as a radical suction. After the publication of the first article on subdermal liposuction, the authors published other studies to clarify that subdermal liposuction is not a method claim-

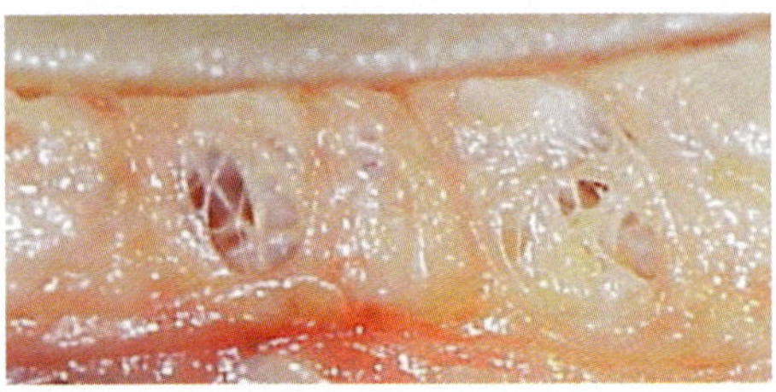

Fig. 2. Detail of the vertical septae of the SFS connecting the skin to the fascia superficialis.

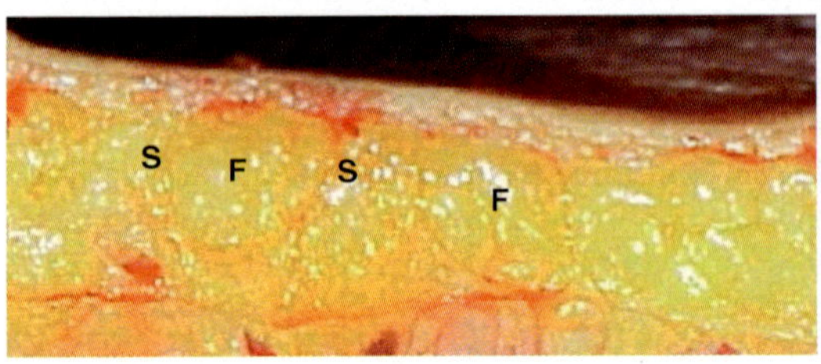

Fig. 3. (*F*) When fat lobules of the areolar layer increase in volume they stretch the fibrous septae of the SFS that pull the dermis, provoking visible dimples on the skin surface, so-called "cellulitis." (*S*) Vertical septae of the SFS.

ing to obtain the same result of "classical" liposuction but rather a way to achieve better results by aspirating whenever necessary both the superficial subdermal layer and the deep lamellar fat [14,15]. As stated previously, not all regions of the body have a thick lamellar layer, but in those areas where it is thick, it must be aspirated to prevent a recurrence of fattening in the future. In women, these areas are the abdomen and flanks, the trochanteric region, the inner thighs, the knees, and the posterior part of the arms.

Some areas of the body may fatten even if a small lamellar layer is present, such as the anterior thighs, the legs, or the dorsal region. In these areas, the areolar fat enhances its volume, but its ability to do so is less than that of the lamellar layer; in a fat subject, the volumes are much bigger in the areas where the lamellar layer is prone to enhance its volume. Suction of areas where the lamellar layer is thin is performed to change the body shape more than to prevent further fattening and gives stable results with no recurrence. The changes made on the areolar layer, which is a structural fat, are considered definitive because, as mentioned previously, this layer poorly changes its volume with fattening or thinning, and the shape achieved with the suction can be considered practically permanent.

In the authors' first publication, the new method was termed *subdermal liposuction* [1]. Later, to stress the fact that the method was a superficial suction, the term *superficial* was added. The term currently used is *superficial subdermal liposuction* (SSL) [13,14, 16,17].

The original technique [1] is still considered by one of the authors (CG) to be the most reliable in his hands and is still used, preceded in some conditions by external ultrasound application [13,17]. External ultrasound is becoming increasingly used since being proposed by Sielberg [18]. The authors apply external ultrasound to enhance the results in areas where the fat is stiff; to render the suction more even in the subdermal layer, improving the cellulitic aspect of the skin; and in secondary cases where the superficial fat has been left irregular [13,17].

Patient selection

The patient must be in good health with normal laboratory values. An evaluation of heart function and other possible pathologic states such as diabetes or coagulation disorders is mandatory to assess the patient's eligibility for a surgical procedure.

The skin condition and adiposities must be observed and evaluated when selecting candidates for liposuction. Patients with poor skin tonicity are inadequate candidates for liposuction as well as those with excessive obesity. Weight loss before the operation is discouraged. With dieting, the body shape changes but the results obtained are usually not stable; therefore, it is impossible to evaluate properly the areas to be treated and the amount of fat to be removed to obtain a good and stable result. If suction is performed when the body shape has been changed in an unstable way by dieting, the effect achieved by the liposuction will not be definitive. If the patient suspends the dieting, the fat that was not seen and not removed may increase again in volume.

Diets induce weight loss, reducing the fat content of fat cells. Fat cells of the lamellar (deep) layer are more affected by diets than are cells of the areolar (superficial) layer. In weight loss obtained with diets, the lamellar layer is reduced, but the skin is unable to retract effectively because the areolar fat that is located immediately under the skin surface, maintaining most of its volume, is an obstacle to skin retraction. Defatting skin is a common procedure in plastic surgery to help skin retraction. It is performed in many occasions as part of techniques for breast reduction, to reduce "dog ears," and so on. When body mass is to be reduced, defatting just under the skin permits a better skin retraction owing to subdermal liposuction as stressed in the authors' publication in 1990 [5]. The esthetic quality of the weight loss obtained with liposuction when compared with that obtained with a diet is better since the advent of subdermal liposuction, because, beyond weight loss, there is less skin redundancy. An SSL attempted after a conspicuous weight loss is impossible to perform well, because it is manually difficult to work under a flaccid skin. Moreover, after liposuction, skin retraction is favored by the slow and progressive reduction of edema that takes place over many months, facilitating the skin retraction that takes place progressively. This favorable feature is not present if the suction is performed after weight loss. The skin is unable to redrape progressively without becoming too flabby. For all of these reasons, it is preferable to perform a suction before a diet.

Patient examination

Patients are examined to assess the areas to be treated and to evaluate the skin tone. Contraction of the abdominal muscles permits detection with palpation of any possible defects of the abdominal muscular wall. If an excessive fat thickness impairs the reliability of the palpation maneuver, a CT scan can be performed to visualize the muscular layer and to detect possible muscular diastasis or the presence of hernias. Performing a liposuction when one of these pathologic conditions is present can be dangerous owing to the risk of abdominal perforation.

When the inferior limbs are examined and edema is observed, a differential diagnosis must be made between edema and lipedema [19]. In lipedema, the foot is not edematous. Lipedema may be treated successfully by liposuction, whereas the cause of edema should be investigated, and liposuction is probably not indicated. To evaluate the fat layer in the calves, the patient is asked to stand on the tip of the toes, and the skin is grasped, permitting one to assess whether the muscle is hypertrophic or the fat thickness is disproportionate.

Scheduling the operation and safety parameters

Safety parameters for liposuction vary in the literature. The authors' postures are as follows:

- If the amount of fat to be removed is expected to be more than 4 kg, an autologous blood transfusion should be considered, or the operation should be scheduled in two or more stages to lessen the amount of trauma [15].
- If large volumes must be aspirated, the number of areas to be treated must be reduced to lessen the amount of trauma. Multiple adiposities can be treated in the same operation if the total amount of aspirated fat will not exceed 4 kg. This quantity may vary depending on the bleeding during the procedure, being less in patients who show a tendency to bleed and more when bleeding is limited.

Care should be taken not to inject excessive lidocaine. The authors prefer to maintain its level under 20 mg/kg to avoid the risk of lidocaine toxicity [13], despite reports in the literature of dosages as high as 35 mg/kg [20] and more. In average weight patients, 1g of lidocaine is sufficient to give a complete analgesia in slight or moderate adiposities when two to three areas will be treated under local anesthesia plus sedation. If is estimated that this amount will need to be exceeded to obtain a proper analgesia, the aspiration is performed under general or peridural anesthesia.

When irregularities are visible on the skin surface, the use of external ultrasound is indicated to render easier and smoother the fat aspiration of the subdermal layer. Skin irregularities may be due to underlying fat irregularity. In that situation, external ultrasound is used to soften the fat, crushing it with the mechanical impact of its waves [13,17, 18,21–23] and permitting an easier control of the aspiration maneuvers. Skin irregularities may also be due to underlying localized traction exercised by the SFS or by scarring consequent to previous liposuction or trauma. In these situations, a liberation of the traction should be accomplished by means of the Toledo dissector [24], and then fat should be injected to replace the missing uniformity of the fat layer [16].

The technique and its rationale

Using a skin marker, the areas to be aspirated are demarcated with the patient in a standing position. More prominent points are signed with a cross and depressed areas with small circles. These markings help the operator to recognize prominences and hollows when the patient lies down [Fig. 4].

The patient is placed on the operating table in the supine or prone position. Other positions may be used depending on the surgeon's preference. To help evaluate the progression of the suction, the position of the limbs may frequently be changed. A patient under local anesthesia may be asked to contract the muscles to appraise the quality of the result obtained in a dynamic situation.

Before beginning the suction, all of the areas are infiltrated with an amount of solution that equals the estimated volume to be aspirated. This method of infiltration has been called the superwet technique [25]. When local anesthesia is planned, the solution is made with saline plus adrenaline in a concentration of 1:500,000 and lidocaine 0.2% to 0.3%. When general anesthesia is used, the solution contains adrenalin in a concentration of 1:1,000,000 and lidocaine 0.05% [13,17]. The infiltration is performed with the Gasperoni multipurpose cannula connected with a 60-mL syringe [Fig. 5]. Other means of infiltration, such as the Klein pump, may be used, but with this

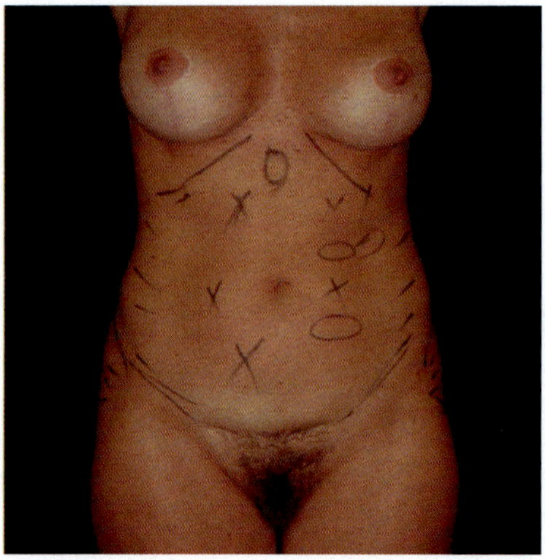

Fig. 4. Preoperative markings with the patient standing up. Dimples are marked with X drawings and hollows with circles.

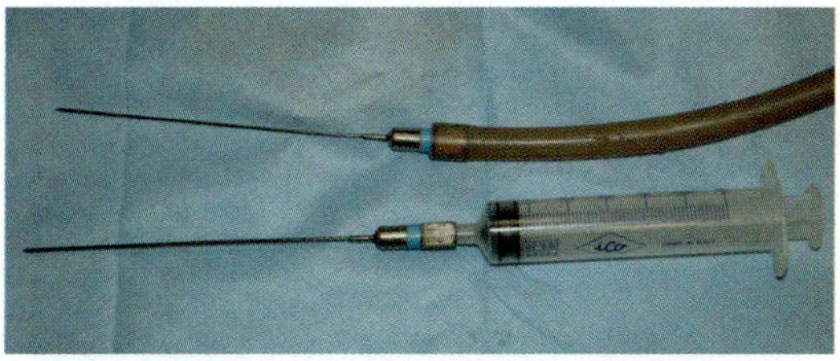

Fig. 5. The Gasperoni multipurpose cannula may be used to aspirate or to infiltrate, connecting it to the tube or to the syringe.

device, there is a tendency to infiltrate more fluids than necessary.

When external ultrasound is used, care should be taken to infiltrate immediately under the dermis to ease the wave propagation in the superficial layer of fat. If the deep fat must be reached by the waves, it must be infiltrated thoroughly to allow a successful cavitation induced by the ultrasound; therefore, the amount of infiltration is more than in the superwet method. A thin layer of ultrasonic gel is spread on the skin of the areas to be treated with external ultrasound, which is delivered through a 3-MHz probe to treat the superficial fat and a 1-MHz probe to treat the deeper layers. A 2-MHz probe may also be used to ensure that the 1- to 2-cm deep layer is effectively reached. The hand-held transducer delivering the external ultrasound is slowly moved on the marked area with slow circular or up and down movements for 10 minutes in each abdominal quadrant, 15 minutes in the flank or dorsal flank, 20 minutes in each external thigh, 15 minutes in each knee, 20 minutes in each ankle, and 15 minutes in each inner arm. The probe must be in constant motion; otherwise, the heat caused by the energy delivered may burn the skin. The use of external ultrasound renders penetration of the cannulas easier because the fat is already somewhat crushed and softened upon insertion [**Fig. 6**].

As mentioned previously, the authors limit the use of external ultrasound as follows: (1) to enhance the results in areas where the fat is stiff; (2) to render the subdermal layer suction more even, improving the cellulitic aspect of the skin; and (3) to treat secondary cases where the superficial fat has been left irregular. There are two reasons for these restricted indications. First, the hand that holds the probe becomes painful after about 20 minutes of continuous use, raising questions about the safety of the application for the surgeon. Second, because the application of external ultrasound to the first area adds 15 to 45 minutes to the procedure time, it increases the operating time and the operating room cost. Subsequent areas are treated when the suction is already in progress, not adding more time to the procedure.

The technique consists of suctioning the superficial subdermal fat through small gauge cannulas (1.8–2 mm diameter) and then proceeding with the same thin cannulas to aspirate the deeper fat before using bigger gauge cannulas. In contrast to other techniques, the authors perform the aspiration progressively, increasing the gauge of the cannulas instead of decreasing it [1,5,6,13–17]. There are many reasons for inverting the gauge order. The use of bigger gauge cannulas at the start of the suction may give rise to irregularities that must be treated afterward with smaller cannulas. One creates defects and then tries to get rid of them! The suction is more progressive and uniform and consequently less painful when using small gauge cannulas first, because the smaller cannulas slide better among the septae of the SFS, reducing their impact with this fibrous structure. Less force is then needed to perform the suction.

Advantages of the SSL technique include the following:

- The suction of the subdermal fat layer reduces the fat just under the skin, making it possible to obtain an effective skin retraction [1,5].
- The progressive treatment of all the layers of fat permits the removal of it in such an even way that good results are predictable.
- It is possible to treat patients with slight adiposities as well as areas with small thickness of the fat layers, such as the ankles.
- The cellulitic aspect of the skin surface may improve as the result of a decompression of the areolar layer that releases the tension on the vertical septae of the SFS that are superficial to the fascia superficialis.
- The procedure is similar for patients with big adiposities and those with small ones.

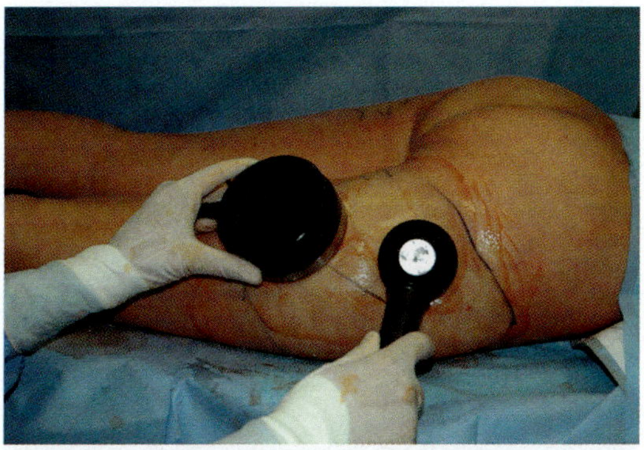

Fig. 6. External ultrasound is delivered with the 3-MHz probe to reach the subdermal fat layer and the 1-MHz probe to reach the deeper layers. A thin layer of ultrasonic gel is applied on the skin surface to permit transmission to the tissues.

The cannula is introduced through 2-mm stab incisions. Their locations should allow the surgeon to do his or her best work. The authors start SSL with treatment of the subdermal layer of fat with a 1.8- to 2-mm Gasperoni Multipurpose Mercedes tip cannula [Fig. 7]. The small gauge allows its superficial use with an effective suction of the subdermal fat layer. The Mercedes tip cannula has a three-fissure tip that permits a 360-degree oriented liposuction and produces an effective aspiration all around it. Cannulas with only downward facing orifices are not suitable for suctioning the subdermal fat, because the suction is made in one direction, whereas the defatting immediately under the dermis must be as uniform as possible. After the subdermal layer of fat is treated, the same cannulas are oriented to the deeper layers. The gauges of the cannulas are subsequently increased up to 2.5 to 3 mm to speed the suction. These cannulas have two or three orifices and remove the fat already crushed but still not aspirated; therefore, they are called "scavenger cannulas" [Fig. 7] [5]. The suction is as progressive and uniform as possible. A spray bottle is used to sprinkle cold saline on the cannulas to reduce the friction through the stab incision. This friction is responsible for inflammation during the healing phase of the wound and causes hyperpigmentation of the scars and surrounding tissues [Fig. 8] [26]. Stitches are not needed to close the small stab incisions that are made to introduce the thin cannulas.

The technique must be adapted to the various areas of the body because of their different characteristics. In the abdomen, a massive all layer liposuction (MALL) [14] is performed to aspirate as much fat as possible, expecting a conspicuous cutaneous retraction. The authors begin with the 2-mm Mercedes cannula in the subdermal layer to ensure that the skin may shrink without forming waves. The cannulas are then directed toward the deeper layers, progressively increasing their gauges.

The best candidates for inner thigh suction are patients with good elasticity of the skin; however, if the amount of fat to be removed is not excessive, patients with less tonic skin may also be treated successfully.

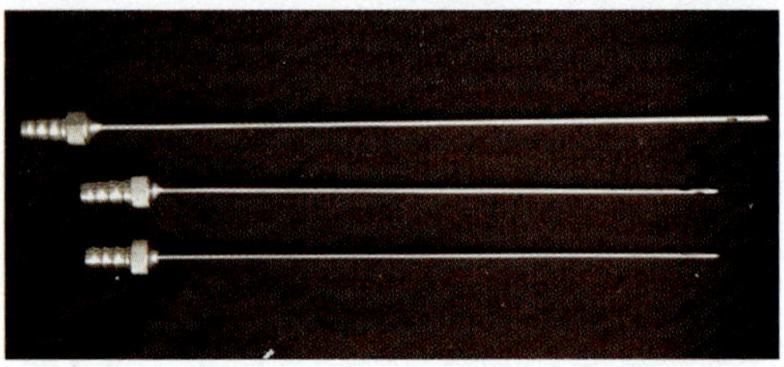

Fig. 7. The 2-mm Mercedes tip cannula has three fissures. The 2.5-mm cannula has two holes at 180 degrees, and the 3-mm cannula has three holes at 120 degrees.

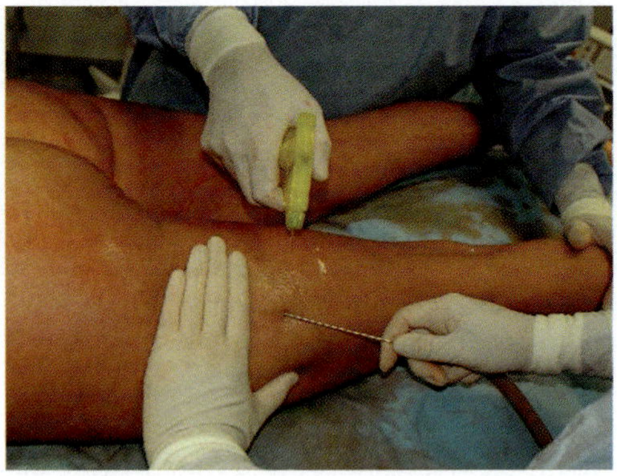

Fig. 8. Saline is sprayed to prevent friction of the cannula on the stab incision.

In the trunk, subdermal liposuction is recommended to promote skin retraction, and the use of external ultrasound aids in the aspiration of fat from this frequently fibrous area [13,17].

In the external thigh, the skin must shrink smoothly, but the fat is usually more fibrous than in other areas. External ultrasound is of utmost benefit to soften it, allowing a smoother penetration of the cannulas and facilitating a uniform aspiration. The extraction of fat after the delivery of external ultrasound is simpler, more even, and less traumatic. In fact, when the subcutaneous tissue is already somewhat crushed by the external ultrasound, the cannula encounters less resistance when pushed through the fat, sliding easier among the fibrous septae with less trauma to them and to blood vessels. Dimples and hollows on the skin surface are smoothed, reducing the tension on the vertical septae of the areolar layer using small gauge Mercedes cannulas (1.8–2 mm) in the subdermal fat. Its firmness is reduced, decreasing the superficial fat resistance to the retraction force and favoring skin retraction. To proceed with the suction as uniformly as possible, it is necessary to change the points of introduction of the cannula along with the position of the limbs to vary the direction of their penetration. After the Mercedes cannula has been used in the subdermal layer, it is directed toward the deeper fat [Fig. 9A,B].

In the flank region, cellulitis is never present. The fat is loose with a soft consistency; therefore, it has a spontaneous tendency to accommodate. For this reason, in this area suction of the subdermal layer is not necessary. The procedure is started with a 2.5-mm two opposite hole tip cannula, and the gauge is increased until 3 mm.

In the anterior thighs, the lamellar layer is thin. The aspiration practically involves just the areolar

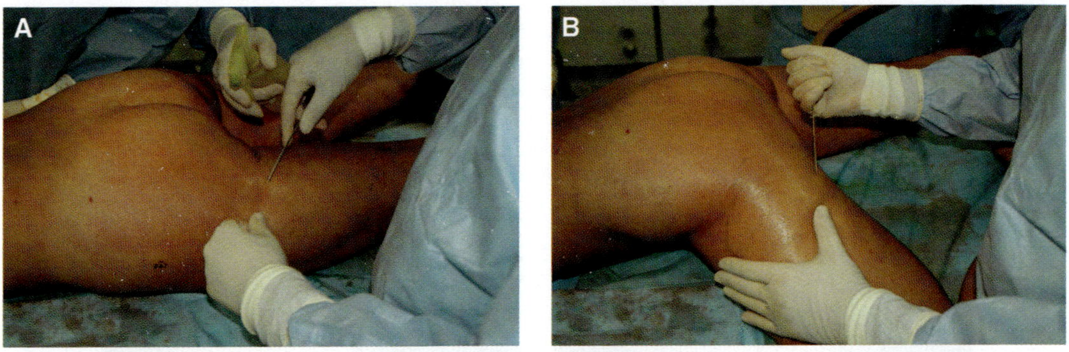

Fig. 9. (*A*) The suction begins in the subdermal fat. (*B*) After the suction has been performed in the subdermal layer, the cannula is directed toward the deeper fat, and the position of the limbs is changed many times to ensure a progressive and even suction.

layer and may be started with slightly bigger cannulas than the ones used in most other areas (2.5 mm). In fact, it is not necessary in this area to perform a careful subdermal defatting because the skin normally accommodates well. As always during the procedure, the gauge is gradually increased. Care must be taken to proceed gradually, because any irregular suction of the anterior thigh becomes evident after the edema has subsided.

In the knee, the suction involves the superficial and deep layers. Because the retraction during the operation is conspicuous, it is possible to judge immediately the result obtained.

In the ankles and calves, as in the anterior thighs, the areolar layer is the only one present for the most part. The aspiration is usually circular on the whole leg and is performed leaving only a thin layer of fat.

Dressings

Every stab incision is covered with an adhesive bandage. Elastic garments for the trunk and elastic stockings for the inferior limbs are applied at the end of the procedure in the operating room.

Postoperative care

Prophylactic antibiotic therapy is prescribed. The recovery time depends on the amount of aspirated fat and the type of anesthesia. When a small liposuction is performed, especially under local anesthesia, the recovery time is a few days. After a large fat extraction, the patient will feel asthenic owing to the surgical trauma and the acute anemia consequential to blood loss, and normal activities must be resumed gradually in a few weeks. Bruises and edema are always present in a variable amount. Bruises subside in about 3 weeks, and swelling lasts for months. The use of elastic stockings and garments is prescribed for approximately 6 weeks. They are worn day and night for the first week and only during the daytime starting from the second week. Abundant fluid intake and a well-balanced diet including proteins to build up hemoglobin are prescribed [27]. Walking is mandatory, particularly for patients who have been operated on at the inferior limbs. Early mobilization the subsequent day is required for prevention of venous thrombosis. Exercising may be beneficial, avoiding strenuous activities. Postoperative physiotherapy such as endermologie and lymphatic vein massage may be started after 3 weeks.

Errors of technique and complications

In a correctly performed SSL, the suction is progressive; therefore, it is easier to control than in the classical technique. Irregularities owing to uneven suction are rare if the progression of the cannula's

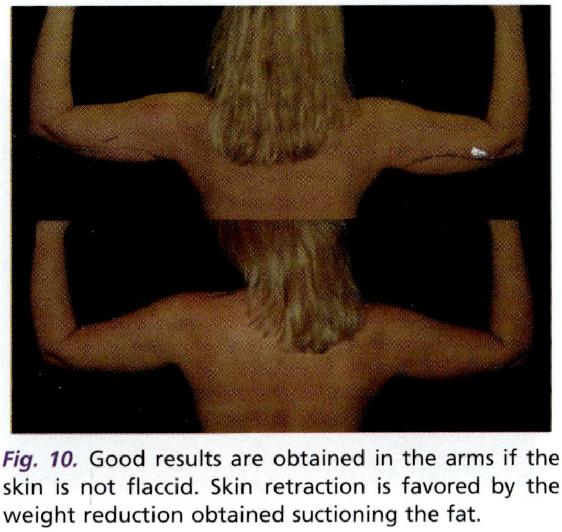

Fig. 10. Good results are obtained in the arms if the skin is not flaccid. Skin retraction is favored by the weight reduction obtained suctioning the fat.

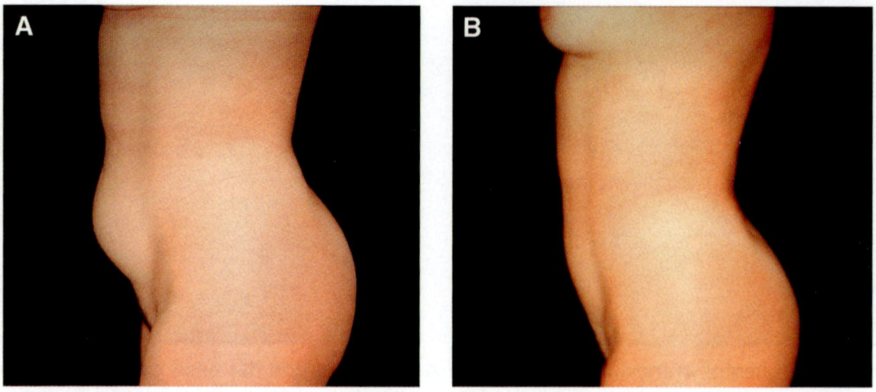

Fig. 11. (*A*) Preoperative view of the abdomen. (*B*) Same patient 7 months after 800 g of fat has been aspirated.

gauge is kept from small to big as recommended, a fundamental feature of the SSL technique. If too much fat is aspirated from a localized point and this is visible during the procedure, it is possible to correct the depression by injecting some fat taken with a syringe. It is advisable to wash the collected fat with saline and to let it separate from the fluids present in the syringe before injecting it. The fat temporarily stored in the syringes must be aspirated from an area where external ultrasound has not been applied, otherwise the fat to be grafted will be less vital after being crushed by the ultrasonic wave.

After many months, at least 6, when it is possible to evaluate whether waves and irregularities are truly present after the liposuction, touch ups may be undertaken. If great irregularities are present before the suction, it is impossible to obtain a smooth result. SSL permits one to obtain better results than in the classical technique, reducing irregularities and rarely being their cause. Skin irregularities should not be considered a complication but rather a limitation of any suction technique and are less conspicuous and less frequent in SSL. Besides skin irregularities, which the authors estimate as a possible outcome in 3% of patients, in more than 2600 cases of SSL several rare complications have occurred. Paresthesias were seen owing to nerve injury (0.5%), which sometimes were permanent and were more frequent in the limbs. Infections (0.15%) included two cases of slight inflammation with erythema of the skin that healed in a few days after antibiotic therapy. Two patients who received a graft of 200 to 300 mL had an inflammation after the first week and were successfully treated with antibiotics. Seromas occurred in 0.07% of patients. Two seromas formed in patients undergoing abdominal liposuction after an attempt to use bigger gauge (1 cm) cannulas to speed the suction time. This observation confirms that if the SSL technique is correctly performed, there is no seroma formation and the procedure is highly reliable. No antithrombotic drugs were used, and no cases of thrombosis have occurred. No skin slough and no deaths were seen.

The SSL technique proposed by the authors in 1989 remains, after 15 years, the most reliable method [**Figs. 10–15**]. Complications are usually

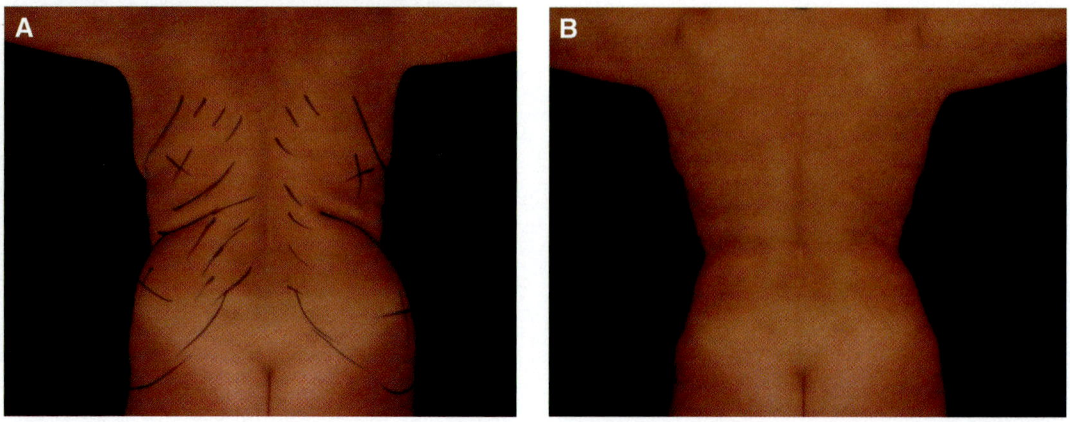

Fig. 12. (*A*) Preoperative view of the dorsal region and flanks. (*B*) Postoperative aspect after 4 months.

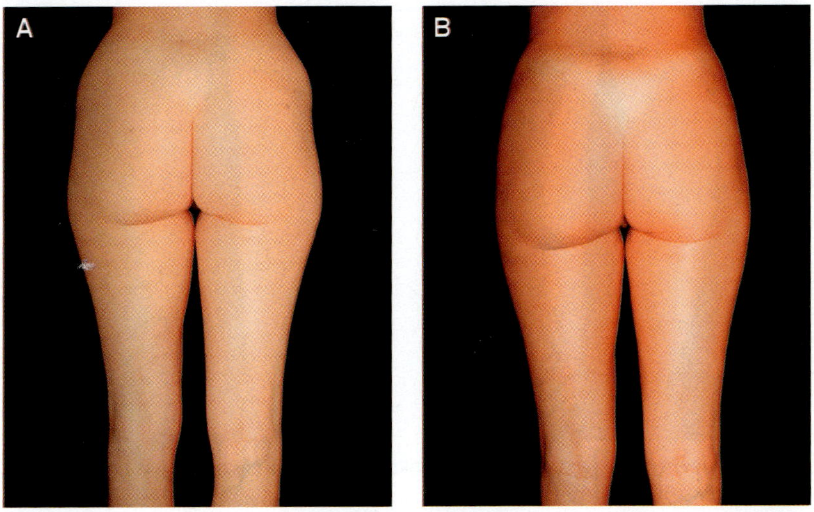

Fig. 13. (*A*) Preoperative view of the flanks and trochanteric region. (*B*) Postoperative aspect after 6 months.

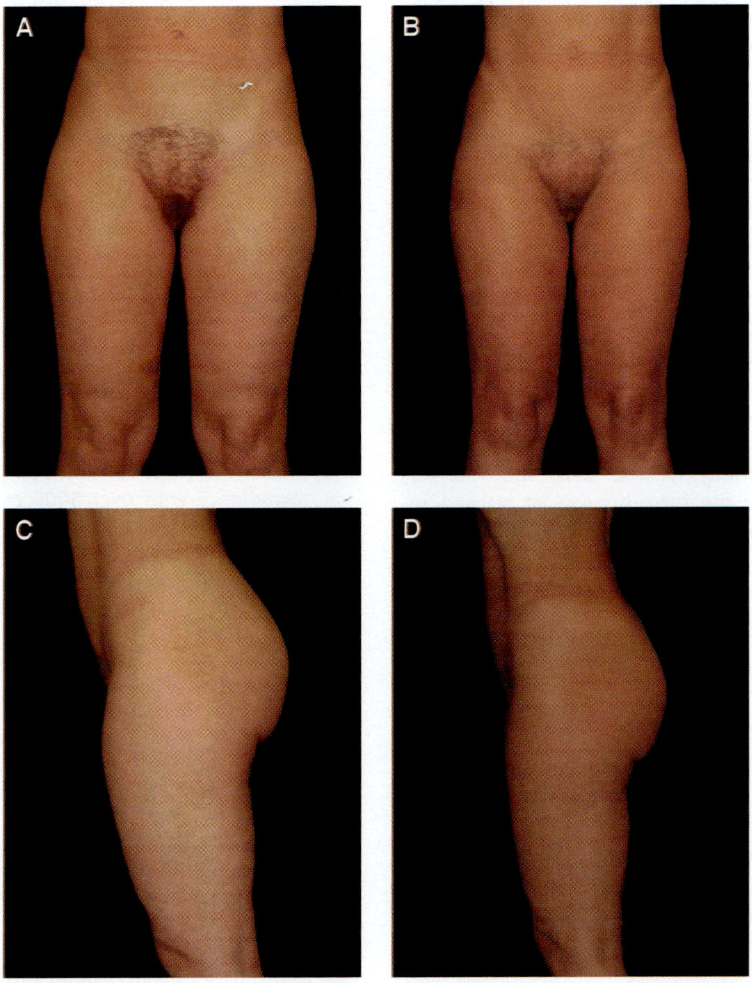

Fig. 14. (*A*) Preoperative view of anterior part of the thighs and knees. (*B*) Postoperative aspect after 8 months. (*C*) Same patient in lateral view. (*D*) Postoperative aspect after 8 months in lateral view.

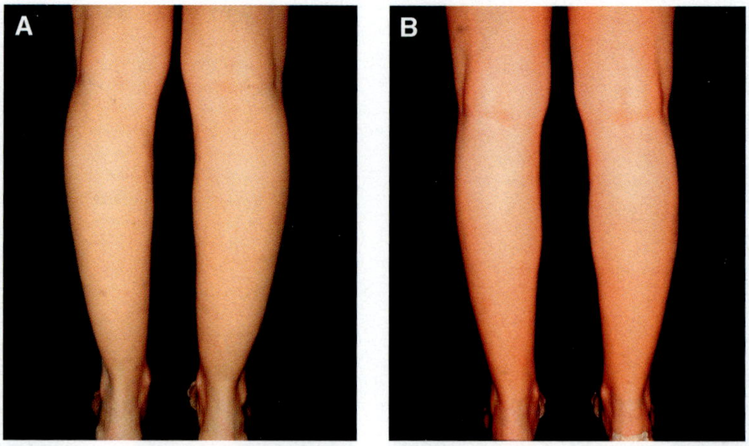

Fig. 15. (*A*) Preoperative view of the legs. Calves and ankles are routinely aspirated, and lipedema is successfully treated. (*B*) Postoperative aspect after 6 months.

transitory and their rate low (0.72%). When indicated, the use of external ultrasound is helpful to further enhance the quality of the results of SSL, but the suction method is still the same, with the identical concepts and steps exposed in the original publication.

Summary

Since its first description, the liposuction technique has greatly changed. Originally, the superficial fat was left untouched because of the fear of producing visible irregularities of the skin surface. In 1989, the authors presented at the International Society of Aesthetic Plastic Surgery congress in Zurich a new way of performing liposuction named subdermal liposuction. In this new technique, the superficial fat that the classical technique imposed to respect was finally treated. This method was made possible by the introduction of refined instruments. The cannula's gauge was reduced, ranging from 1.8 to 3 mm compared with the smallest gauge of 5 mm in the classical technique presented by Illouz.

The advantages of treating the superficial fat are many. Very small adiposities can be suctioned, and skin retraction is favored by defatting immediately under the skin. In fact, fat removal to favor skin accommodation is a common procedure in plastic surgery that, since the introduction of subdermal liposuction, can be accomplished by suctioning and not with sharp instruments. The cellulitic aspect of the skin may also improve, because the suction of the subdermal fat reduces the tension on the vertical septae of the SFS, responsible for the dimples of cellulitis. The use of thin cannulas permits a more progressive suction with better control of the evolution of the procedure. To stress the fact that the superficial subdermal fat was addressed by the authors' procedure, the original name "subdermal liposuction" was changed to "superficial subdermal liposuction." Knowledge of anatomic features and functional distinction of the subcutaneous fat as described herein are crucial to obtain permanent and good quality results. The introduction of external ultrasound has permitted the treatment of difficult cases and is performed in selected patients to enhance the quality of the results.

References

[1] Gasperoni C, Salgarello M, Emiliozzi P, et al. Subdermal liposuction [abstract]. In: Programs and Abstracts of the 10th Congress of the International Society of Aesthetic Plastic Surgery, Zurich, September 11–14, 1989. p. 95.

[2] Illouz YG. Body contouring by lipolysis: a 5-year experience with over 3000 cases. Plast Reconstr Surg 1983;72(5):591–7.

[3] Fischer A, Fischer G. First surgical treatment for molding body's cellulite with three 5 mm incisions. Bull Int Acad Cosmet Surg 1976;3:35.

[4] Kesselring UK. Regional fat aspiration for body contouring. Plast Reconstr Surg 1983;72(5):609–10.

[5] Gasperoni C, Salgarello M, Emiliozzi P, et al. Subdermal liposuction. Aesthetic Plast Surg 1990;14:137–42.

[6] Gasperoni C, Salgarello M. Suction-assisted lipectomy of the subdermal fat layer: a new way of performing liposuction. In: Annals of the International Symposium Recent Advances in Plastic Surgery, São Paulo, Brazil, March 28–30, 1990. p. 477–91.

[7] Gasparotti M. Superficial liposuction for flaccid skin patients. In: Annals of the International Symposium Recent Advances in Plastic Surgery, Sao Paulo, Brazil, March 28–30, 1990. p. 441–5.

[8] Toledo LS. Superficial syringe liposculpture. In: Annals of the International Symposium Recent Advances in Plastic Surgery, Sao Paulo, Brazil, March 28–30, 1990. p. 446–53.
[9] Souza Pinto EB. Lipoinjerto y liposuction superficial. In: Memoria XVI Congreso Nacional de Chirurgia, Santa Cruz de la Sierra, Bolivia. JICA; 1991. p. 325–30.
[10] Goddio AS. Skin retraction following suction lipectomy by treatment site: a study of 500 procedures in 458 selected subjects. Plast Reconstr Surg 1991;87(1):66–75.
[11] Souza Pinto EB. Superficial liposuction and fat graft cellulitis. Presented at Recent Advances in Plastic Surgery International, VI Annual. Beverly Hills, CA, July 20–21, 1991.
[12] Avelar JM, Illouz YG. Lipoaspiraçao. Sao Paulo (Brazil): Editoria Hipocrates; 1986.
[13] Gasperoni C, Salgarello M, Gasperoni P. External ultrasound used in conjunction with superficial subdermal liposuction: a safe and effective technique. Aesthetic Plast Surg 2000;24:253–8.
[14] Gasperoni C, Salgarello M. MALL liposuction: the natural evolution of the subdermal superficial liposuction. Aesthetic Plast Surg 1994;18:253–7.
[15] Gasperoni C, Salgarello M. La lipoaspirazione totale: l'evoluzione della lipaspirazione subdermica [abstract]. In: Programs and Abstracts of the 41st National Congress of the Italian Society of Reconstructive and Aesthetic Plastic Surgery, Genova, December 6–9, 1992. p. 235.
[16] Gasperoni C, Salgarello M. Rationale of subdermal superficial liposuction related to the anatomy of subcutaneous fat and the superficial fascial system. Aesthetic Plast Surg 1995;19: 13–20.
[17] Gasperoni C, Salgarello M. The use of external ultrasound combined with superficial subdermal liposuction. Ann Plast Surg 2000;45(4): 369–73.
[18] Sielberg BN. The technique of external ultrasound-assisted lipoplasty. Plast Reconstr Surg 1998; 101:552.
[19] Rudkin GH, Miller TA. Lipedema: a clinical entity distinct from lymphedema. Plast Reconstr Surg 1994;94:841–7.
[20] Klein JA. Tumescent technique for regional anesthesia permits lidocaine dose of 35 mg/kg for liposuction surgery. Am J Cosmet Surg 1987; 4:263.
[21] Cook WR. Utilizing external ultrasonic energy to improve the results of tumescent liposculpture. Dermatol Surg 1997;23:1207–11.
[22] Havoonjian HH, Luftman DB, Menaker GM, et al. External ultrasonic tumescent liposuction: a preliminary study. Dermatol Surg 1997; 23:1201–6.
[23] Kinney BM, and the Plastic Surgery Educational Foundation DATA Committee. Body contouring with external ultrasound. Plast Reconstr Surg 1999;103:728–9.
[24] Pitman GH, Grazer FM, Lockwood TE, et al. Liposuction: problems and techniques. Perspect Plast Surg 1993;7(1):73.
[25] Bela Fodor P. Defining wetting solutions in lipoplasty. Plast Reconstr Surg 1999;103:1519.
[26] Gasperoni C, Salgarello M, Cimino A, et al. A new tool to eliminate hyperpigmentation in liposuction scars. Ann Plast Surg 2000;45(2):214–5.
[27] Fournier PF. Liposculpture: the syringe technique. Paris: Arnette Blackwell; 1991.

ELSEVIER
SAUNDERS

CLINICS IN
PLASTIC
SURGERY

Clin Plastic Surg 33 (2006) 75–77

Sequential (Serial) Suction

Robert G.W. Girling V, Mark A. Salisbury, MD,
Robert A. Ersek, MD, FACS*

When Illouz first described blunt liposuction in 1982 at the Honolulu meeting of the American Society of Plastic Surgery (ASPS), the safe amounts to be taken were in great question [1]. The Lipoplasty Society of North America and the ASPS issued guidelines that strongly suggested 2.5 L was the maximum amount of fat that could be removed safely at one time [2–7]. If larger amounts were required, it was suggested that blood transfusions be available. With the subsequent discoveries of AIDS in the next few years, the idea of blood transfusion became a negative concept. For this reason, the authors began performing serial suctions as a routine [8].

Materials and methods

All surgeries are performed under diazepam (Valium) and ketamine dissociative anesthesia [1,9–11]. When patients enter the facility, they are given 20 mg of diazepam orally, which often calms their fears so that they are more comfortable by the time that the intravenous line is started. Once patients are in the operating room and prepared, they are given more diazepam until their speech is slurred. This amount may be as little as 5 mg in a sensitive patient and as much as 150 mg. A total of 75 mg of ketamine is given over 1 to 2 minutes, which subdues patients to a somnolent and completely anesthetic state. Although pain free, all reflexes remain intact so that patients are breathing on their own, still have a cough reflex, and the muscle tone remains normal. The area is then infiltrated with a dilute solution of lidocaine with epinephrine (0.025% lidocaine with epinephrine in Ringer's solution), with the goal of achieving a ratio of about one liter per liter. As an example, if one expects to take 2 L out of the abdomen, 2 L of fluid will be put in. This ratio is not strict and is regarded as an approximation. This protocol renders the patient insensitive in these areas so that the authors can perform liposuction.

The authors use the fewest possible entrance sites and employ extra long cannulas measuring 45 cm in length. The largest cannula is 8 mm in diameter for larger patients; however, most patients need a 5- or 6-mm cannula. Using the long cannulas, a 1-cm site is created in the back at the gluteal crease and reaching down to the knees and all the way up to the shoulders. When operating on arms, an additional incision is made in the crease at the back of the elbow, which enables one to reach 360 degrees around the arm to remove as much as 1 L of fat. In the calves and ankles, a single incision is placed in the crease of the Achilles tendon or in the back of the knee. In the front, one to two incisions are made in the lateral borders of the pubic hair. In small patients in whom small amounts of fat are removed, the entire front is entered from a single incision about 3 mm in length at the midline owing to current trends in pubic grooming. Through these incisions, one can reach from the knees to the neck. The incisions are then closed with one

Personique Surgery Center, 630 West 34th Street, Suite 201, Austin, TX 78705, USA
* Corresponding author.
E-mail address: personique@hotmail.com (R.A. Ersek).

0094-1298/06/$ – see front matter
doi:10.1016/j.cps.2005.08.005
plasticsurgery.theclinics.com

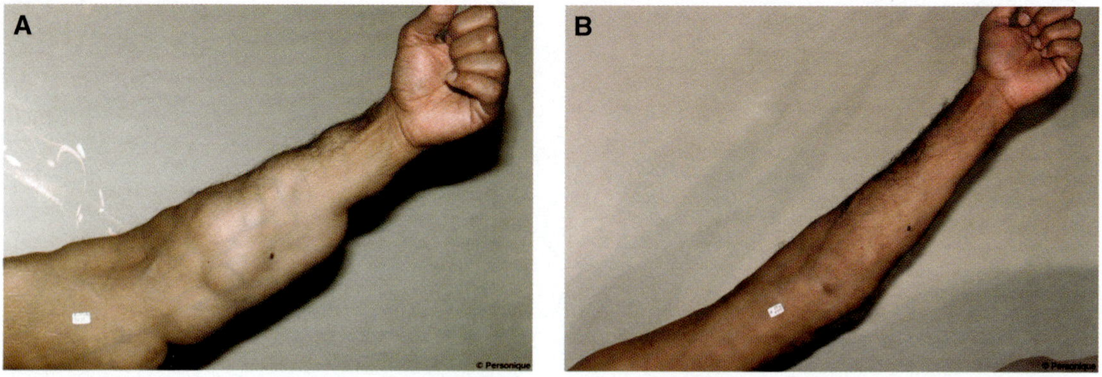

Fig. 1. (*A*) This 50-year-old man was a general surgeon with lipomatosis. From the age of 28 years, the lipomas had increased in size and began to interfere with his daily life. (*B*) Serial suction enabled the authors to remove 10.3 L of fat over a 3-year period without the patient ever missing a day of work.

or two stitches of 4-0 Vicryl and then reinforced with suture-strips.

Serial suction

When large amounts of fat are removed without transfusion, the authors believe it is safest to remove the fat in serial subsequent episodes [8,12,13]. Waiting at least 6 weeks between procedures allows the blood to re-equilibrate and the patient to heal completely. It is always more difficult to perform liposuction in the same area a second time because of scar formation; however, acceptable results can be achieved safely.

Discussion

Using this method of serial suction, the authors have been able to take seemingly lethal amounts of fat over a protracted period of time with no untoward sequelae. One such case is the patient shown in Fig. 1A, a general surgeon, in whom hereditary lipomatosis developed at age 28 years. On Friday afternoons, the authors were able to operate on one area at a time. This arrangement enabled the patient to return to work by Monday; therefore, he never missed a day of work. Over a 3-year period, 10.3 L of lipomas was removed [Fig. 1B]. This liposuction was performed before the tumescent technique was used and was more extensive than anyone would attempt with the dry technique. Recently, the patient has returned after 15 years for the removal of several smaller lipomas. This case represents a 15-year series of serial suction.

Another dramatic case is the patient shown in Fig. 2A who presented with a very thin waist (21 inches), very thin legs, and tremendous buttocks. This liposuction was before the development of tumescent techniques, and serial suction was performed over a 2-year period. The authors were

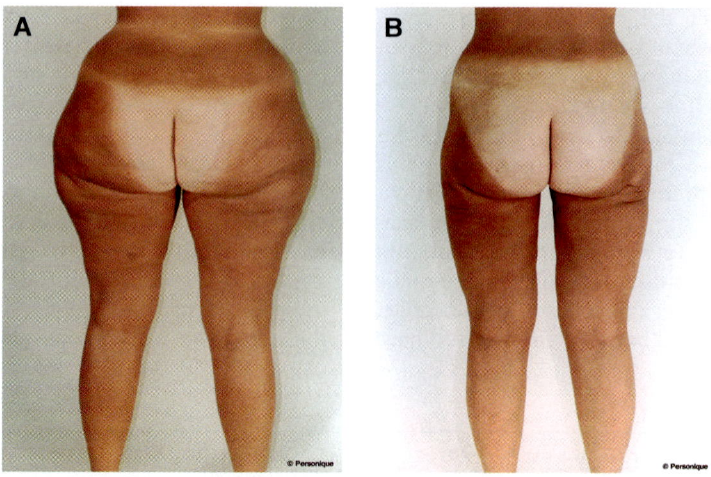

Fig. 2. (*A*) This young woman had a very thin waist and thin legs but was burdened by a tremendous buttocks. (*B*) Over a 2-year period, 10.5 L of fat was removed by serial suction, restoring her proportions.

able to remove 10.5 L without transfusion, providing very reasonable results [Fig. 2B].

Since the development of tumescent or superwet techniques, the authors are able to remove safely more fat at a time. These methods enable the infiltration of large amounts of fluid, mechanically compressing the area and forcing blood out of the capillaries. The small amounts of epinephrine shrink the precapillary arteries so that less blood is contained in the area that is treated. In this manner, the authors have removed as much as 27 L at one time (having the patient donate 2 U of autologous blood beforehand). The authors do not wish to extend this further to discover the median lethal dose (LD_{50}) for liposuction. When faced with a large patient and the knowledge that one cannot safely complete the task in one sitting, it is perfectly reasonable to remove only a safe amount at one time. Any method can be completed successfully by waiting 6 weeks for a full recovery and repeating the procedure. Having done this as many as five times for a patient, it is uncertain what the limit would be, as long as the amount taken each time is kept within reasonable parameters. Serial suction provides a way to achieve large results over a protracted period safely.

References

[1] Ersek RA. Dissociative anesthesia for safety sake: ketamine and diazepam—a 35-year personal experience. Plast Reconstr Surg 2004;113(7):1955–9.

[2] Courtiss EH. Suction lipectomy: a retrospective analysis of 100 patients. Plast Reconstr Surg 1984;73:780–94.

[3] Ersek RA. Severe and mortal complications. In: Hetter GP, editor. Lipoplasty: the theory and practice of blunt suction lipectomy. 2nd edition. Boston: Little, Brown; 1990. p. 223.

[4] Ersek RA. Obesity can be treated by suction lipoplasty when combined with other procedures. Aesthetic Plast Surg 1991;15:67–71.

[5] Hetter GP. Lipoplasty: the theory and practice of blunt suction lipectomy. Boston: Little, Brown; 1984.

[6] Illouz YG. Body sculpturing by lipoplasty: the cannulae. New York: Churchill Livingstone; 1989. p. 98–103.

[7] Teimourian B, Rogers III WB. A national survey of complications associated with suction lipectomy: a comparative study. Plast Reconstr Surg 1989;84(4):628–31.

[8] Ersek RA. Serial suction lipectomy. Clin Plast Surg 1989;16(2):313–7.

[9] Ersek RA. A new magnetic board for medication monitoring during outpatient anesthesia. Lipoplasty 1989;6(2):56–7.

[10] Ersek RA. Lipoplasty in the nineties. Travis County Med Soc J March 1990:27–9.

[11] Ersek RA, Belton IV HN, Salisbury AV. Serial and superficial suction for staetopygia (Hottentot bustle). Aesthetic Plast Surg 1994;18:279–82.

[12] Illouz YG. The origin of lipolysis. In: Hetter GP, editor. Lipoplasty: the theory and practice of blunt suction lipectomy. Boston: Little, Brown; 1984. p. 30.

[13] Illouz YG. Body sculpturing by lipoplasty: anesthesia. New York: Churchill Livingstone; 1989. p. 114–9.

ELSEVIER
SAUNDERS

CLINICS IN PLASTIC SURGERY

Clin Plastic Surg 33 (2006) 79–90

Abdominoplasty Combined with Lipoplasty Without Panniculus Undermining: Abdominolipoplasty—a Safe Technique

Juarez M. Avelar, MD

Abdominoplasty is one of the most frequent procedures in plastic surgery. There are two important components—an esthetic and a reconstructive approach—that provide a wide variety of options in abdominoplasty. The esthetic component is inherent to the surgical act, because it aims to create a new silhouette harmonizing the abdomen with the other segments of the body contour. The reconstructive component is related to the need for reinforcement of the musculoaponeurotic wall during abdominoplasty, which, in some cases, is a mandatory procedure to treat extensive alterations caused by repeated pregnancies, unesthetic and retracted scars secondary to previous surgeries, or many other etiologies.

History

Since the nineteenth century, esthetic treatment of the abdominal wall has been performed by abdominal lipectomy, first described by Kelly [1] in 1899 through an elliptical horizontal skin resection including adipose tissue and the umbilical area. This procedure was the beginning of a long and rich history of surgery performed by many other surgeons using a horizontal incision [2–8], vertical incision [9–11], circular incision [12–14], submammary incision [15–17], and, recently, a half-moon skin resection bilaterally on the submammary fold introduced by the author [18–22].

Work for this article was supported by the Brazilian Scientific Institute of Aesthetic and Reconstructive Plastic Surgery.
Alameda Gabriel, Monteiro da Silva, 620, São Paulo 01442-000, Brazil
E-mail address: juarezavelar@bol.com.br

doi:10.1016/j.cps.2005.08.007
plasticsurgery.theclinics.com

In 1980, liposuction was a remarkable improvement that was presented and popularized by Illouz [23–25]. It was the first surgical method for esthetic treatment of the abdominal wall that did not perform full-thickness panniculus resection. Nevertheless, the use of lipoplasty enabled removal of only localized adiposity, because the skin excess and plication of the muscle-aponeurotic disturbances required traditional techniques. Several complications occurred during and after operation [26,27], such as hematoma, seroma formation, skin necrosis, wound ischemia, and severe infection of the neighboring areas, as described by D'Assumpção [28] among others [29–31]. In an extensive survey of 10,940 abdominoplasties performed by 958 plastic surgeons from all over, Grazer and Goldwyn [32] found complications that included thromboembolism (1.9%), infection and skin necrosis (5.4%), and wound dehiscence (5.4%). Mélega [33] reported vascular coagulation disturbances and other systemic situations that might increase the risk of thromboembolism [34–36]. Concerning the combination of traditional abdominoplasty with lipoplasty, Shestak [37] reported that the most frequent complication was panniculus necrosis (5%). Such combined procedures were complex and controversial, with a high incidence of complications, and were not performed routinely by many surgeons. To avoid complications, Matarasso [38–40] proposed that the procedures should not be performed during the same operation. In an important analysis, Stocchero [41] found a 2.6% rate of necrosis and a 15.1% rate of seroma formation that required aspiration by syringe.

New technique with minimal trauma on subcutaneous panniculus

In the author's practice, a similar incidence of complications occurred. These complications discouraged the author from recommending and performing the operation and led to a radical decision of not performing traditional abdominoplasty or abdominoplasties in association with lipoplasty. Nevertheless, we continued to study the anatomy of the panniculus based on previously published work [42,43]. In addition to performing anatomic dissections on cadavers and analyzing all aspects of the problems experienced by our patients, we were looking for adequate concepts that could lessen the risk of intraoperative and postoperative complications. After a long period of research, we concluded that trauma on the tissue during traditional abdominoplasty inflicted on the vascular network of the abdominal panniculus was the essential origin of the complications. Our anatomic research [42,43] and the behavior of the panniculus after lipoplasty [44] provided fundamental information from which we developed a new technique of abdominoplasty that combined excess skin excision with lipoplasty without panniculus undermining and resection.

Our first presentations were in November 1999 at the International Symposium of Aesthetic Plastic Surgery in Mexico [19] and the Brazilian Congress of Plastic Surgery in Rio de Janeiro [20], where we described new concepts for abdominoplasty. In our original publication [18,45], we demonstrated that the perforating vessels of the abdominal panniculus were not cut; consequently, the arterial, venous, and lymphatic circulation was preserved, maintaining normal vascularization to the abdominal panniculus and avoiding major complications during and after surgery. Afterward we accepted several invitations to present our technique [46–48] in Brazil and other countries, and we organized two courses during which surgical demonstrations were performed for the participants. After our presentation in Canada [49], Matarasso's publication [40] described these new concepts for abdominoplasty and emphasized the importance of the method. Latter, we published [50] an analysis and 3-year follow-up of 97 consecutive cases in which a more esthetic result with fewer complications and less patient discomfort was achieved. Currently, several surgeons employ this technique with good results [51,52].

Selection of patients and indication for surgery

Several abnormalities on the abdominal wall, such as unesthetic and retracted scars, cutaneous striae, excess tissue, adipose skin flaccidity, and weakness and diastasis of the muscle-aponeurosis caused by distension or enlargement of the abdominal volume and weight, such as in obesity, repeated pregnancies, excessive weight loss, hernias, and eventrations, require adequate esthetic and reconstructive treatment [4,53]. During abdominoplasty, all disorders of the abdomen must be treated to reinstate the harmony of the body contour [**Fig. 1**].

Adequate physical examination during consultation is an important step before planning the operation. Measurement of three levels of the circumference of the abdomen with the patient in a standing position is performed. Even more important is measurement of the vertical distance from the xyphoid bone to the umbilicus (XU) and from the umbilicus to the pubis (UP). Usually, when a patient presents with the XU more than 20 cm or the UP less than 12 cm, he or she is a good candidate for full abdominoplasty [**Figs. 2 and 3**]. Of course, all mea-

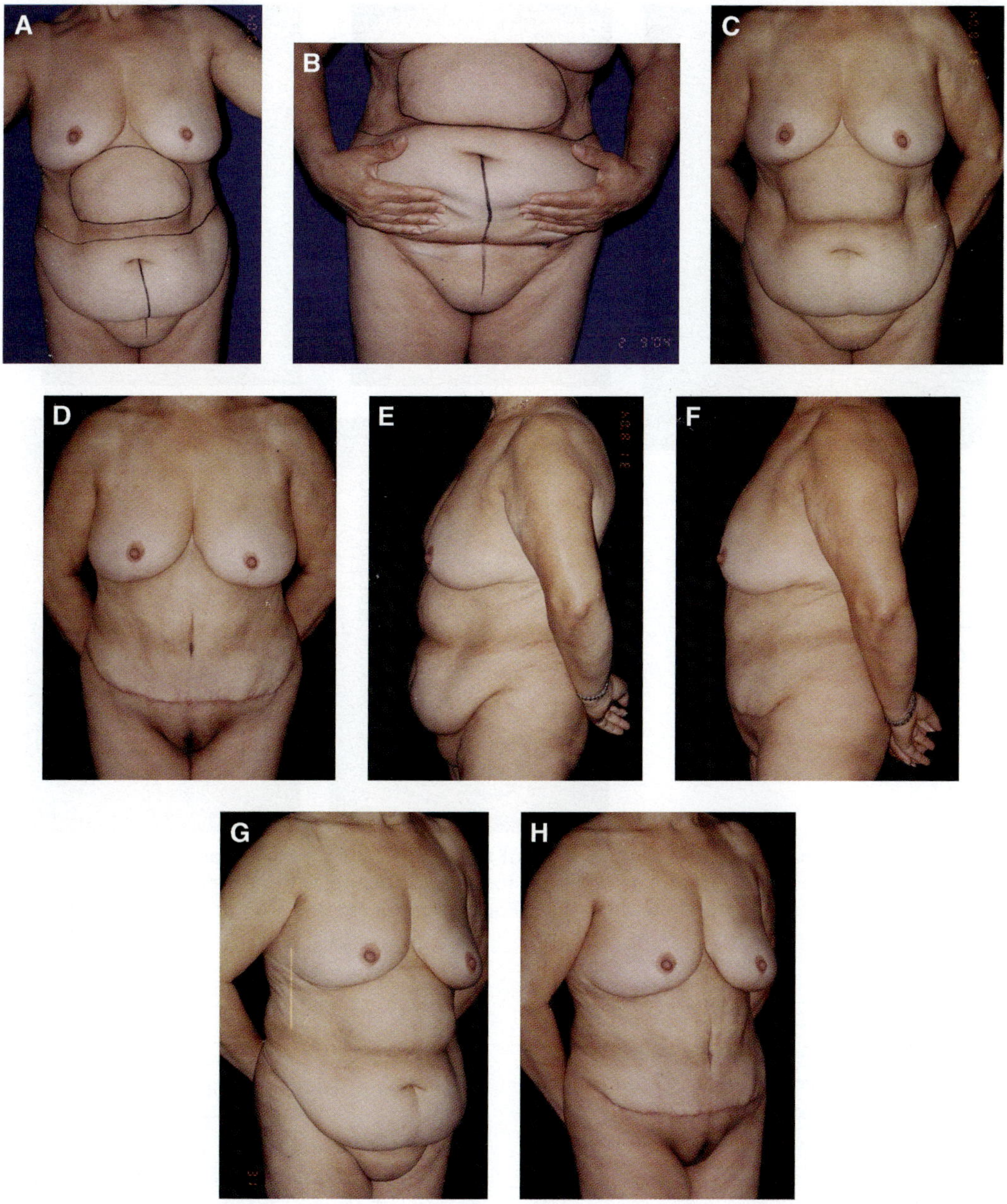

Fig. 1. A 62-year-old woman presented with an unesthetic body contour with localized adiposity on the upper and lower abdomen. (*A*) Demarcation of the operation. The lower abdomen is hanging, and the area of skin resection is drawn. (*B*) The abdomen is pulled upward to show the demarcation. (*C,E,G*) Preoperative photographs. (*D,F,H*) Photographs 5 months after abdominolipoplasty.

surements have a relative value, because they may change according to several circumstances [48]. In fact, the sense of beauty and the surgeon's esthetic judgment in evaluating the level of the umbilicus are very important. One must evaluate whether all skin below the umbilicus may be resected and whether the cutaneous covering of the upper abdomen may be pulled downward to cover the anterior abdomen wall after a full abdominoplasty.

When diastasis of the rectus abdominalis is identified, we routinely ask patients to undergo tomography of the abdominal wall to evaluate and measure the distance of the muscles and the level of the diastasis above and below the umbilicus.

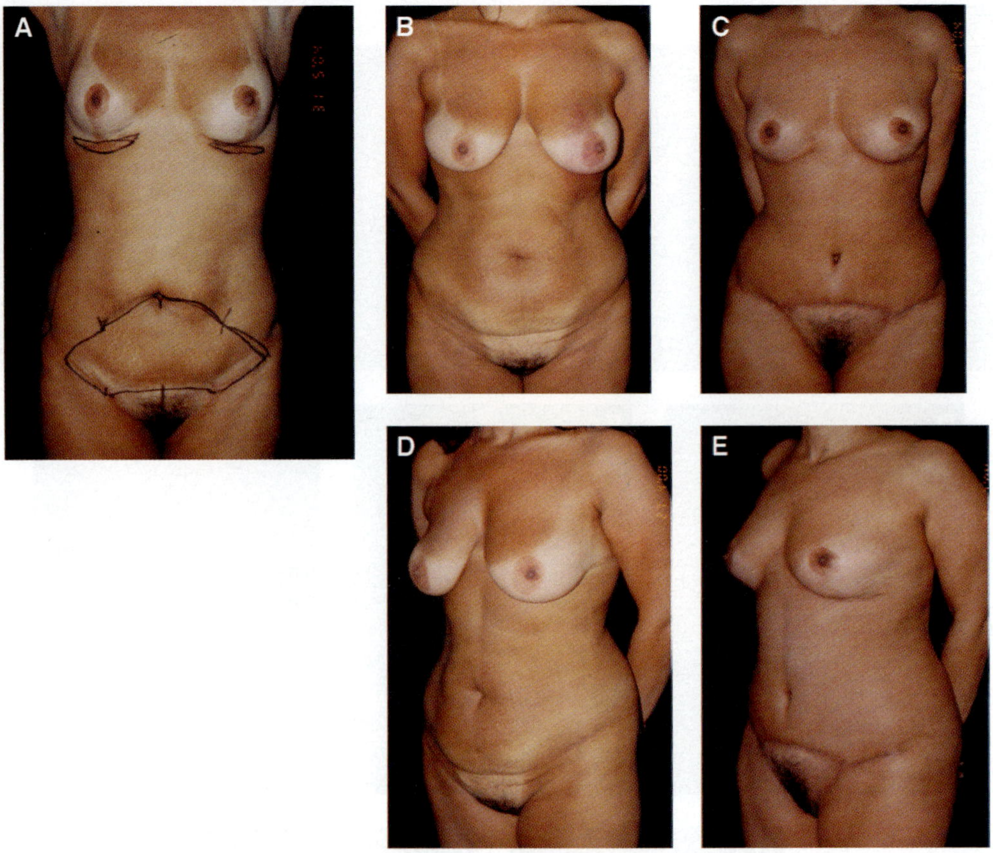

Fig. 2. A 43-year-old woman presented with flaccidity of the abdomen and localized adiposity with irregularities owing to previous lipoplasty. (*A*) Surgical demarcation for abdominolipoplasty and scar revision on the submammary folds. (*B,D*) Photographs before operation. (*C,E*) Photographs 5 months after abdominolipoplasty.

Tomography is not a method of diagnosis but a useful examination to certify what is found during the clinical examination. It has been very useful in the author's practice and is well accepted by patients [Fig. 3].

Surgical demarcations

Surgical demarcations are made 1 day before the operation with the patient in a standing position in front of a mirror to follow the surgeon's work. The cutaneous incisions are similar to those described by Callia [2]. Two areas must be well demarcated for adequate orientation during operation: (1) the areas for skin resection corresponding to the whole segment that is below the umbilicus on the suprapubic region, and (2) the area for liposuction on the abdominal wall and the lateral and posterior aspects of the torso [**Figs. 1A,B, 2A, and 4A**]. All deformities (localized adiposity and skin excess) must be drawn and shown to the patient 1 day before the operation.

The operation

When only abdominoplasty is performed, the author's preference is for epidural anesthesia combined with intravenous sedation under the care of an anesthesiologist. Afterward, local infiltration is performed according to surgical planning. Deep infiltration is performed on the supramuscular level on all regions selected for liposuction, and superficial and deep infiltration on areas for skin resection. Sequential steps of the operation are as follows: (1) skin incisions, (2) lipoplasty, (3) full-thickness skin resection, (4) reinforcement of the musculoaponeurotic abdominal wall, (5) traction of the remaining abdominal panniculus flap, (6) transposition of the umbilicus, (7) closure of the surgical wound, and (8) bandaging.

Incisions

Cutaneous incisions are made following the previous demarcations without damage to the subder-

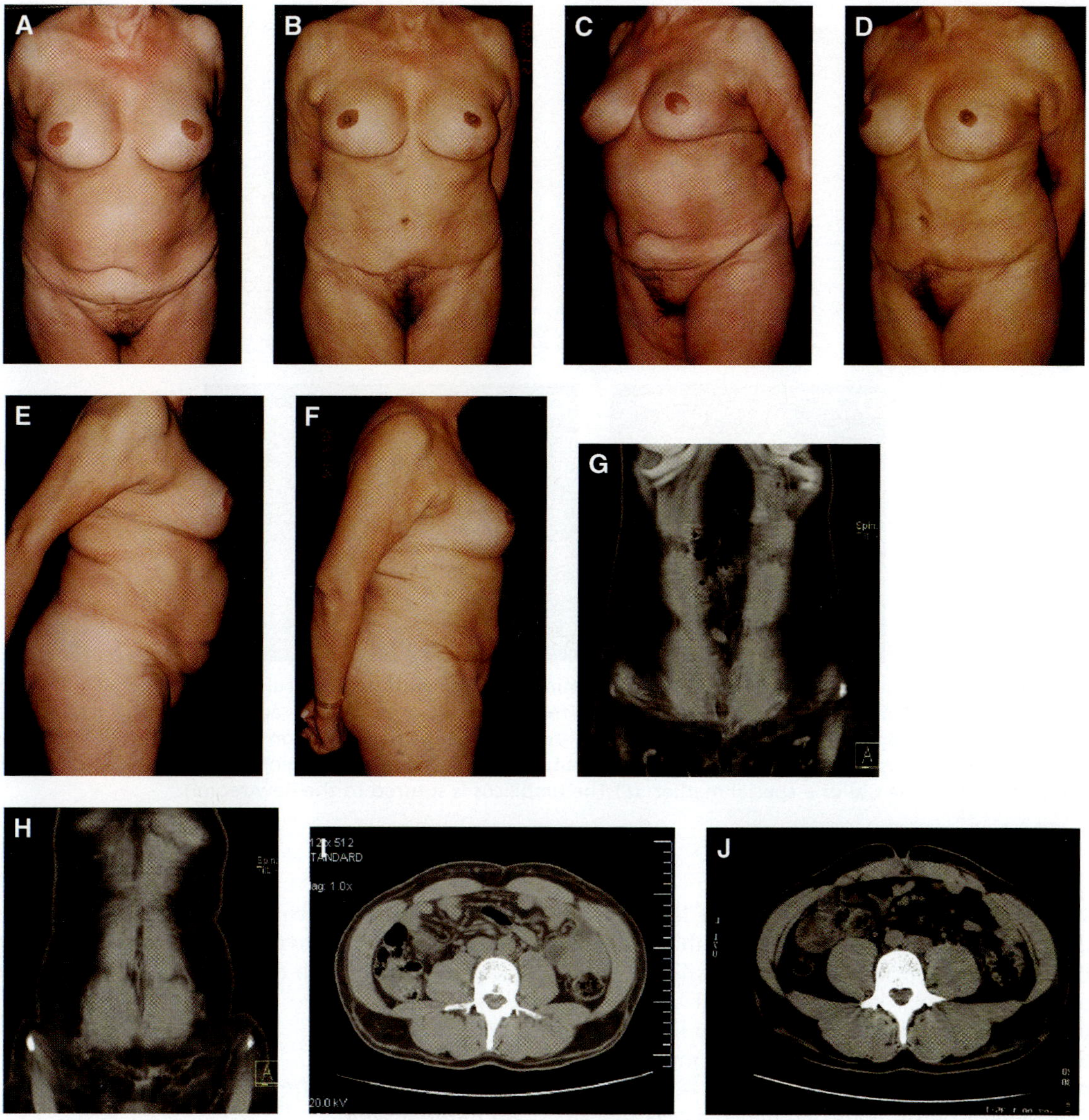

Fig. 3. A 72-year-old woman presented with an unesthetic abdomen with severe distension of the supraumbilical region and diastasis of the musculoaponeurotic wall. (*A,C,E*) Photographs before operation. (*B,D,F*) Photographs after abdominolipoplasty with plication of the musculoaponeurotic wall. (*G*) Tomography before surgery in front view. (*H*) Tomography after abdominolipoplasty with plication of the aponeurosis. (*I*) Transverse section before surgery. (*J*) Transverse section after surgery.

mal fat layer [Fig. 5A]. To create a natural and esthetic umbilical region during abdominoplasty, the author's personal technique is employed [54,55]. A star-shaped drawing is made inside the umbilicus, and cutaneous incisions are performed on the umbilical cavity [Figs. 4D,E and 5B,C].

Lipoplasty

Lipoplasty is performed using two different approaches on two areas—the infraumbilical area (lower abdomen) and the supraumbilical area (upper abdomen). In the infraumbilical area where skin resection will be done, liposuction is performed on the full thickness of the panniculus [Fig. 5D,E]. The superficial and deep adipose layers must be aspirated below the skin. All perforating vessels (arteries, veins, and nerves), connective tissue, and fascia superficialis are preserved. All fat tissue is removed by liposuction, and the skin lies on that structure above the muscular wall. In the supraumbilical area where the skin will not be resected, deep lipo-

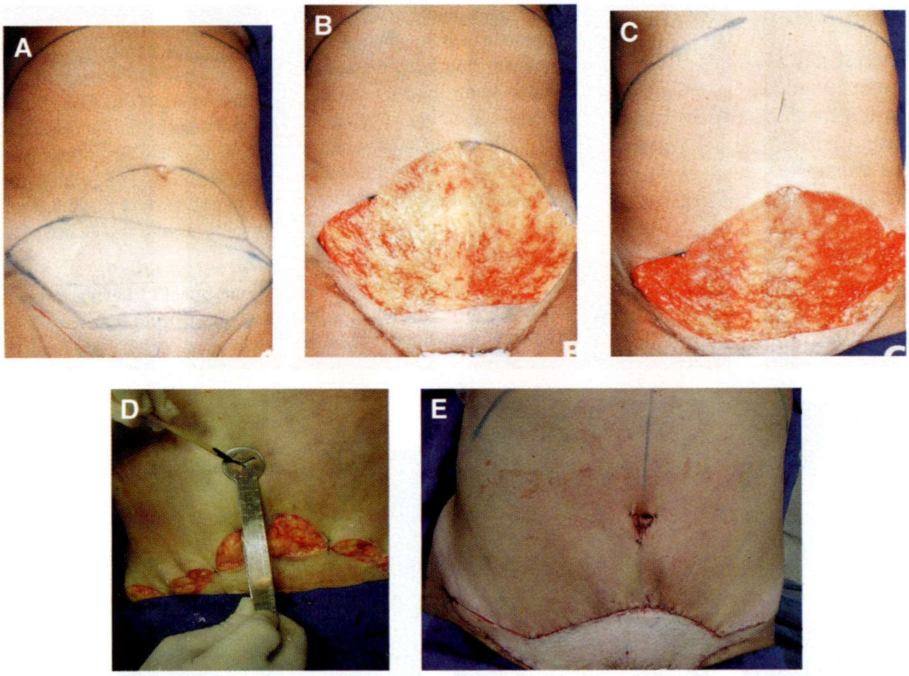

Fig. 4. Sequential perioperative photographs of abdominolipoplasty without panniculus undermining. (*A*) Surgical demarcation. (*B*) Skin resection was performed and the umbilicus incision made according to the star-shaped demarcation. (*C*) Lipoplasty was performed on the full-thickness of the panniculus on the raw area. (*D*) The upper abdominal panniculus flap is pulled downward and sutured to the suprapubic region. The new umbilical area is demarcated with the use of a special marker. (*E*) The umbilicus is sutured to the new region.

suction is performed on the lamellar layer below the fascia superficialis. At the end of this step, the thickness of the remaining panniculus will be formed only by the areolar layer. As described in our anatomic dissection of cadavers, after deep liposuction, the panniculus slides easily over the musculoaponeurotic wall [42,43]. This situation is similar to that found in dissections on child cadavers in that the panniculus does not have adiposity in the lamellar layer.

In previous publications [55,56], we have emphasized that the areolar layer must be preserved to achieve regular thickness of the remaining panniculus, giving a harmonious result and smooth balance to the body contour.

Full-thickness skin resection

Full-thickness skin resection is performed with a knife that goes just beneath the skin, following the previously made cutaneous incisions [see Fig. 4B, C]. All of the structures underneath that have been preserved during liposuction should not be damaged. Because the vascular network is empty, there is no bleeding during skin resection. Such skin resection is a new concept for abdominoplasty, because all previously described techniques perform panniculus undermining and resection according to Kelly's surgical principles, which damage the perforator vessels during surgery.

Reinforcement of the musculoaponeurotic abdominal wall

As described previously, plication of the muscles was not a routine procedure when the author and his colleagues performed traditional abdominoplasty [55,56]. It is a useful step when the patient presents with moderate or severe muscular flaccidity, diastasis of the rectus abdominalis, or herniation of the abdominal wall as mentioned by Pontes [53] and emphasized and popularized by Pitanguy [57]. Appiani [58] and Psillakis [59] introduced lateral plication of the oblique muscles. Nahas [60], when studying cadavers, performed advancement of the external oblique muscle to improve the waistline, and Jackson [61] emphasized plication according to classification of the abdomen by Bozola [62] and Nahas [63].

Although the abdominal panniculus is not undermined during full abdominolipoplasty, it is possible to perform plication of the abdominal aponeurotic

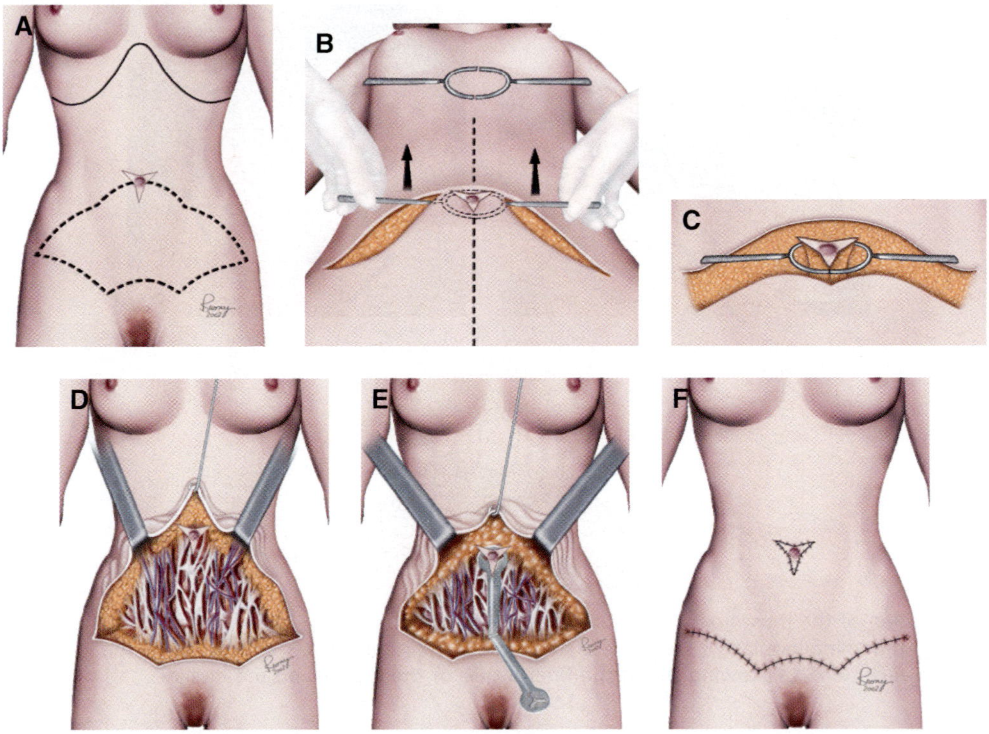

Fig. 5. Sequential drawings show the technique of abdominolipoplasty. (*A*) Demarcation. The dotted line denotes the area below the umbilicus to be resected. The line on the upper abdomen is the limit of the lipoplasty. (*B*) The new umbilical region is created with a special instrument introduced around the umbilicus and pulled upward to perform cutaneous incisions. (*C*) One can see the umbilicus already incised with the instrument around it. (*D*) Lipoplasty is performed all over the abdomen. The skin is already resected after full-thickness lipoplasty on the lower abdomen. On the raw area, the connective tissue and perforator vessels remain. (*E*) A special instrument with two segments is used to mark the new umbilical region on the abdominal flap. One segment is placed on the umbilicus and the other on the abdominal flap where the new area is marked. (*F*) The remaining abdominal flap is pulled downward and sutured. One can see the new umbilicus with a star-shaped surface, the final aspect of abdominolipoplasty.

structures to reinforce the muscular wall and to treat diastasis of the rectus abdominalis. This surgical step was not performed in our first publication [18] because there was no indication for it in our first 22 patients. We mentioned that it could be done by a videoendoscopy approach as described by Ferraro and coworkers [64], Correa [65], and others [66]. Afterward, we found a good indication for plication in some patients who underwent abdominolipoplasty. The plication may be performed on the anterior layer of the aponeurosis, on the midline [Figs. 6A–C and 7A], and on each side laterally to the umbilicus [Fig. 7B]. We do not perform plication on the posterior layer of the aponeurosis nor oblique muscular rotation, as described by some authorities [59,60].

We developed new surgical instruments to perform dissection on the midline without damaging the perforating vessels that are preserved during lipoplasty [Fig. 8A,B]. When using these instruments, it is not necessary to perform panniculus undermining, because the perforator vessels indicate the correct location of the aponeurosis of the rectus abdominalis [see Fig. 6]. In our anatomic dissections on cadavers, we found that the perforating vessels ran perpendicularly from the muscles to the panniculus [42,43]. In fact, after deep lipoplasty beneath the fascia superficialis, it is easy to identify that most of these vessels course from the rectus abdominalis on each side to the remaining panniculus [Fig. 6].

Isolated stitches or a running suture is performed from the inner border of a muscle to the other [Fig. 6A–C] according to the surgical plan based on the physical examination and clearly demonstrated on preoperative tomography [see Fig. 3].

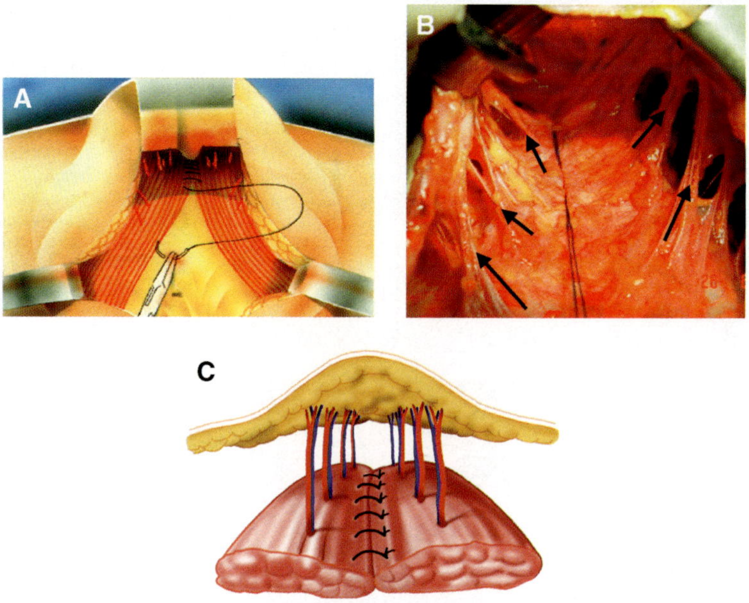

Fig. 6. (*A*) Plication of the musculoaponeurotic wall on the midline without panniculus undermining. (*B*) Photograph during abdominolipoplasty. The arrows show the perforator vessels coming from the muscles to the panniculus on each side. (*C*) Drawing shows the final suture of the muscles on the midline.

The plication is performed all the way from above until the umbilicus and even below it if necessary [Fig. 8C]. Although shortening of the umbilical pedicle is not a routine procedure, it may be performed if it is too long, as occurs in a thick panniculus [54,67].

Traction of the remaining abdominal panniculus flap

The next step of the operation is to pull downward the remaining abdominal flap. The perforating vessels follow the traction of the flap, and their length increases up to four times [Figs. 6B,C and 9A,B]. If necessary, the table is bent to place a temporary stitch on the midline from the upper abdominal flap to the pubic region. Using the author's surgical instrument, the new umbilical area is marked [Figs. 4D and 5E] [56].

Transposition of the umbilicus

The first transposition of the umbilicus during abdominoplasty was described by Vernon [68]. It is a mandatory procedure when full abdominoplasty is performed. After demarcation of the new umbilical area, we employ our personal approach [67,69] to create a natural umbilicus. A circle is drawn and three incisions are marked to create three small cutaneous flaps on the abdominal

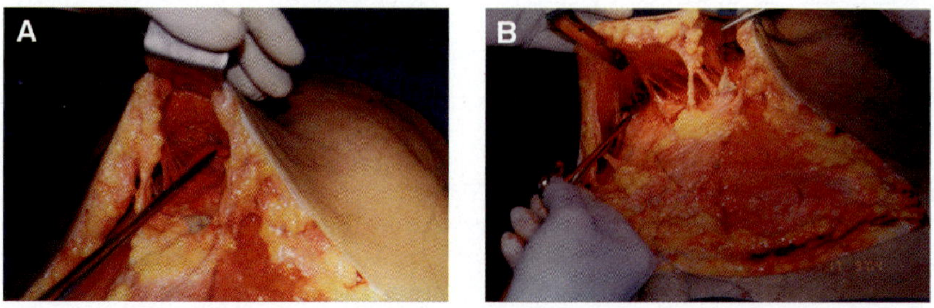

Fig. 7. Plication of the musculoaponeurotic wall during abdominolipoplasty without panniculis undermining. One can see the perforator vessels preserved after lipoplasty below the fascia superficialis. (*A*) Photograph shows medial plication above the umbilicus. (*B*) Lateral plication on right side of the abdomen.

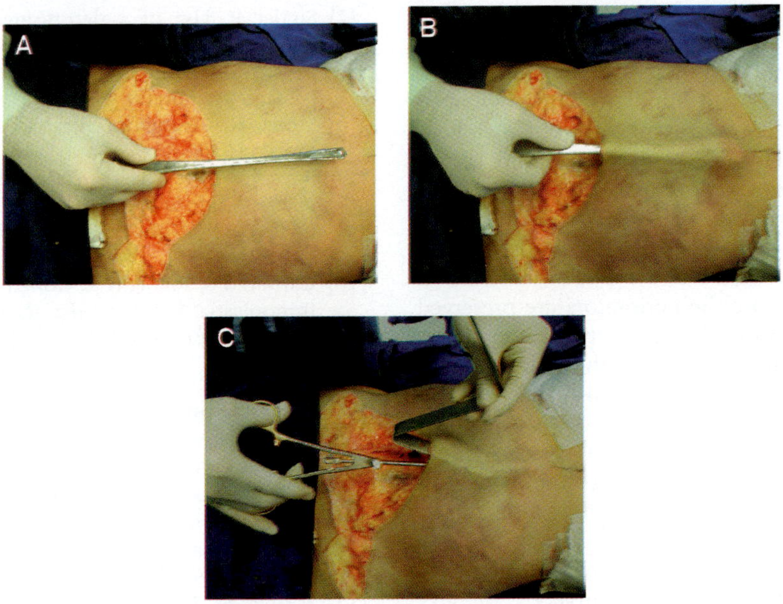

Fig. 8. Perioperative photographs show the abdomen after lipoplasty on the full-thickness of the raw area below the umbilicus. Deep lipoplasty was performed on the remaining panniculus to perform plication of the rectus abdominalis and the aponeurosis of the abdomen without panniculus undermining. (*A*) Special instrument used for tunnelization without cutting the perforator. (*B*) The instrument is introduced below the panniculus, creating a tunnel on the upper abdomen. (*C*) Plication of the musculoaponeurotic wall.

flap [Fig. 4D]. The umbilicus is then pulled and sutured to the panniculus [54].

Closure of the surgical wound

Suturing is performed using absorbent material with isolated stitches in three or four layers. In the raw areas where full-thickness skin resection is performed, the connective tissue is preserved and is folded over, including the fascia superficialis and all perforator vessels. The fascia superficialis must be sutured from the border of the upper panniculus flap to that of the lower border where liposuction is not performed [Figs. 4E and 5F] [70].

After suture of the subdermal layers, a running intradermal suture is placed using absorbable material. When this type of suture is used, there are no external stitches needing removal during postoperative care.

Bandaging

It is not necessary to use drainage after surgery because there is no bleeding during or after operation. No vessels are damaged during operation because the surgical principles of the technique are that of a closed vascular system.

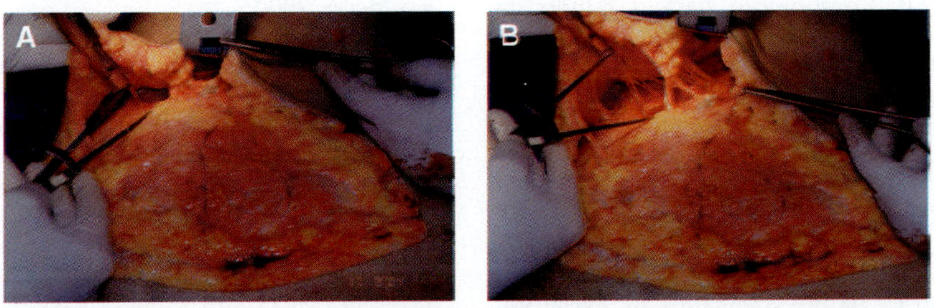

Fig. 9. Elongation of the perforator vessels after deep lipoplasty below the fascia superficialis. (*A*) The perforator with its natural length. (*B*) After traction of the flap, the length of the perforator vessel is four times longer than before.

Discussion

The method described herein is a combination of abdominoplasty and lipoplasty. Although such associated procedures are controversial owing to the risk of a high incidence of severe complications, our technique presents peculiar surgical principles that avoid damage to the neurovascular pedicle of the perforator vessels during operation. Consequently, the arteries, veins, lymphatic vessels, and nerves that compose the perforators are preserved because the abdominal panniculus is not undermined. Anatomic research on the subcutaneous panniculus performed by the author has demonstrated that, when adequate lipoplasty is performed on the lamellar layer, the perforator vessels work as multiple pedicles to the remaining abdominal panniculus. The arteries provide a regular blood supply and the venous blood and lymph drain naturally from the panniculus to the deep vessels, maintaining normal vascularization after surgery.

Most patients report that the postoperative recovery is comfortable. They do not complain about pain and can walk normally without banding the body, as usually occurs after traditional abdominoplasty. Patients also appreciate the fact that no drainage is used because there is no bleeding during or after operation.

We have had no severe complications such as skin necrosis, panniculus ischemia, wound dehiscence, hematoma, or thromboembolism. In our earlier series, two patients had small seroma formation (30 mL each), which was solved by a single aspiration with a syringe without discomfort.

Patients can walk and return home the day after surgery. For a period of 7 days, they wear a garment constantly around the body. After that period, they can remove the garment to shower but must continue wearing it at other times for 30 days.

References

[1] Kelly HA. Report of gynecological cases. John Hopkins Med J 1899;10:197.

[2] Callia WEP. Contribuição para o estudo da correção cirúrgica do abdome pêndulo e globoso-técnica original. Presented at the Tese de Doutorado Fac Med USP, São Paulo, 1965.

[3] Malbec EF. Lipectomia abdominal. La Prensa Méd Arg 1948;35:26.

[4] Pitanguy I. Abdominoplastias. O Hospital Rio de Janeiro 1967;71(6):1541–56.

[5] Regnault P. Abdominoplasty by the W technique. Plast Reconstr Surg 1975;55(3):265–74.

[6] Sersonneto D. Técnica geométrica. In: Avelar JM, editor. Anais do Simp Bras Abdomin. São Paulo: Soc Bras Cir Plast; 1982. p. 25.

[7] Sinder R. Use of a decorticated dermo-adipose flap in abdominoplasty [abstract]. Presented at the 6th International Congress of Plastic and Reconstructive Surgery, Paris, August 24–29, 1975.

[8] Sinder R. Cirurgia plástica do abdome. Niteroi, Brazil; 1979.

[9] Babcock WW. The correction of the obese and relaxed abdominal wall, with special reference to the use of buried silver chain. Am J Obstet 1916;74:596.

[10] Carreirão S, Pitanguy L, Correa WE, et al. Abdominoplastia vertical: uma técnica a ser relembrada. Ver Bras Cir 1983;73(3):184–94.

[11] Fischl RA. Vertical abdominoplasty. Plast Reconstr Surg 1973;51(2):139–43.

[12] Gonzalez-Ulloa M. Belt lipectomy. Br J Plast Surg 1967;13:179–86.

[13] Somalo M. Dermolipectomia circular del tronco. La Semana Méd 1940;1:1435.

[14] Vilain R, Dubourret J. Technique et indications de Ia lipectomie circulaire: 150 observo. Ann Chir 1984;18:289–300.

[15] Thorek M. Plastic reconstruction of the female breasts and abdomen. Ann J Surg 1939;43: 269–78.

[16] Rebello C, Franco T. Abdominoplastia por incisão submamária. Rev Bras Cir 1972;62(7–8): 249–52.

[17] Rebello C. Abdominoplastia por incisão submamária. In: Avelar JM, editor. Anais Simp Bras Abdomin. São Paulo: Soc Bras Cir Plast; 1982. p. 52.

[18] Avelar JM. A new technique for abdominoplasty: closed vascular system of subdermal flap folded over itself combined to liposuction. Rev Bras Cir 1999;88/89(1/6):3–20.

[19] Avelar JM. Abdominoplasty: new concepts for a new technique. Presented at the XXVI Annual International Symposium of Aesthetic Plastic Surgery, Puerto Vallarta, Jalisco, México, November 10 to 13, 1999.

[20] Avelar JM. New concepts for abdominoplasty—a new technique. Presented at the 36th Brazilian Congress of Plastic Surgery, Rio de Janeiro, November 12 to 16, 1999.

[21] Avelar JM. I Course of abdominoplasty. Presented at Municipal Hospital, São Paulo, March 10, 2000.

[22] Avelar JM. II Course of abdominoplasty. Presented at Hospital do Coração, São Paulo, October 6, 2000.

[23] Illouz Y-G. Une nouvelle technique pour les lipodystrophies localisées. Rev Chir Esth Franc 1980; 6:9–14.

[24] Illouz Y-G. My technique of selective suction lipectomy. Presented at the Annual Meeting of the American Society of Plastic and Reconstructive Surgeons, Honolulu, Hawaii, October 1982.

[25] Illoux Y-G. A new safe and aesthetic approach to suction abdominoplasty. Aesthetic Plast Surg 1992;16:237–45.

[26] Baroudi R. Cuidados pós-operatórios, locais e sistêmicos, para lipoaspiração. In: Avelar JM, Illouz

YG, editors. Lipoaspiração. São Paulo: Hipócrates; 1986. p. 105–9.
[27] Baroudi R, Ferreira CAE. Seroma: how to avoid it and how to treat it. Aesthetic Surg J 1998;18: 439–41.
[28] D'Assumpcao EA. Três complicações comuns em abdominoplastias: infecção, discência e seroma. In: Avelar JM, editor. Anais do Simp Bras de Abdomin. Sao Paulo: Soc Bras Cir Plast; 1982. p. 77.
[29] Dellerud E. Abdominoplasty combined with suction lipoplasty: a study of complication, revisions, and risk factors in 487 cases. Ann Plast Surg 1990;25(5):333–8.
[30] Flageul G, Elbaz JS, Karcenty B. Complications of plastic surgery of the abdomen. Ann Chir Plast Esthet 1999;44(4):497–505.
[31] Guerrerosantos J, Spaillat L, Morales E, et al. Some problems and solutions in abdominoplasty. Aesthetic Plast Surg 1980;4:227.
[32] Grazer EM, Goldwyn RM. Abdominoplasty assessed by survey, with emphasis on complications. Plast Recontr Surg 1977;59(4):513–7.
[33] Melega M. Tromboembolismo como Complicação da Abdominoplastia: Etiologia, Profilaxia e Tratamento. In: Avelar JM, editor. Anais do Simpósio Brasileiro de Abdominoplastias. São Paulo: Soc Bras Cir Plástica; 1982. p. 73–6.
[34] Hetter GP, et al. Abdominoplasty combined with other major surgical procedures: safe or sorry? Plast Reconstr Surg 1989;June:997.
[35] Mohammad JA, et al. Ultrasound in the diagnosis and management of fluid collection complications following abdominoplasty. Ann Plast Surg 1998;41(5):498–502.
[36] Pontes R. Plástica abdominal: resultados insatisfatórios. In: Avelar JM, editor. Anais do Simp Bras Abdomin. São Paulo: Soc Bras Cir Plast; 1982. p. 47–51.
[37] Shestak KC. Marriage of abdominal and liposuction expands abdominoplasty concept. Plast Reconstr Surg 1999;103(3):l027.
[38] Matarasso A. Liposuction as an adjunct to a full abdominoplasty. Plast Reconstr Surg 1995; (April):829.
[39] Matarasso A. Awareness and avoidance of abdominoplasty complications. Aesthetic Surg 1997; 17:256, 258–61.
[40] Matarasso A. Liposuction as an adjunct to full abdominoplasty revisited. Plast Reconstr Surg 2000;106:1197–206.
[41] Stocchero IN. Systemic and local complications after traditional abdominoplasty. In: Avelar JM, editor. Abdominoplasty without panniculus undermining and resection. São Paulo: Hipócrates; 2002. p. 123–36.
[42] Avelar JM. Surgical anatomy and distribution of the subcutaneous fat tissue on human body. In: Avelar JM, Illouz YG, editors. Lipoaspiração. São Paulo: Hipócrates; 1986. p. 45–57.
[43] Avelar JM. Regional distribution and behavior of the subcutaneous tissue concerning selection and indication for liposuction: the best scientific work presented in Zurich, Suiss. Aesthetic Plast Surg 1989;13:155–65.
[44] Batuir A, Tournieux AT, Callia WEP, et al. Comportamento do tegumento dermo-adiposo pós lipoaspiração. Presented at the XXI Cong Bras Cir Plast, November 1984.
[45] Avelar JM. Abdominoplasty: a new technique without undermining and fat layer removal. Arq Catarinense de Med 2000;29:147–9.
[46] Avelar JM. A new technique for abdominoplasty subdermal flap folded over itself. Presented at the XV ISAPS Congress, Tokyo, Japan, April 2000.
[47] Avelar JM. Abdominoplasty without lipectomy. Minicourse presented at the ISAPS Aesthetic Plastic Surgery Congress, Valladolid, Spain, March, 2001.
[48] Avelar JM. The new abdominoplasty and derived technique. Presented at the ASAPS and ASERF Annual Meeting, The Aesthetic Meeting, New York, May 2001.
[49] Avelar JM. Abdominoplasty: a new technique without panniculus undermining and without panniculus resection. Presented at the 57th Instructional Course of ISAPS, Montreal, Quebec, Canada, September 2000.
[50] Avelar JM. Abdominoplasty without panniculus undermining and resection: analysis and 3-year follow-up of 97 consecutive cases. Aesthetic Surg J 2002;22:16–25.
[51] Saldanha OR. Lipoabdominoplasty. In: Avelar JM, editor. Abdominoplasty without panniculus undermining and resection. São Paulo: Hipócrates; 2002. p. 315–22.
[52] Toledo LS. Future perspectives of the skin resection technique without panniculus undermining and resection. In: Avelar JM, editor. Abdominoplasty without panniculus undermining and resection. São Paulo; Hiócrates; 2002. p. 261–78.
[53] Pontes R. Plástica abdominal: importância de sua associação à correção das hérnias incisionais. Rev Bras Cir 1966;52:85.
[54] Avelar JM. Abdominoplasty: technical refinements and analysis of 130 cases in 8 years' follow-up. Aesthetic Plast Surg 1983;7:205.
[55] Avelar JM. Fat-suction versus abdominoplasty. Aesthetic Plast Surg 1985;9:265–76.
[56] Avelar JM. Combined liposuction with traditional surgery in abdomen lipodystrophy. Presented at the XXIV Instructional Course of Aesthetic Plastic Surgery of ISAPS, Madrid, September 19, 1985.
[57] Pitanguy I. Abdominal lipectomy: an approach to it through an analysis of 300 consecutive cases. Plast Reconstr Surg 1967;40(4):384–91.
[58] Appiani E. Muscular plastic for aesthetic conformation of abdominal girdle. Ann Plast Surg 1984;l3:2.
[59] Psillakis J. Abdominoplasty: some ideas to improve results. Aesthetic Plast Surg 1978;2:205.
[60] Nahas FX. Advancement of the external oblique muscle flap to improve the waistline: a study in cadavers. Plast Reconstr Surg 2001;108(2):550–5.

[61] Jackson I. Abdominoplasty: the waistline stitch and other refinements. Plast Reconstr Surg 1978; 61(2):180.
[62] Bozola A, Psillakis J. Abdominoplasty: a new concept and classification for treatment. Plast Reconstr Surg 1988;December:883.
[63] Nahas FX. An aesthetic classification of the abdomen based on the myoaponeurotic layer. Plast Reconstr Surg 2001;108(6):1787–95.
[64] Ferraro FJ, Zavitsanos GP, Van Buskirk ER, et al. Improving the efficiency ease and efficacy of endoscopic abdominoplasty. Plast Reconstr Surg 1977;99:895–8.
[65] Correa MA. Videoendoscopy subcutaneous techniques for authentic and reconstructive surgery. Plast Reconstr Surg 1995;August:446.
[66] Zukowski ML. Endoscopic extracorporeal abdominoplasty: a review of 85 cases. Plast Reconstr Surg 1998;2(2):516.
[67] Avelar JM. Abdominoplasty: systematization of a technique without external umbilical scar. Aesthetic Plast Surg 1978;2:141–51.
[68] Vernon S. Umbilical transplantation upward and abdominal contouring in lipectomy. Am J Surg 1957;94:490–2.
[69] Avelar JM. Umbilicoplastia—uma técnica sem cicatriz externa. Anais do XIII Congr Bras Cir Plast, Porto Alegre, 1976. p.81–2.
[70] Lockwood T. High lateral-tension abdominoplasty with superficial fascial system suspension. Plast Reconstr Surg 1995;96:603–15.

ELSEVIER
SAUNDERS

CLINICS IN PLASTIC SURGERY

Clin Plastic Surg 33 (2006) 91–105

Power-Assisted Liposuction

Ângelo Rebelo, MD

Fischer [1] and Illouz [2] were the first "maîtres" and the pioneers of fat removal from the human body through small incisions using suction machines and large cannulas, known as liposuction. Fournier [3,4], using a syringe, changed and completely revolutionized liposuction with the added advantage of decreasing the cost and with no special maintenance or assistance needed. He taught us that fat could not only be aspirated but could also be used to reshape the body, creating the concept of liposculpture—a method to manage and transfer fat using small cannulas or needles.

Ultrasound-assisted liposculpture was introduced and presented by Zochi [5]. It became the ideal solution for liposuction in difficult or fibrous regions and for correcting classic liposuction. Klein [6–11] was also decisive in liposculpture, introducing the concept of tumescence.

At the end of 1990s, power-assisted liposuction became available, a mechanical technique using compressed air. This new concept in liposculpture was invented by Malak, a Belgium medical doctor, and was developed with the help of the author, who named the technique - "vibroliposuction." Subsequently, several systems were introduced, driven by gas or electricity but working with a turbine.

Materials and methods

Since December of 1997, the author has performed more than 8000 liposuctions using the vibroliposuction technique [Fig. 1]. The vibroliposuction system includes the Lipomatic device [Fig. 2], a small machine that vibrates, cannulas, pressure and aspiration sources.

The Lipomatic device

The Lipomatic device works with compressed air, is easy to handle (weighing less than 600 g), easy to clean and wash, and can be sterilized in an autoclave or any other system. The passage of air induces movements of "go and come," with 10 Hz of frequency at 3 bars and a course of 6 mm. The cannulas vibrate and have a rotational and translational movement called nutation. The frequency of 10 Hz correspond to 600 times the movement of "go and come" in each minute. The goal is to break down the fat so that it is emulsified and aspirated [Figs. 3 and 4] at the same time.

The cannulas

Specific cannulas [Fig. 5] of different lengths, diameters (3 to 5 mm), and holes can be connected.

Clinica Milenio, Rua Manuel Silva Leal, 11C, Lisboa 1600-166, Portugal
E-mail address: clinicamilenio@netcabo.pt

doi:10.1016/j.cps.2005.08.008
plasticsurgery.theclinics.com

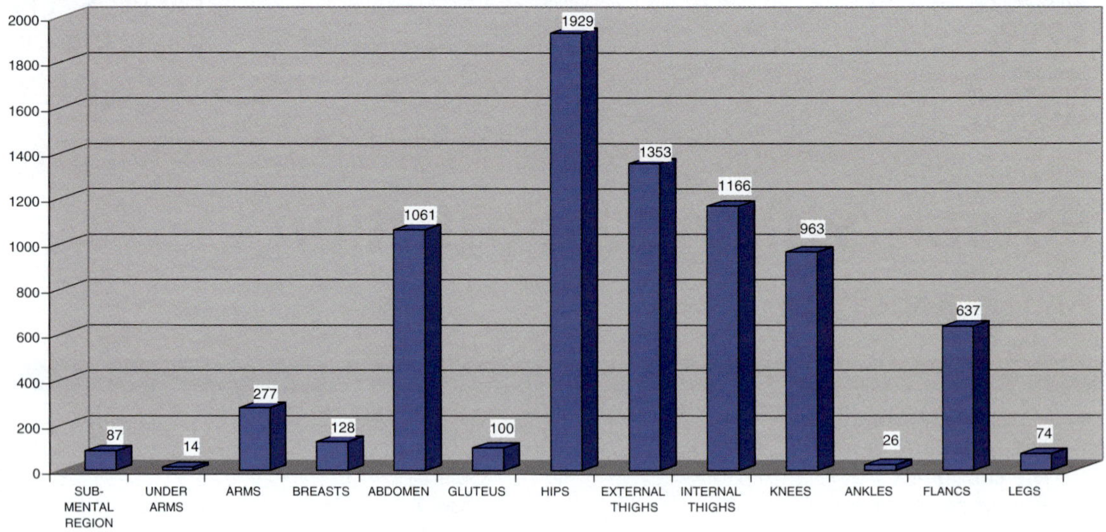

Fig. 1. Vibroliposuction (main areas treated).

The type of cannula used depends on factors such as the region of the body and the quantity of fat.

Two years ago, I introduced a new cannula, the Rebelo type, which permits the use of a smaller diameter, maintaining a good speed [Fig. 6].

The pressure source

Any pressure source can be used, such as a cylinder, an operating room air compressed system, or a compressor. This last source seems to be the best option for economical reasons and operating terms.

The vacuum source

Although commonly available aspirators can be used, I prefer the use of the Lipomatic system vacuum source [Fig. 7] because it is synchronized, and the on/off is the same as that of the Lipomatic device.

Technique

For tumescence, I use the Vibrolipo infiltrator [Fig. 7]. With a special cannula [Fig. 8], this system allows infiltration with the Lipomatic with the advantage of vibration. There is better and easier diffusion of the liquid, especially in difficult areas with fibrosis, and patients report that the infiltration is better tolerated.

The tumescent fluid used is based on Klein's formula. The following agents are added to each 1000 mL of 8.4% saline solution heated up to 37 °C:

- One ampule of adrenaline, 1mg/mL
- 800 mg of lidocaine 2% without adrenaline
- 4 mL of sodium bicarbonate

It is not usual to use more than 2 L per surgery. For good vasoconstriction, one should wait at least 30 minutes.

Discussion

The association of more than one anatomic region in a procedure depends on the total amount of

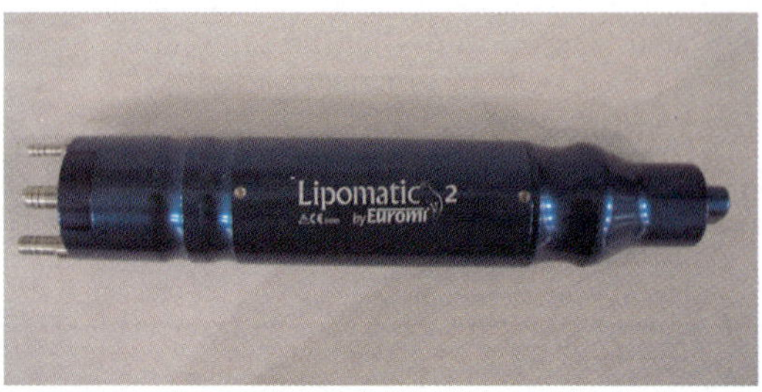

Fig. 2. The Lipomatic device.

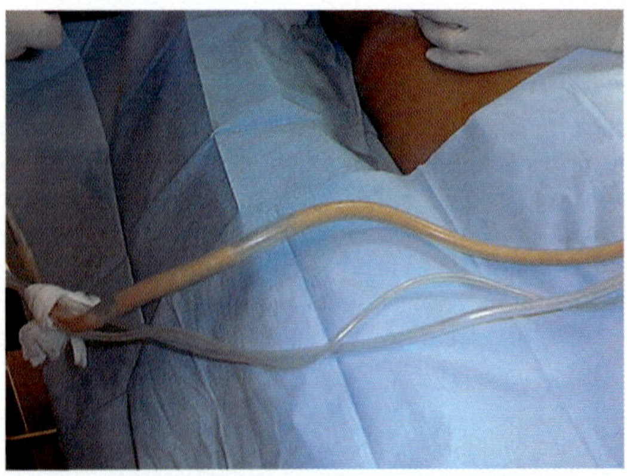

Fig. 3. Aspiration of fat.

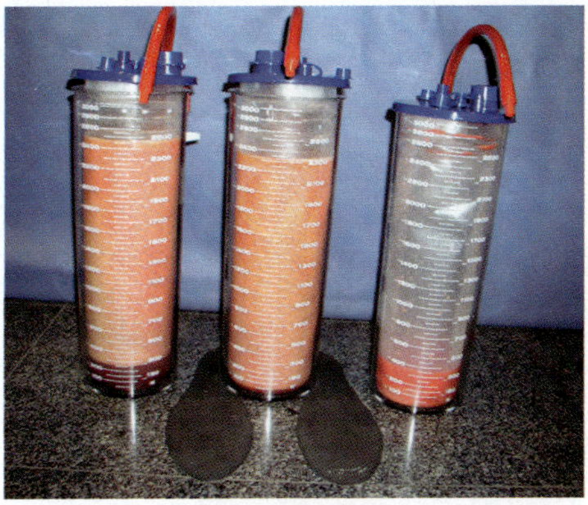

Fig. 4. Emulsified fat.

tumescence and lidocaine to be used. It is safer and more comfortable for the patient to perform the vibroliposuction in more than one session when indicated and necessary. Apart from the recovery being quicker, patients are less limited in their everyday life. Owing to the vibroliposuction technique, it is rare to spend more than 2 hours on a surgery, even in extensive suctions or those associating more than one anatomic region. The average time between administrating the anesthesia and completing the vibroliposuction ranges from 45 minutes to 2 hours.

In the postoperative period, patients undergo a program of manual lymphatic drainage during 1 month three times a week. Patients can take a daily shower and must wear a moderate compression garment [Fig. 9]. Medication after surgery consists of an oral antibiotic, an anti-inflammatory agent, and analgesics (rarely used). A massage with an anti-inflammatory cream is recommended twice a day until the bruising disappears or for a period of about 2 months. Sun block protection is recommended on the small scars and ecchymosis.

One must also emphasize the valuable contribution of prior liposuction in breast reductions with vertical scars, especially in severe hypertrophies or gigantomastias.

Summary

The best indicator for liposuction is localized fat and localized lipodystrophy regardless of size. Such localizations have a genetic cause. In women, the areas of fat are localized in the chin [Figs. 10–12], abdomen [Figs. 13,14], flanks [Figs. 15,16], hips [Fig. 17], thighs [Figs. 18–20], and knees [Figs. 21,22]. In men, the areas of fat are in the chin, hips, and breast [Figs. 23,24]. Other regions and severe lipodistrophies or obesities can be treated by vibroliposuction, but, in my opinion, the results are better in the aforementioned areas.

The surgeons expert in liposuction know very well that the physical effort they expend during the surgery is considerable and limits the number of patients that can be operated on in a working day. The surgery itself, being long and tiring, in the ultimate analysis can jeopardize the results. Many surgeons and physicians refuse to perform liposuction or liposculpture because of the sheer physical effort involved. Age and physical disability are influencing factors.

The vibroliposuction technique using the Lipomatic device solves all of these problems because the surgeon is not fatigued, even after four or five surgeries. This relief permits one to perform more daily surgeries.

The vibroliposuction technique is without doubt an important development. It is safe and efficient, has no counterindications, requires no special maintenance, and is easy to execute. The author and his colleagues have experienced good results, fewer problems and risks, and an easier execution with no technical problems. There is less swelling and bruising, with faster and better recovery for the patient.

Important advances have occurred in liposuction and liposculpture over the past few years in the syringe, the tumescence method, the diameter of cannulas, the level of depth, and the technology. Technology will undoubtedly have an important role in the future of this and other treatments. Nevertheless, some aspects of the procedure will remain fundamental regardless of the technique used, including the clinical history, preoperative examinations, a correct and recent diagnosis, the surgical proposal, and good planning.

The vibroliposuction technique has the following advantages for the patient:

- Less traumatic
- Less swelling
- Less ecchymoses
- Quicker recovery

Advantages for the surgeon are as follows:

- Less tiring
- More versatile
- Easy to execute
- Technically easy

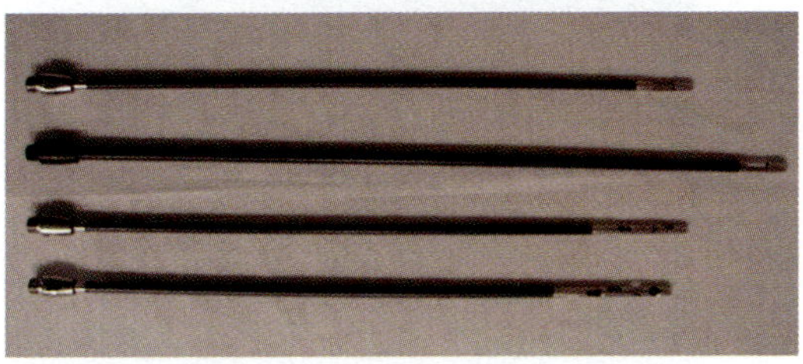

Fig. 5. Aspiration cannulas.

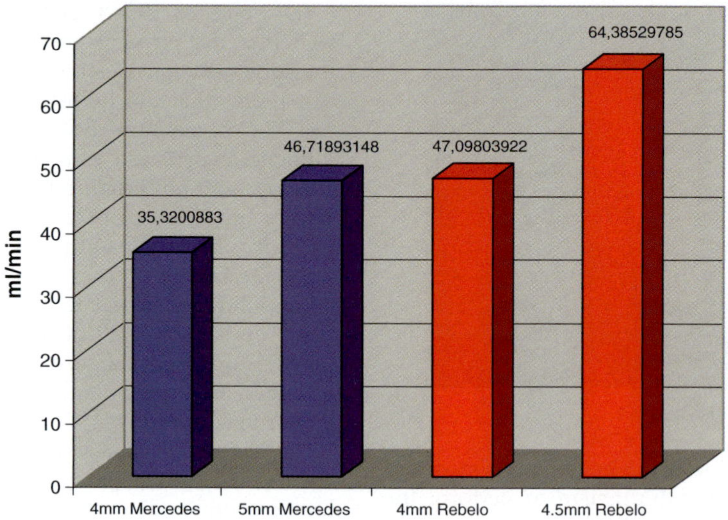

Fig. 6. Aspiration speed of different cannulas.

Good results combine happiness of the patient and surgeon with a realistic expectation by both. Technology cannot replace the surgeon but can help to resolve situations with better results and fewer complications.

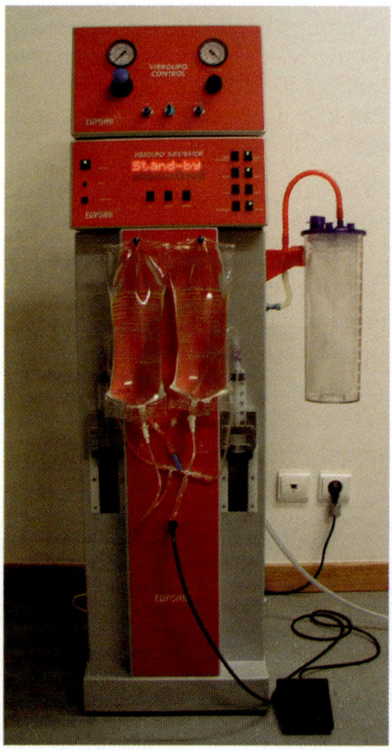

Fig. 7. Lipomatic system and Vibrolipo infiltrator.

Case reports

Case 1

A 67-year-old woman underwent vibroliposuction of the submental region. A total of 50 mL of emulsified fat was removed in one session [Fig. 25].

Case 2

A 42-year-old woman underwent vibroliposuction of the arms. A total of 100 mL of emulsified fat was removed in one session [Fig. 26].

Case 3

A 31-year-old man underwent vibroliposuction of the abdomen and hips. A total of 2600 mL of emulsified fat was removed in one session [Figs. 27–29].

Case 4

A 35-year-old woman underwent vibroliposuction of the abdomen, hips, and flanks. A total of 2700 mL of emulsified fat was removed in two sessions [Figs. 30–32].

Case 5

A 42-year-old woman underwent vibroliposuction of the abdomen, hips, and flanks. A total of

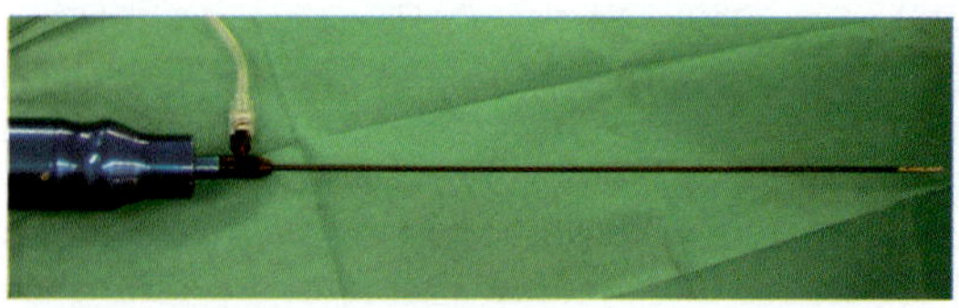

Fig. 8. Infiltration cannula.

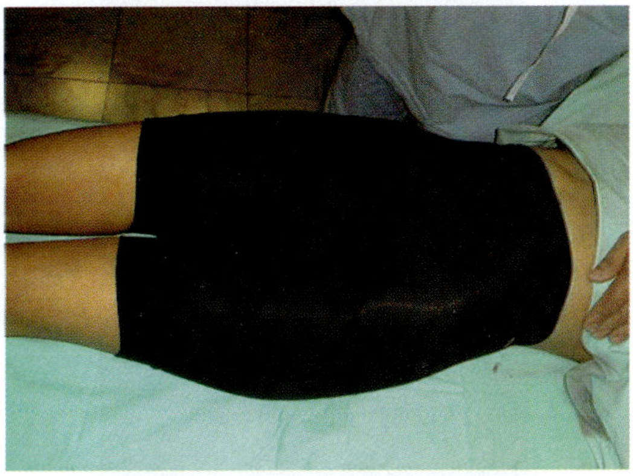

Fig. 9. Compression garment.

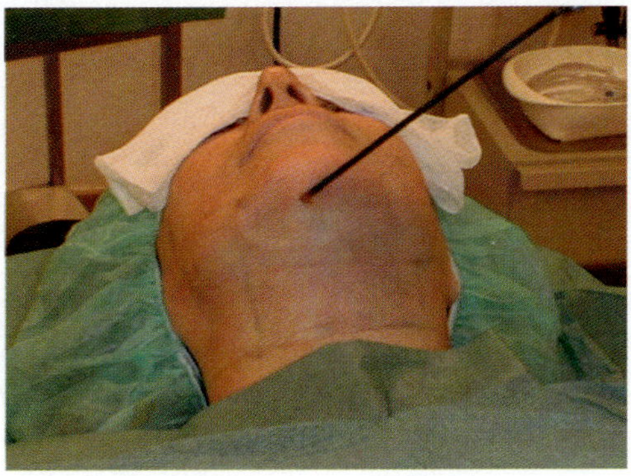

Fig. 10. Vibroliposuction of the chin.

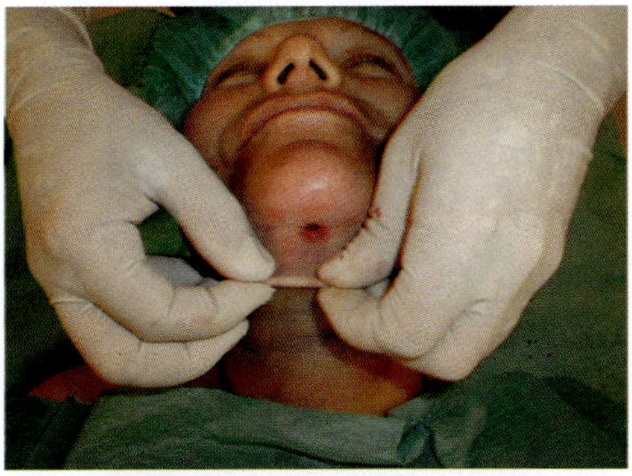

Fig. 11. Vibroliposuction of the chin.

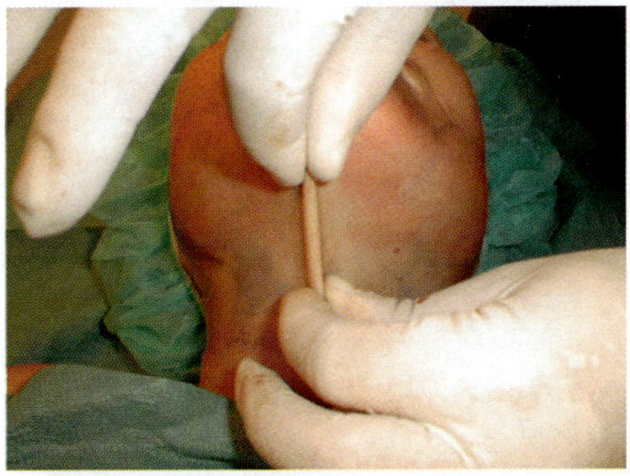

Fig. 12. Vibroliposuction of the chin.

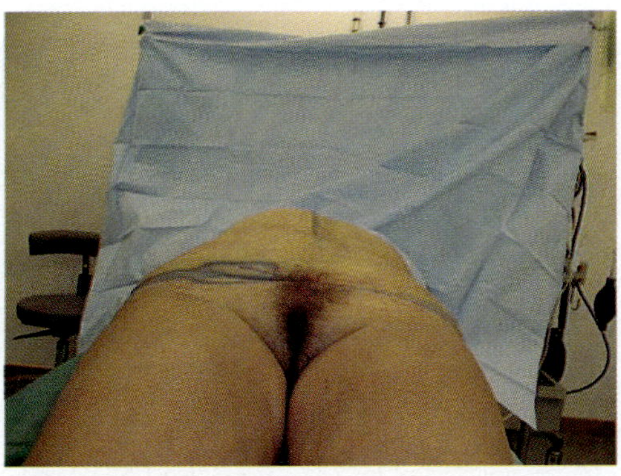

Fig. 13. Vibroliposuction of the abdomen.

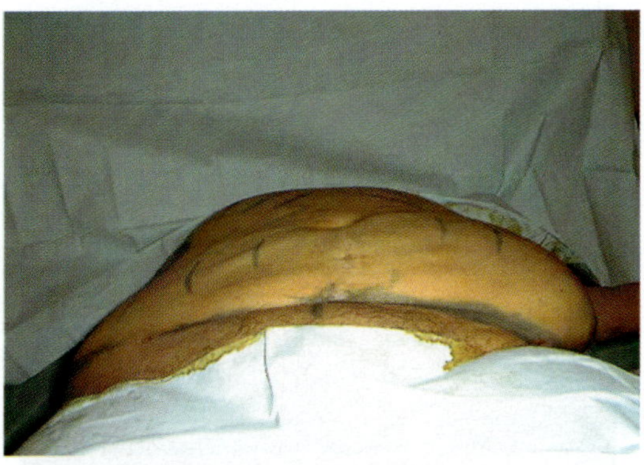

Fig. 14. Vibroliposuction of the abdomen.

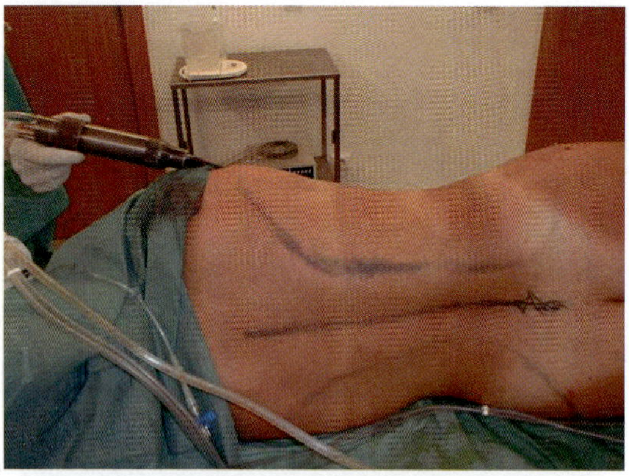

Fig. 15. Vibroliposuction of the flanks.

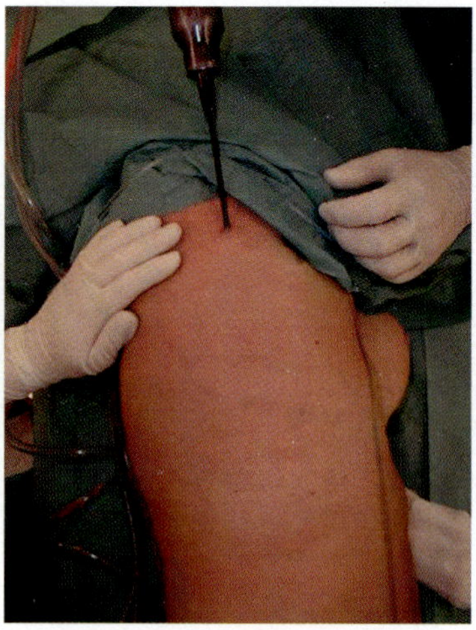

Fig. 16. Vibroliposuction of the flanks.

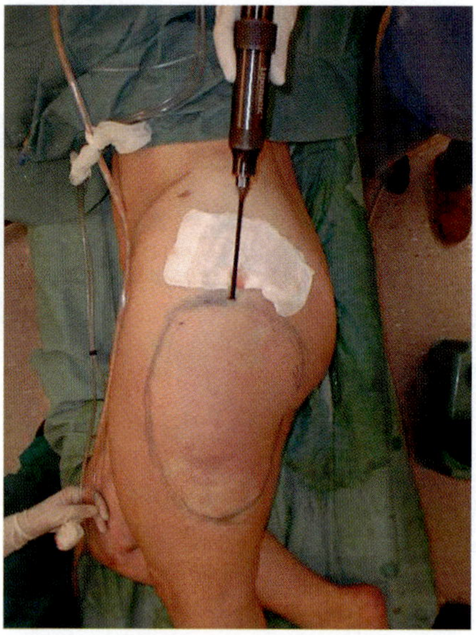

Fig. 17. Vibroliposuction of the hips.

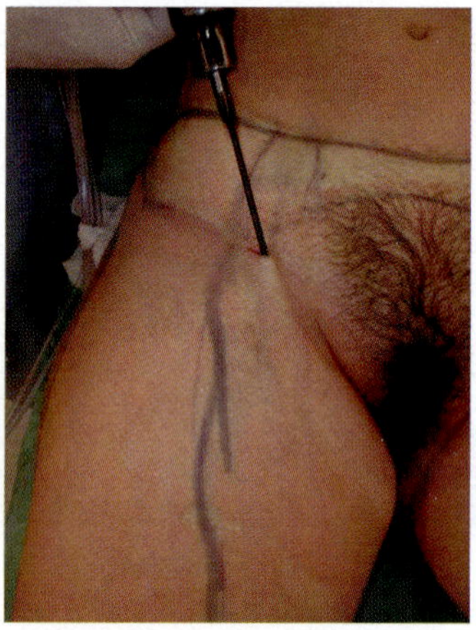

Fig. 18. Vibroliposuction of the thighs.

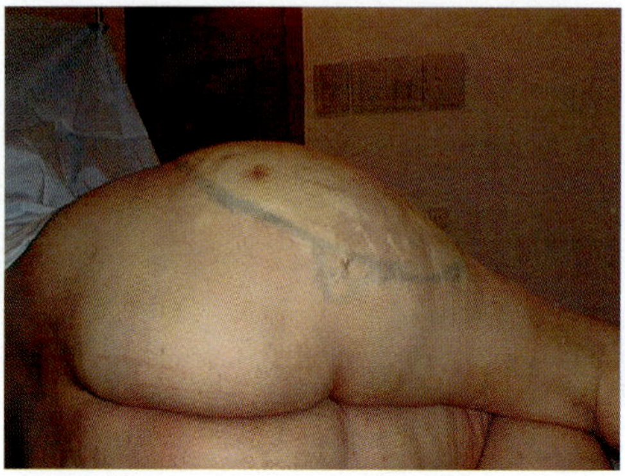

Fig. 19. Vibroliposuction of the thighs.

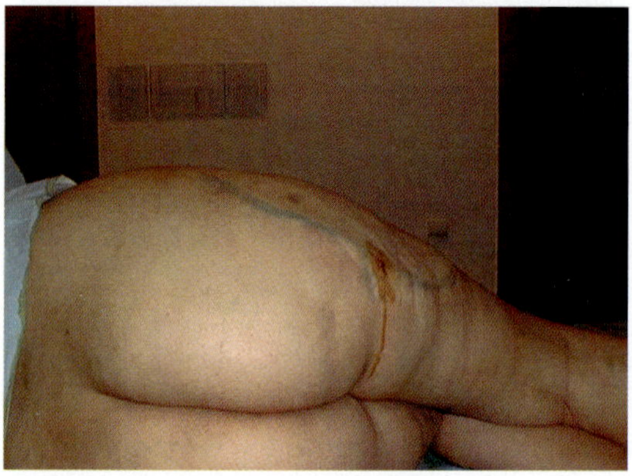

Fig. 20. Vibroliposuction of the thighs.

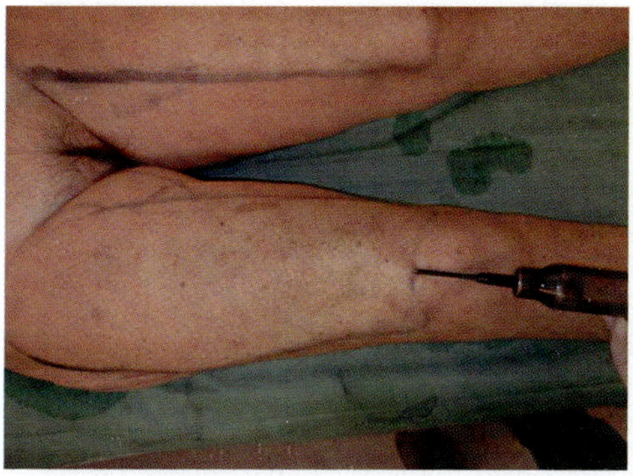

Fig. 21. Vibroliposuction of the knees.

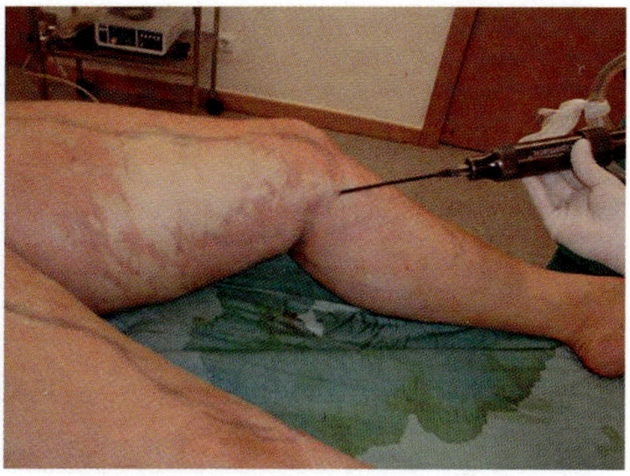

Fig. 22. Vibroliposuction of the knees.

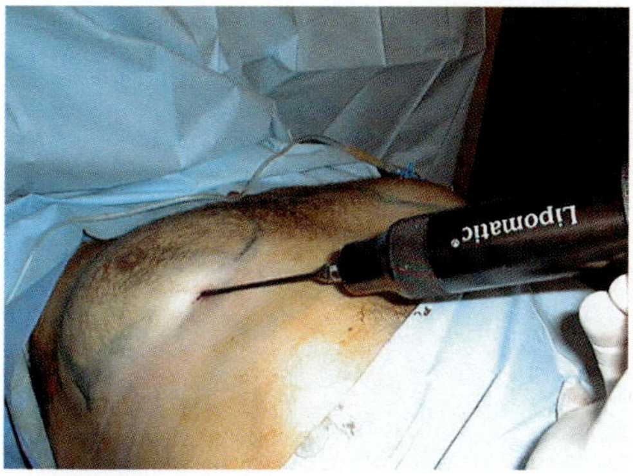

Fig. 23. Vibroliposuction of the breasts.

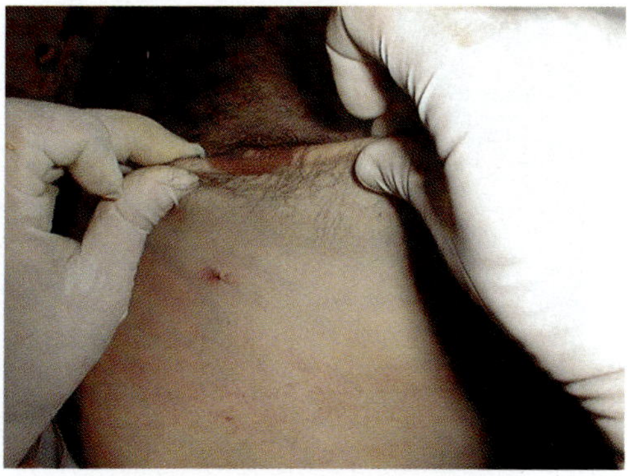

Fig. 24. Vibroliposuction of the breasts.

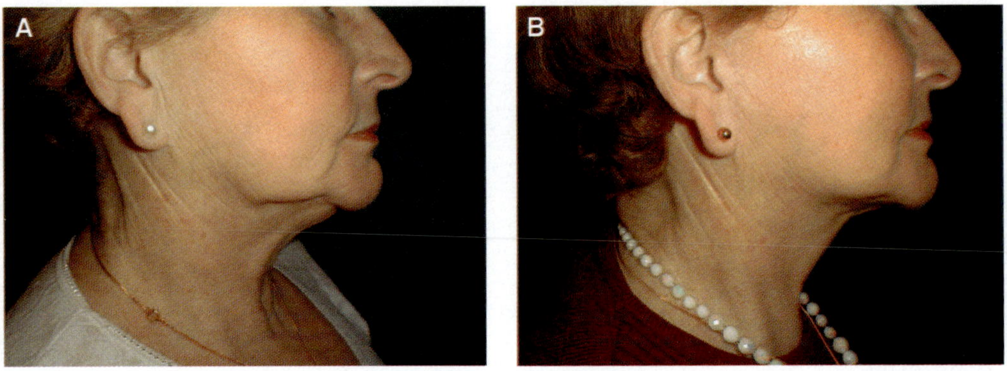

Fig. 25. (*A*) Preoperative appearance. (*B*) Postoperative appearance at 3 months.

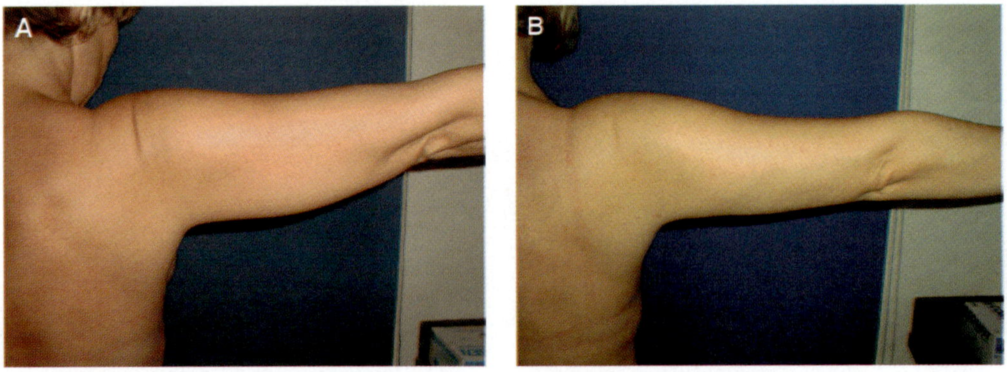

Fig. 26. (*A*) Preoperative appearance. (*B*) Postoperative appearance at 3 months.

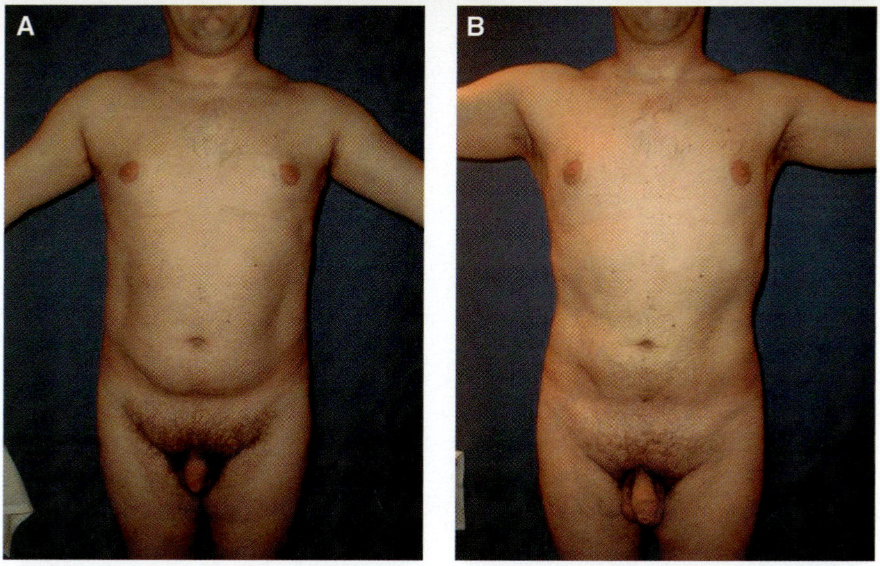

Fig. 27. (*A*) Preoperative appearance (frontal view). (*B*) Postoperative appearance at 3 months (frontal view).

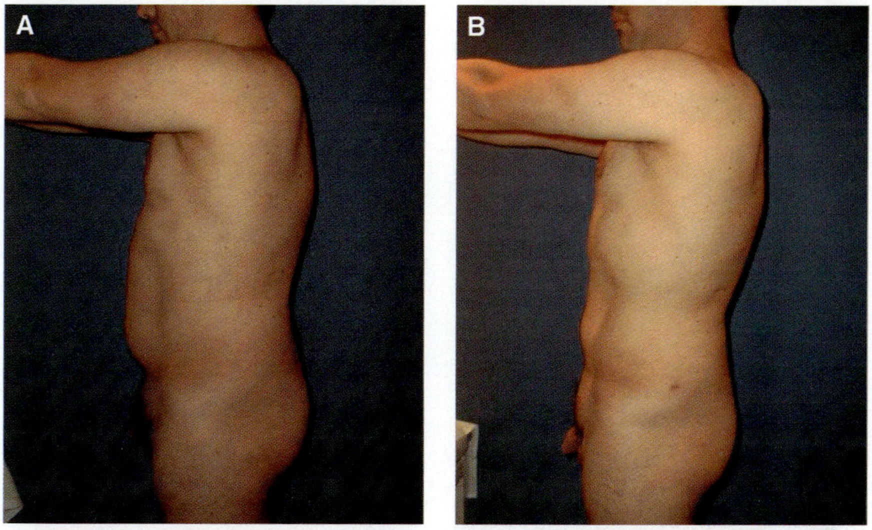

Fig. 28. (*A*) Preoperative appearance (lateral view). (*B*) Postoperative appearance at 3 months (lateral view).

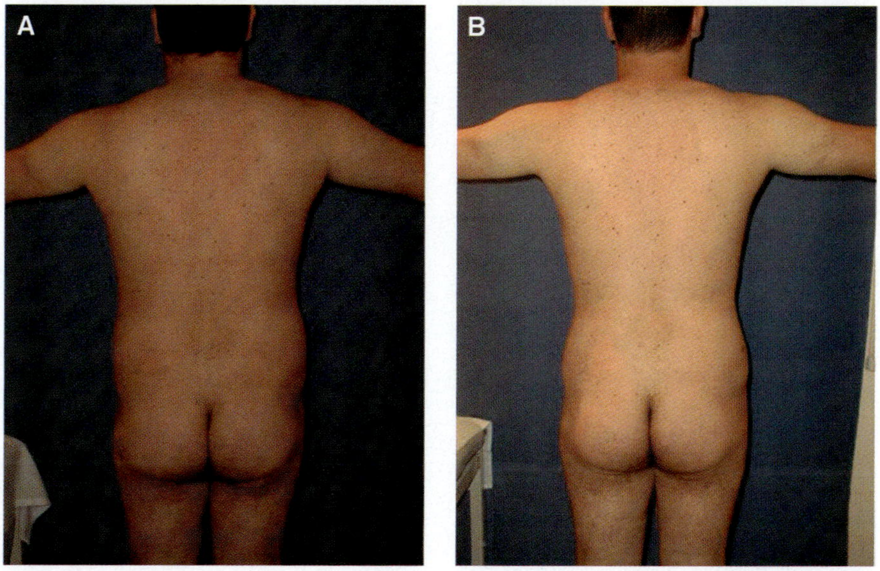

Fig. 29. (*A*) Preoperative appearance (back view). (*B*) Postoperative appearance at 3 months (back view).

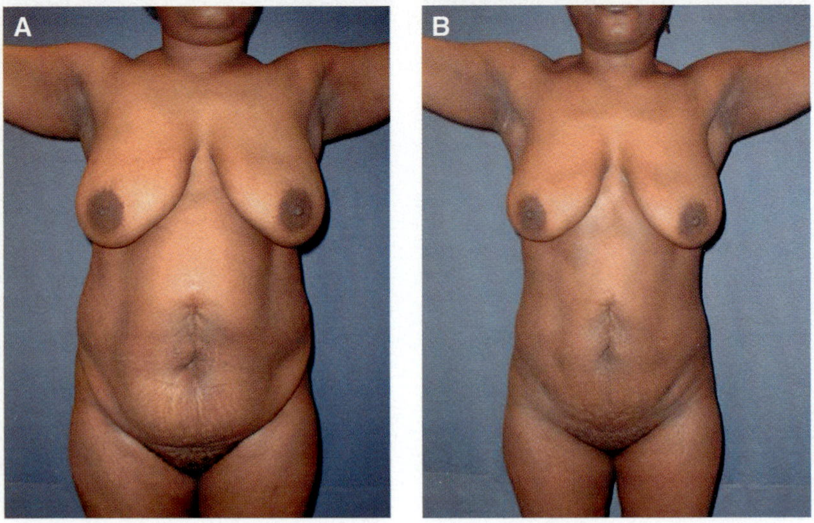

Fig. 30. (*A*) Preoperative appearance (frontal view). (*B*) Postoperative appearance at 24 months (frontal view).

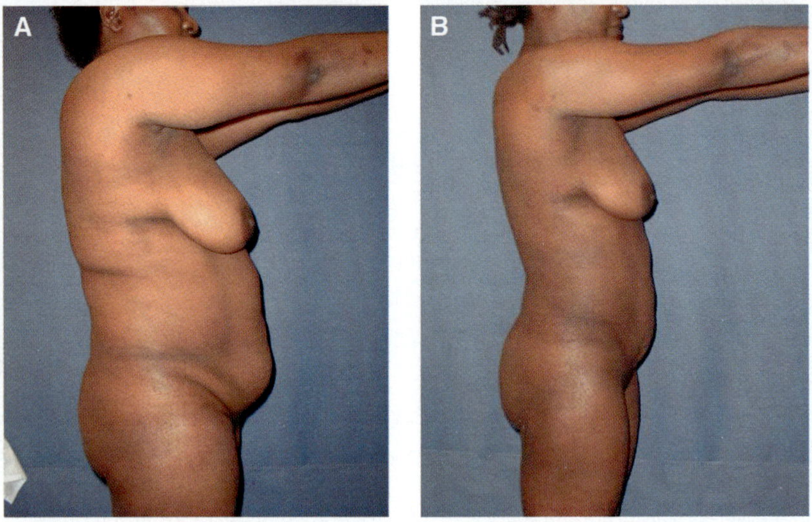

Fig. 31. (*A*) Preoperative appearance (lateral view). (*B*) Postoperative appearance at 24 months (lateral view).

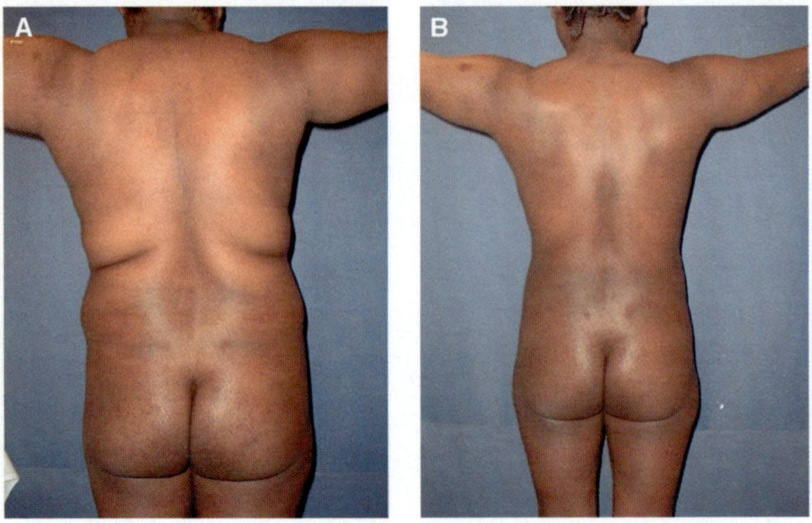

Fig. 32. (*A*) Preoperative appearance (back view). (*B*) Postoperative appearance at 24 months (back view).

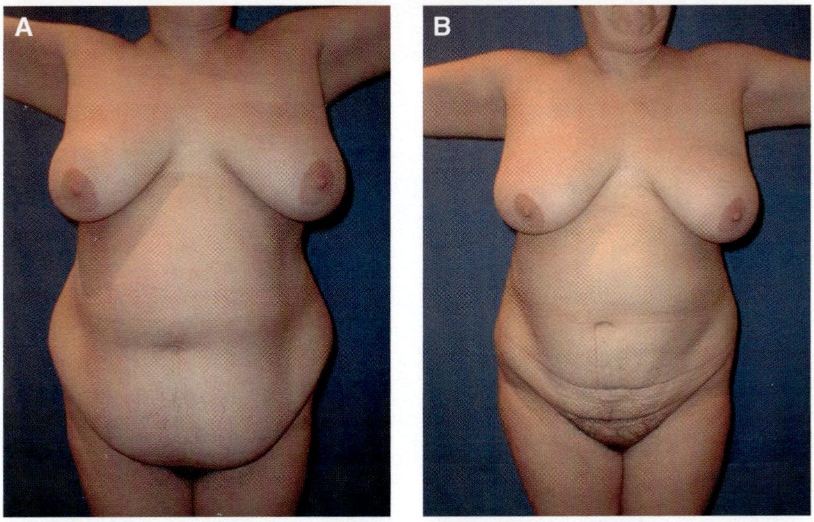

Fig. 33. (*A*) Preoperative appearance (frontal view). (*B*) Postoperative appearance at 7 months (frontal view).

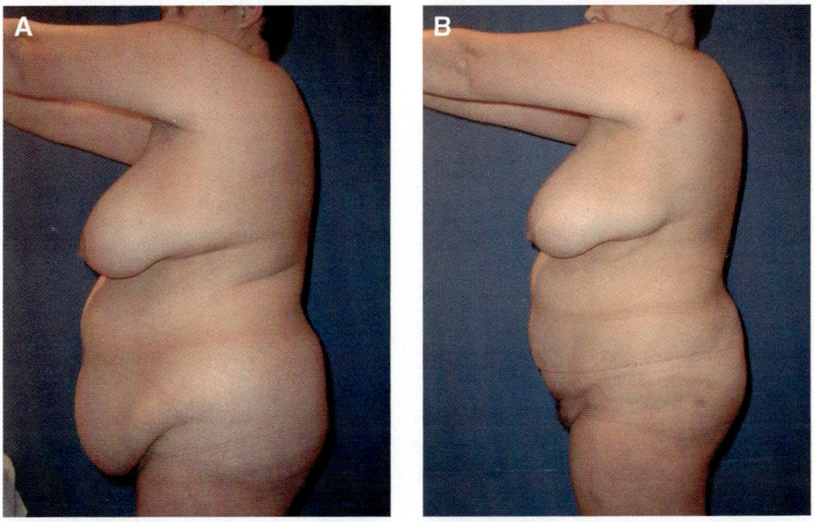

Fig. 34. (*A*) Preoperative appearance (lateral view). (*B*) Postoperative appearance at 7 months (lateral view).

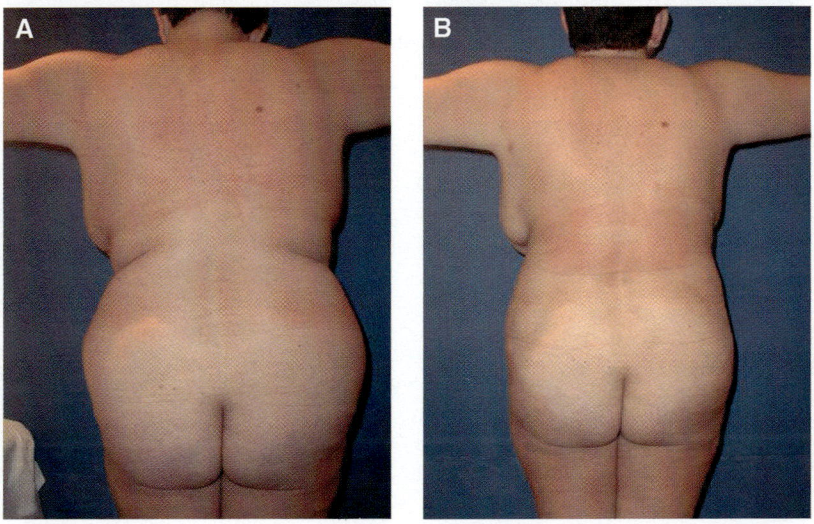

Fig. 35. (*A*) Preoperative appearance (back view). (*B*) Postoperative appearance at 7 months (back view).

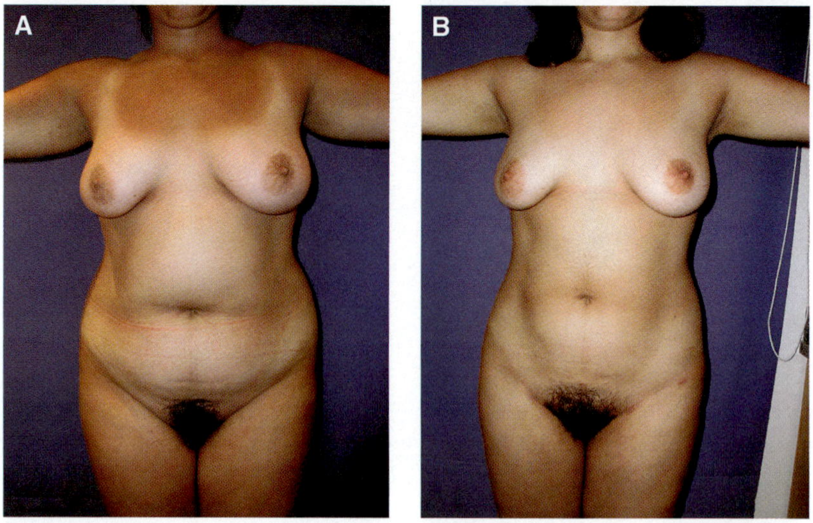

Fig. 36. (*A*) Preoperative appearance (frontal view). (*B*) Postoperative appearance at 6 months (frontal view).

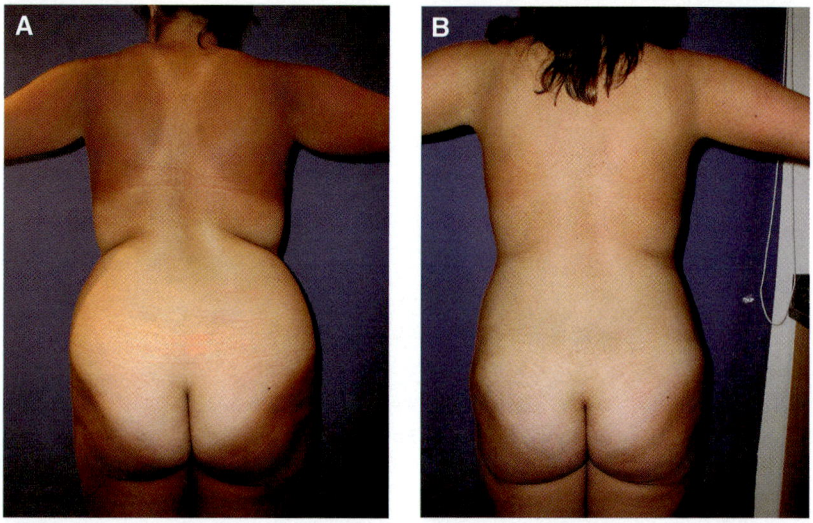

Fig. 37. (*A*) Preoperative appearance (back view). (*B*) Postoperative appearance at 6 months (back view).

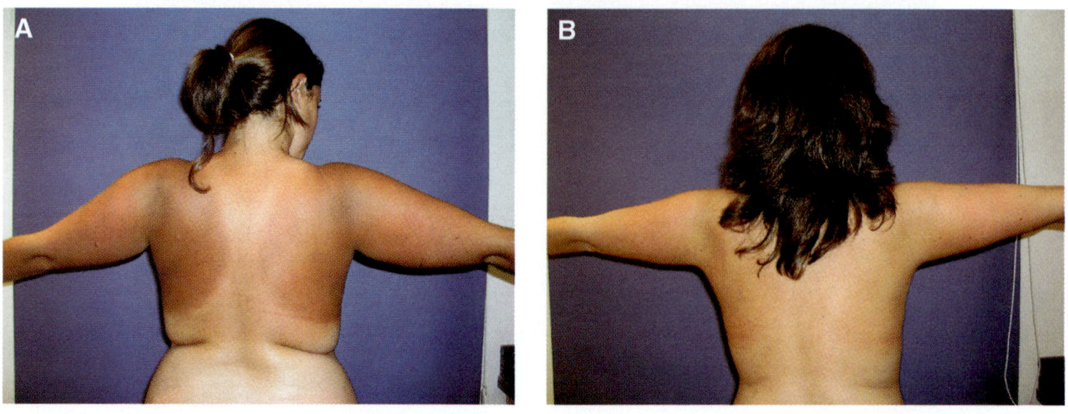

Fig. 38. (*A*) Preoperative appearance (back view). (*B*) Postoperative appearance at 6 months (back view).

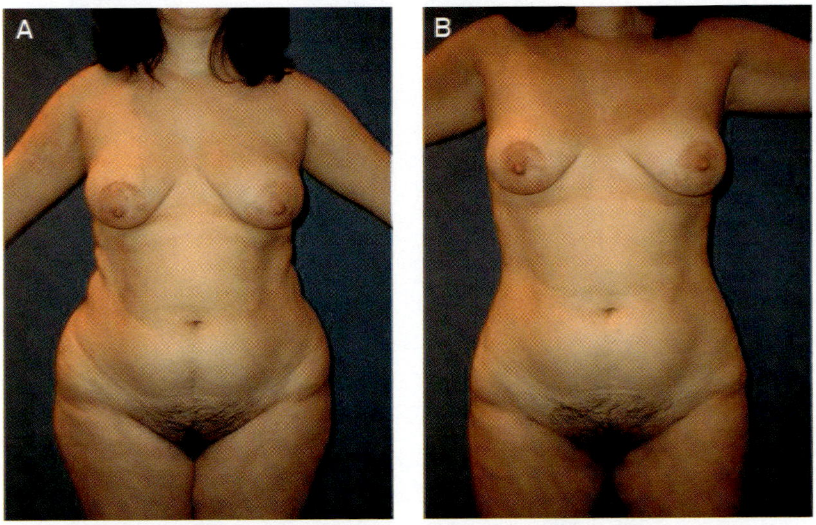

Fig. 39. (*A*) Preoperative appearance (frontal view). (*B*) Postoperative appearance at 11 months (frontal view).

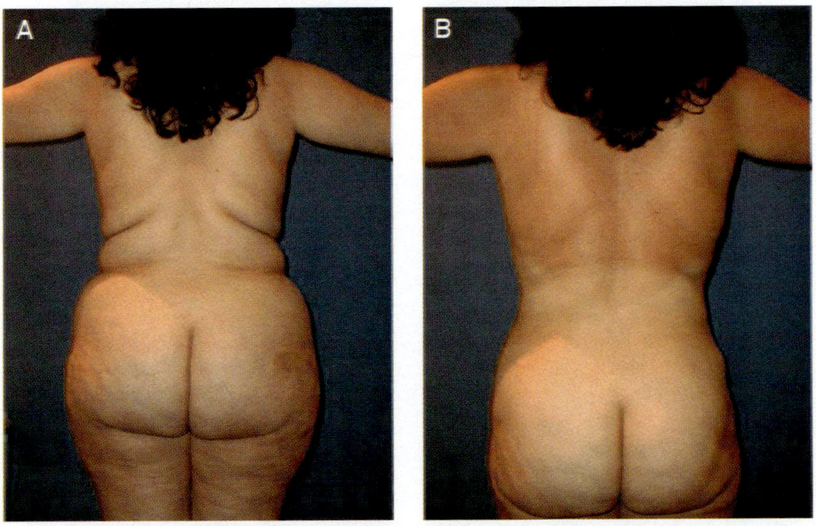

Fig. 40. (*A*) Preoperative appearance (back view). (*B*) Postoperative appearance at 11 months (back view).

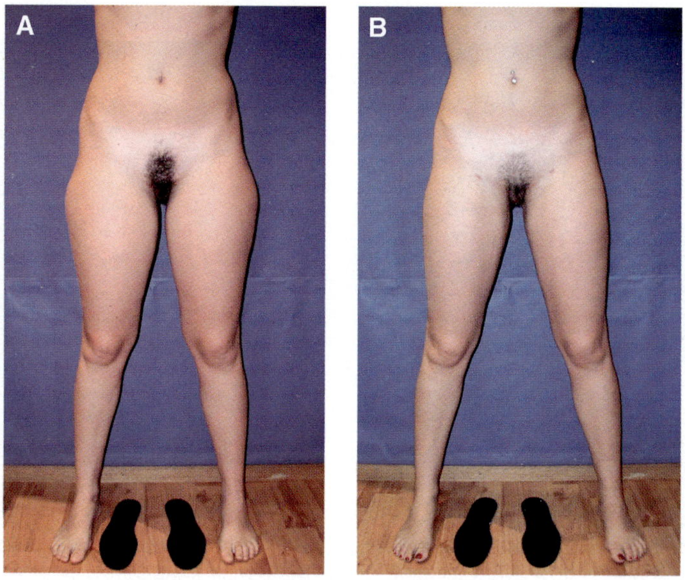

Fig. 41. (*A*) Preoperative appearance (frontal view). (*B*) Postoperative appearance at 3 months (frontal view).

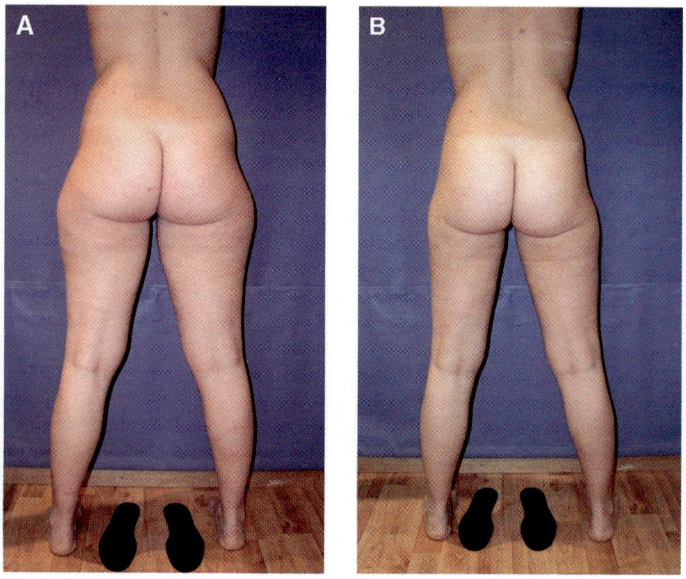

Fig. 42. (*A*) Preoperative appearance (back view). (*B*) Postoperative appearance at 3 months (back view).

7700 mL of emulsified fat was removed in two sessions [Figs. 33–35].

Case 6

A 22-year-old woman underwent vibroliposuction of the abdomen, hips, flanks, and arms. A total of 8350 mL of emulsified fat was removed in three sessions [Figs. 36–38].

Case 7

A 34-year-old woman underwent vibroliposuction of the hips, external thighs, internal thighs, and knees. A total of 7700 mL of emulsified fat was removed in one session [Figs. 39,40].

Case 8

A 26-year-old woman underwent vibroliposuction of the hips, external thighs, internal thighs, and knees. A total of 3200 mL of emulsified fat was removed in one session [Figs. 41,42].

References

[1] Fischer G. Liposculpture—ma technique. 2nd edition. Paris: Arnette; 1996.
[2] Illouz YG. Body contouring by lipolysis: a 5-year experience with over 3000 cases. Plast Reconstr Surg 1983;72:591.
[3] Pierre F. Fournier liposculpture—ma technique. Paris: Arnette; 1989.
[4] Pierre F. Fournier liposculpture—ma technique. 2nd edition. Paris: Arnette; 1996.
[5] Zochi M. Ultrasound-assisted lipoplasty. Adv Plast Reconstr Surg 1998;11:197–221.
[6] Klein JA. Anesthesia for liposuction in dermatologic surgery. J Dermatol Surg Oncol 1988;14: 1124–32.
[7] Klein JA. The tumescent technique: anesthesia and modified liposuction technique. Dermatol Clin 1990;8(3):425–37.
[8] Klein JA. The tumescent technique for liposuction surgery. Am J Cosmetic Surg 1987;4:263–7.
[9] Klein JA. Tumescent technique for regional anesthesia permits lidocaine doses of 35 mg/kg for liposuction. J Dermatol Surg Oncol 1990; 16:3.
[10] Klein JA. Tumescent technique for local anesthesia improves safety in large-volume liposuction. Plast Reconstr Surg 1993;92:1085–98.
[11] Klein JA. Anesthesia for dermatologic cosmetic surgery: principles and techniques. In: Coleman WP, Hanke CW, Alt TH, et al, editors. Cosmetic surgery of the skin. Philadelphia: BC Decker; 1991. p. 39–45.

ELSEVIER
SAUNDERS

CLINICS IN PLASTIC SURGERY

Clin Plastic Surg 33 (2006) 107–115

Liposuction and VASER

Ewaldo Bolivar de Souza Pinto, MD*,
Priscila Chiarello de Souza Pinto Abdala, MD,
Christovam Montecinos Maciel, MD,
Fabiana de Paula Turchiari dos Santos, MD,
Rodrigo Pessoa Martello de Souza, MD

The idea of removing excess fat from localized deposits is not new. Since the beginning of the twentieth century, many surgeons have tried to model the body contour to fit it to the running concept of beauty of each time period. Historically, various approaches have been used to evacuate fatty deposits during lipoplasty. In 1921, Charles Dujarrier attempted to remove subcutaneous fat from a dancer's calves and knees using a uterine curette. A tragic complication occurred, probably because of an injury to the femoral artery, which led to the amputation of one of the dancer's legs [1]. The following decades brought nothing different from en bloc resections of fat and skin, like those performed by Pitanguy, which resulted in great scars and poor outcomes and diminished the popularity of this technique [2]. In the 1970s, Joseph Shcrudde used a delicate curette to remove fat from the lower leg through a small incision, taking the first of three steps of liposuction evolution as it is currently known [1,3].

The second step came with the technique and instruments of Arpad and Giorgio Fisher in 1976. They developed a fat-removing system by means of hollow cannulas equipped with suction (motor-driven suction cannula). They also developed the criss-cross tunnel formation technique, which consisted of tunneling from multiple incisions—a technique that is used currently for more uniform results [1,4]. In 1978, Meyer and Kesserling developed the sharp curettage aided by suction technique, but this technique was not widely accepted because of the frequent residual seroma that caused irregularities [1,3,4].

In 1977, Dr. Ives Gerard Illouz took the third step in the field of modern liposuction. He used a negative pressure device with high suction power connected to a cannula. He developed the wet technique in which a hypotonic saline solution that contained hyaluronidase was infiltrated in the subcutaneous tissue before aspiration. He believed that solution would perform a dissecting hydrotomy that facilitated the removal of fat and diminished the blood loss and surgical trauma. This technique is known worldwide as standard lipoplasty [1,3–5].

Hetter reported that the use of diluted epinephrine solutions reduced blood loss to 15% to 30% of the aspirate [6]. Fodor expanded the concept of wetting solutions to the superwet technique, in which larger volumes of infiltration in a 1:1 infiltration-to-aspiration ratio were used [6]. In 1987, Jeffery Klein reported his development of the tumescent technique, in which even higher

Department of Plastic Surgery, Santa Cecilia University, Brazil
* Corresponding author. Av. Ana Costa, n° 120 Vila Mathias, Santos – SP, Brazil CEP: 11060-000.
E-mail address: ewaldo@desouzapinto.com.br (E.B. de Souza Pinto).

doi:10.1016/j.cps.2005.09.001
plasticsurgery.theclinics.com

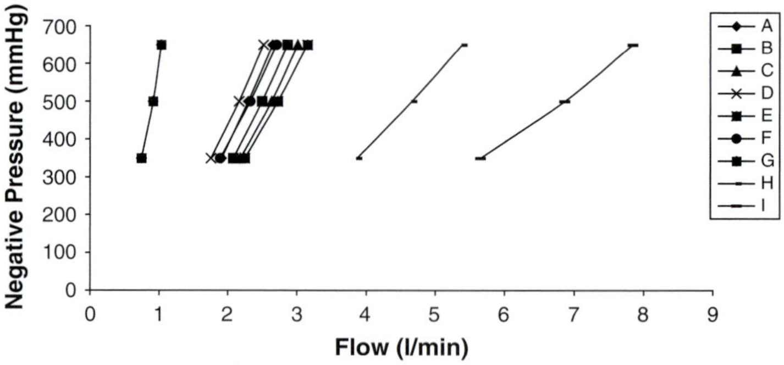

Fig. 1. Characteristic surves of the studied cannulas considering their diameter, length, and number of hole in the tip. A, Robbles type, 4 × 25; B, 4 × 25, *n* = 1; C, 4 × 25, *n* = 2; D, 4 × 25, *n* = 3; E, 4 × 15, *n* = 3; F, 4 × 30, *n* = 3; G, 3 × 25, *n* = 3; H, 5 × 25, *n* = 3; I, 6 × 25, *n* = 3.

volumes were infiltrated until the point that the tissue developed significant turgor (infiltration-to-aspiration ratio of 3–6:1) [6].

Historically several different approaches have been used to evacuate fatty deposits during lipoplasty. Initially, improvements in standard lipoplasty outcomes were linked to advances in aspiration cannula tip design and changes in diameter. Such interest is valid currently, as seen in many publications worldwide. De Souza Pinto and colleagues [7] recently published a paper that described the relation among the number of holes on the tip of the liposuction cannulas, their diameter and length, and the aspiration efficiency for a given suction negative pressure [**Fig. 1**]. Despite these improvements, limitations of the technique include blood loss, postoperative ecchymosis, limited effectiveness in fibrous areas of the body, and surgeon fatigue.

Another major advance in lipoplasty involved the addition of techniques that used energy-based devices, such as external ultrasonic-assisted lipoplasty, ultrasonic-assisted lipoplasty (UAL), and power-assisted lipoplasty [6].Other technologic approaches, such as the application of laser and microwave energy for fat fragmentation, have been tried experimentally, but they have not been clinically applied widely. Power-assisted lipoplasty devices seem to work in a similar way to that of traditional lipoplasty with a blunt avulsion/aspiration mechanism, but the procedures are performed by mechanically reciprocating cannulas [6]. In the late 1980's, Zocchi [8] developed the UAL, which was based on the emission of continuous ultrasound energy that aimed the selective fragmentation/emulsification of fat before its aspiration. This technology was first popularized by Scuderi after his experience with a first-generation UAL device, which delivered continuous ultrasound through blunt, solid, thick probes (4–6 mm diameter) to pretreat fat [6,9]. Second-generation machines featured hollow cannulas for simultaneous fat fragmentation and aspiration, but the internal narrow lumen diameter (only 2 mm) did not allow an efficient evacuation of the fragmented tissue [6]. In the meantime, several complications arose, especially related to the inadvertent excessive exposure of the treated tissues to ultrasound energy. This misuse of the technique was mistakenly related to the method itself. Such situations made surgeons name the guidelines for the development of a more efficient and safe ultrasound-based lipoplasty technology [6].

The VASER

The VASER device was developed as an answer to the search for an enhanced ultrasonic device that might overcome the limitations of the first- and second-generation UAL machines [**Fig. 2**]. Like the previous devices, it uses a method for pretreating the fatty tissue with ultrasonic energy, which causes fragmentation/emulsification by three biologic effects [10–12]. (1) Micromechanical effect, which is the damage caused directly by the unidirectional action of the ultrasonic waves in the

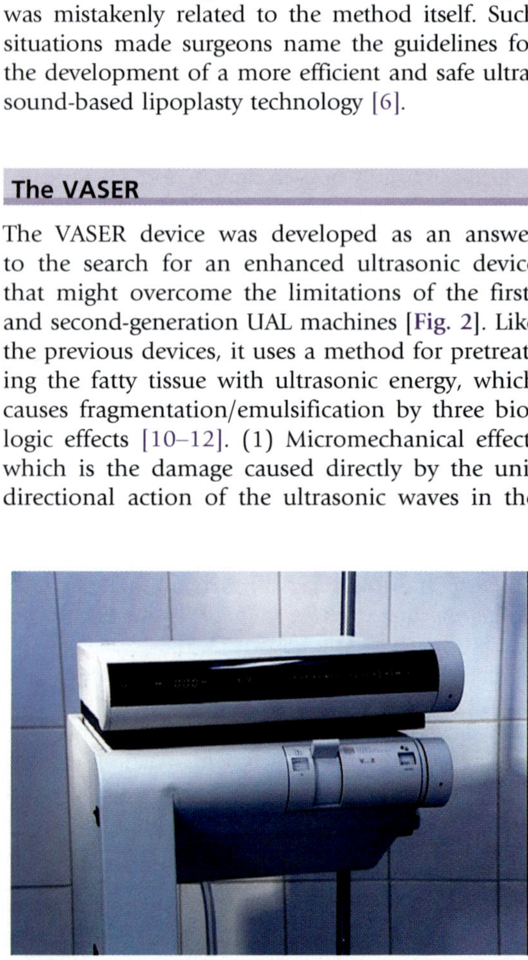

Fig. 2. The VASER ultrasound device.

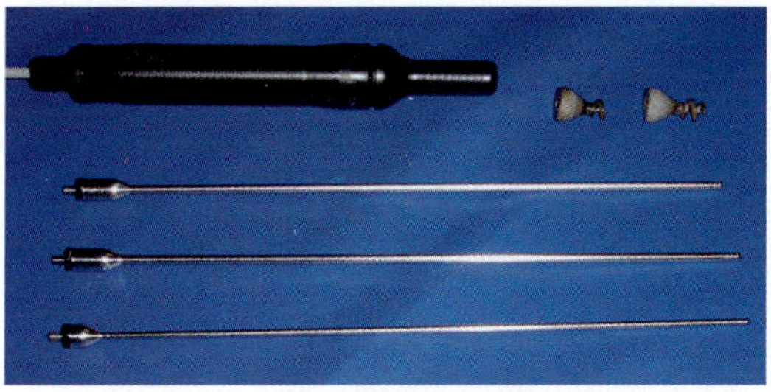

Fig. 3. VASER accessories: probes and ports.

intracellular organic molecules. This effect is minimal. (2) Thermal effect, which is a byproduct that originates from the friction of the cannulas passing through the fat and by the conversion of the ultrasonic waves into heat by the surrounding tissues. (3) Microcavitation effect, which involves gaps between the molecules of the cellular membrane. When the ultrasonic waves are in their higher amplitude plateau and reach such gaps, they cause expansion. Expansion is followed by the passive contraction of the gaps when the ultrasonic waves reach their lower amplitude plateau, establishing repetitive cycles of active expansion and passive contraction. The frequency with which the cycles happen, however, does not allow the contraction phase to be carried out before expansion happens again. The result is the increasing size of the gaps until they reach 120 μm and implode, which causes the rupture of the cellular membrane and the release of the lipid content to the extracellular environment [10–12].

The VASER system uses small diameter titanium solid probes (ie, 2.9 and 3.7 mm) with grooves near the tip to increase fragmentation efficiency [Fig. 3]. The positioning of the grooves near the tip redistributes the ultrasound energy and transfers some of the vibration from the tip to a region just proximal to tip. Thanks to the enhancement of the efficiency of the ultrasound energy achieved with the grooves on the tip of the probes, less energy is necessary to reach the desired fragmentation of the fatty tissue when compared with the previous devices. The probe design can result in a nearly 50% reduction of applied power with improved fragmentation capability in the continuous mode. Such a gain in efficiency allowed the development of the VASER mode, which works with pulsed ultrasonic energy delivery to reduce the applied power even further while maintaining efficiency. It carries a nearly two-thirds reduction of power with a slight loss of efficiency when compared with second-generation devices. It is important to emphasize that simply turning down the power in first- and second-generation equipment does not achieve the desired results once the efficiency of fragmentation falls together with the decreased amplitude [6]. Another major difference is that the VASER system's handpiece and its instrumentation are lighter, smaller, less cumbersome, and handy than those of earlier devices [6,13–15].

VASER lipoplasty technique

Preoperative marking is mandatory and should be done with the patient standing in front of a tridimensional mirror [Fig 4]. Appropriate amounts of wetting solutions should be used with the superwet technique (1:1 infiltrate/aspirate ratio) [6]. In our service, a solution that contains 0.4 mg/mL of lidocaine and epinephrine (1:500,000 epinephrine/solution ratio) is used. The surgeon must be sure

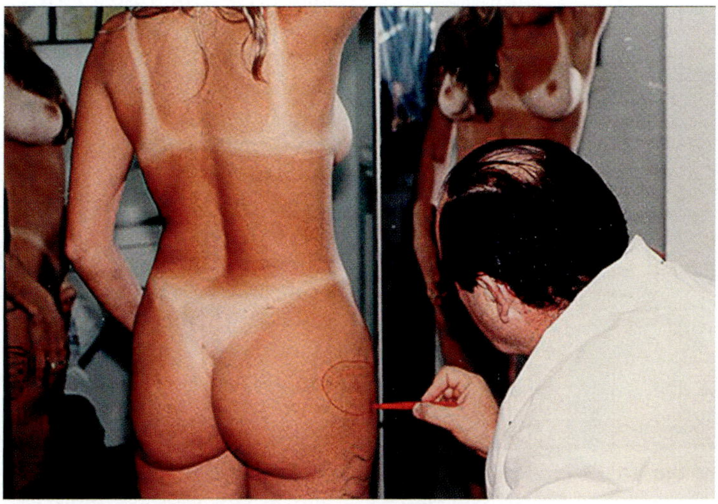

Fig. 4. Preoperative marking in front of a tridimensional mirror.

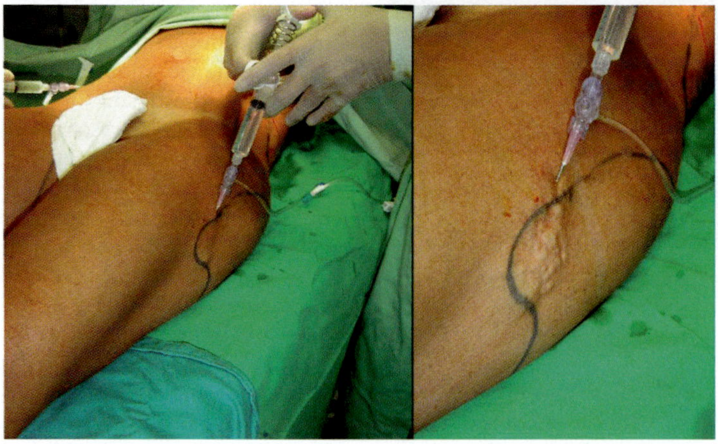

Fig. 5. Infiltration using the super-wet technique.

that the solution is uniformly and evenly distributed over the area to be treated. A gentle fullness and firmness is desired [Fig. 5]. The deep and superficial layers should be infiltrated. The wetting solution should be applied slightly beyond the boundaries of the areas marked for treatment, as should the potential port locations. Sufficient time must be allowed for the vasoconstrictive effects of the solution to take place before emulsification—usually 10 minutes minimum. The amount of lidocaine infused should not exceed 35 mg/kg of body weight [6].

Access incisions are 3 to 4 mm in length, and skin protectors are placed. They are specially designed to protect incision edges during the fragmentation phase without extending their length. Such protectors always must be used to guarantee the safety of the method [6]. The skin near the port should be protected with a wet towel so as to avoid accidental lesions in the unfortunate event that a probe touches exposed skin [Fig. 6]. This protection is especially important in curved areas, in which the maneuvers of the surgeon to reach the area to be treated may expose the skin to contact with the probe. For such reasons, extreme maneuvers should be avoided and the probe must never be placed on exposed skin. The probe must be introduced through the port; simple axial back-and-forth movements should be used and the probe should not be levered to the sides or up and down. The probe should be moved smoothly at a speed that the tissue and the VASER settings can allow without excessive pushing. A speed similar to standard suction cannula movement or a bit slower is appropriate. The probe should be kept moving and never stay in one location.

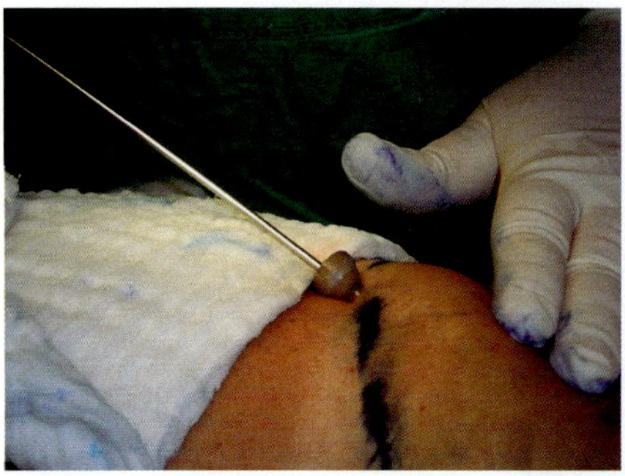

Fig. 6. Introduction of the VASER probe through the skin port. Notice the protection of nearby skin with a wet towel.

Cross-tunneling is highly desirable and should be done whenever possible for more uniform emulsification and to improve subsequent aspiration. The probe must never be vibrated in the air, or damage may occur. The distal 1 or 2 cm of the probe—at least—must be kept in contact with tissue or fluids and inside the skin port and patient before vibration is started. Punching the dermis from below and end-hits should be avoided, and the probe movements must be generally parallel to the skin.

The VASER probe selection must consider the characteristics of the localized fat deposit to be treated and the region of the body. As described by de Souza Pinto [16], the disposal and characteristics of the fat cells in the many areas of the body, as much as the collagen structure and density of the conjunctive septi among the fat cells, are different in each site. The knowledge of these differences allows the right probe to be used for fragmentation on each body site and enables the surgeon to establish the expected skin retraction in that area [Table 1].

Table 1: **Conjunctive septi in the different body sites and relation to skin retraction**

Body site	Conjuntictive septi in the superficial layer of the subcutaneous tissue	Skin retraction after liposuction
Sacral region	90% of the septi are thick	High
Dorsum	80% of the septi are thick	High
Lateral part of the thigh	70% of the septi are thick	High
Flanks	50% of the septi are thick	Medium
Lower abdomen	70% of the septi are thick	Medium
Submentonian	40% of the septi are thick	Medium
Front part of the thigh	50% of the septi are thick	Medium
Upper abdomen	50% of the septi are thick	Medium
Inner part of the thigh	30% of the septi are thick	Low
Buttocks	90% of the septi are thick	Low

The probe diameter and number of grooves on the tip influence how the probe penetrates any given tissue. For a given diameter, probes with more grooves emulsify fat tissue more efficiently, although they do not penetrate fibrous tissues easily because of the significant amount of vibratory energy that is transferred to the sides of the probe as opposed to the front surface. Probes with fewer grooves are more appropriate for fibrous tissues. Smaller diameter probes also penetrate fibrous tissues more easily besides the number of grooves. The 3.7-mm probes are meant for rapid debulking and contouring of medium to large volumes of soft to fibrous tissues. The number of grooves on the tip should vary according to the more or less fibrous areas. The 2.9-mm probes are intended for treating smaller soft to extremely fibrous localized fat deposits and sensitive areas and are used for fine contouring.

In general terms, the continuous mode should be used in fibrous tissues, for faster fragmentation, and when tissue emulsification is not readily achieved with the VASER mode. The VASER mode is better for more delicate work, finer sculpting, or softer tissues. The device must be adjusted in such a way that the probe moves smoothly through the tissue. If the probe is struggling or dragging, the amplitude should be raised or a different probe with fewer grooves or a smaller diameter should be selected.

Initial application times are suggested as maximum 1 minute per 200 mL of infused solution with the VASER or the continuous mode, but this approach usually results in only partial fragmentation of a targeted area. These parameters are suggested by the manufacturer, but experience and practice allow the use of up to 1 minute per 100 mL infused. The parameters vary according to the different regions treated and the time taken to achieve a loss of resistance to the probe movement in all areas intended for fragmentation, which can be considered as an indicator of surgical endpoint. In general, the surgical endpoint occurs somewhere between the loss of resistance of the tissues to the probe and the time guidelines.

After emulsification of the targeted localized fat deposits, aspiration can be accomplished by suction-assisted lipoplasty or power-assisted lipoplasty [6,12,14,15,17,18]. Additional aspiration can be performed for optimal aesthetic refinement if necessary, and the probe can never be reapplied after aspiration because the site is dry. Incisions are closed with sutures, and the conventional postoperative care for liposuction begins.

Results and clinical outcomes

The VASER system works in a complementary fashion when used with suction-assisted lipoplasty or power-assisted lipoplasty. It is a pretreatment method for the fatty tissue that uses ultrasound energy to fragment/emulsify fat before its aspiration. With its smaller diameter and specially designed probes, it uses the minimum amount of ultrasound power necessary to precondition fatty tissue for subsequent aspiration and prevent damage to other elements of the tissue matrix and

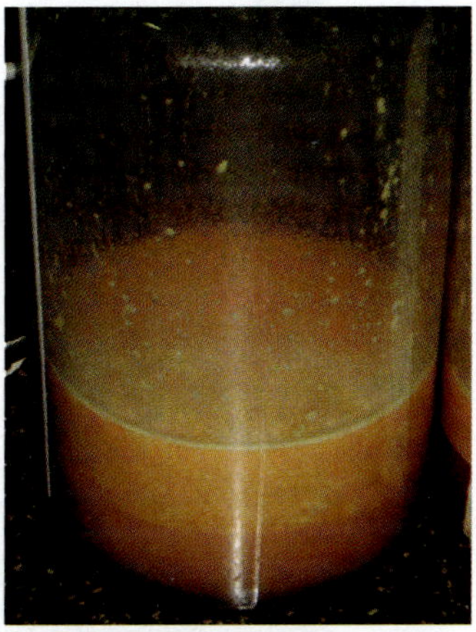

Fig. 7. Fat aspirated with power-assisted lipoplasty device after previous treatment with VASER.

surrounding tissues. It is possible to treat a greater number of areas and create more crossing tunnels for more uniform fragmentation without extending the operative time to hazardous periods [6,12,14, 15,17,18].

When evaluating the supernatant, fat exceeds 80% in all publications and in some of them was as high as 95% of the total volume of aspirate [**Fig. 7**] [6,19]. Histochemical analysis of the aspirate confirmed 70% to 90% cellular disruption when using the VASER device. Ultrasound energy breaks the cellular membrane and releases the lipid content to the extracellular environment but does not cause the release of fatty acids from the triglyceride molecular structure, which means that the remaining fat tissue is not damaged [19].

The clinical outcomes mentioned in the literature are satisfactory and range from good to excellent in most series [**Figs. 8–10**] [6,12,14,15,17,18]. There is a smaller incidence of revisionary lipoplasties and the need for secondary body countouring procedures when the VASER device is used [6]. When the features of VASER are analyzed and compared with earlier UAL equipment, patient and surgeon satisfaction is good, pain is average for lipoplasty procedures, and bruising and swelling are minimal [6,12,14,15,17,18].

Complications

The most recent series that compared the VASER device to first- and second-generation UAL devices

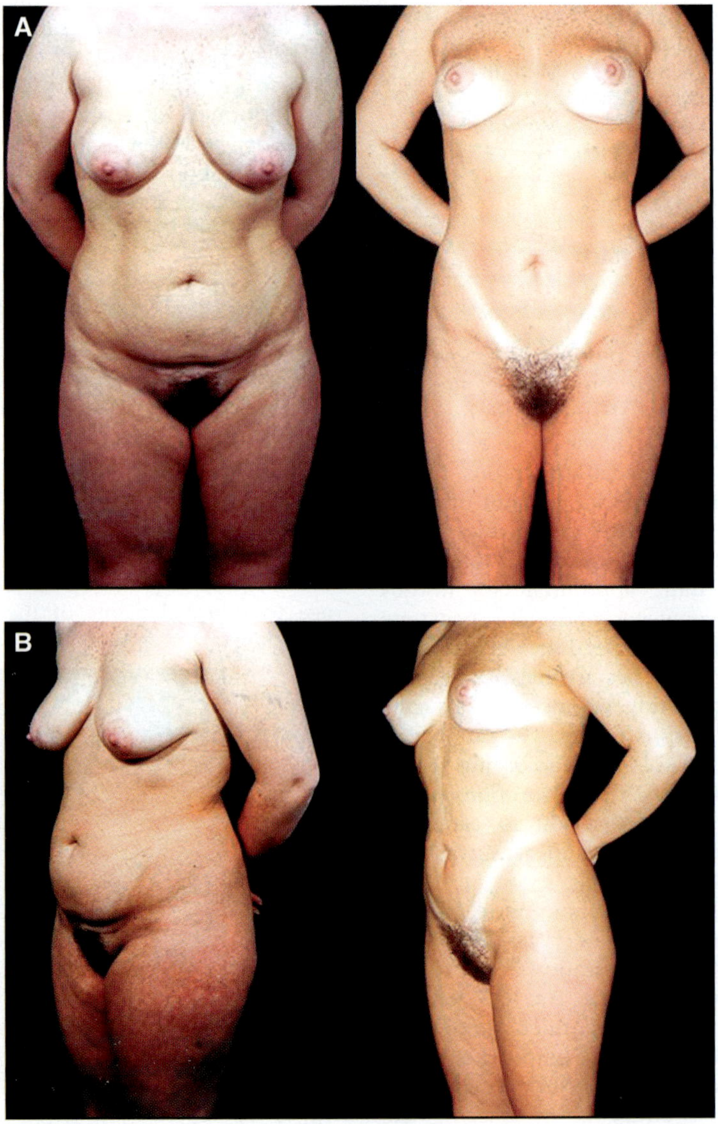

Fig. 8. Before (*A*) and after (*B*) VASER-assisted liposuction.

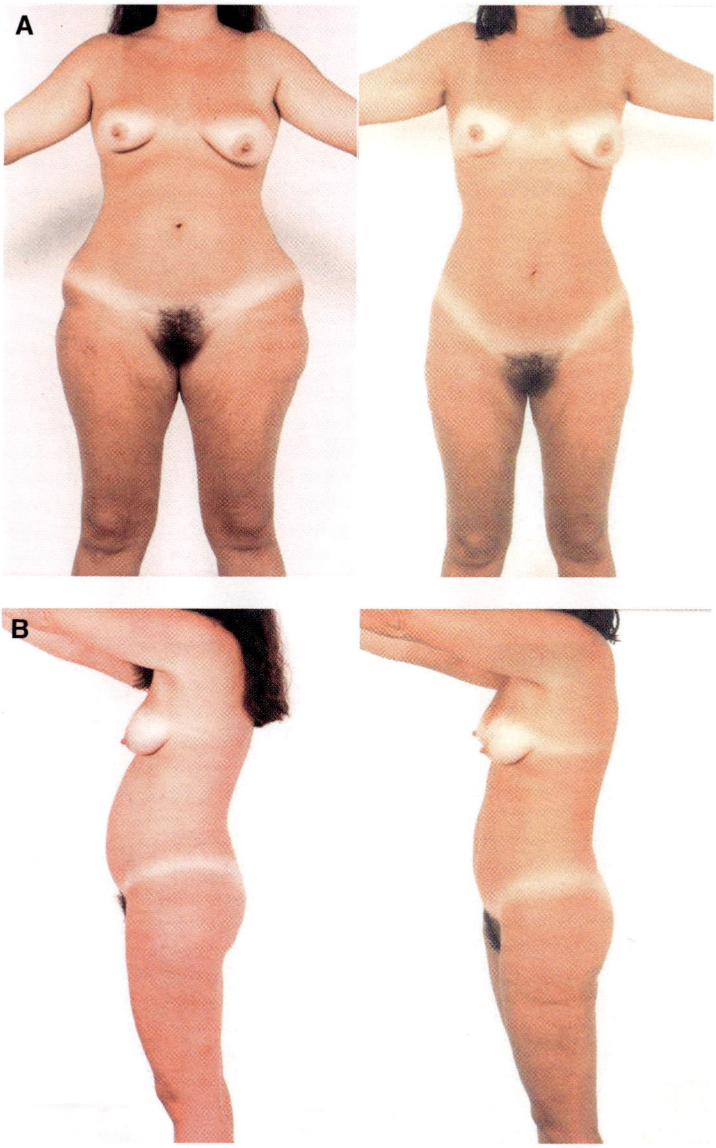

Fig. 9. Before (*A*) and 1 year after (*B*) VASER-assisted liposuction.

showed a minimal to null incidence of complications with the use of VASER, whereas the average incidence of complications with earlier UAL devices is approximately 5% [6]. The most common complications related to UAL are seromas, prolonged dysesthesias, burns, induration, contour irregularities, hyperpigmentation, cellulitis, and prolonged swelling, but these have been reported as being related to the use of excess energy or extended application. When it comes to neural injury, reports have shown that it is actually related to the exposure period rather than the use of ultrasound energy itself [20,21].

The decreased incidence of such complications with the use of VASER can be explained by the lower need for energy demanded for emulsification because of the optimization of the applied energy by the grooved probes and the pulsed emission of energy in the VASER mode. Reports in the literature of burns and ischemic injuries related to UAL systems seem to be related to execution problems, such as end-hitting and intimate contact with the dermis from below [6]. The application of UAL to the undersurface of the dermis seems to be hazardous and unpredictable at best. Research also has demonstrated that the core body temperature remains stable during the UAL application and the subcutaneous tissues experience a gradual increase of temperature during the time of application of ultrasonic region; however, it remains below the

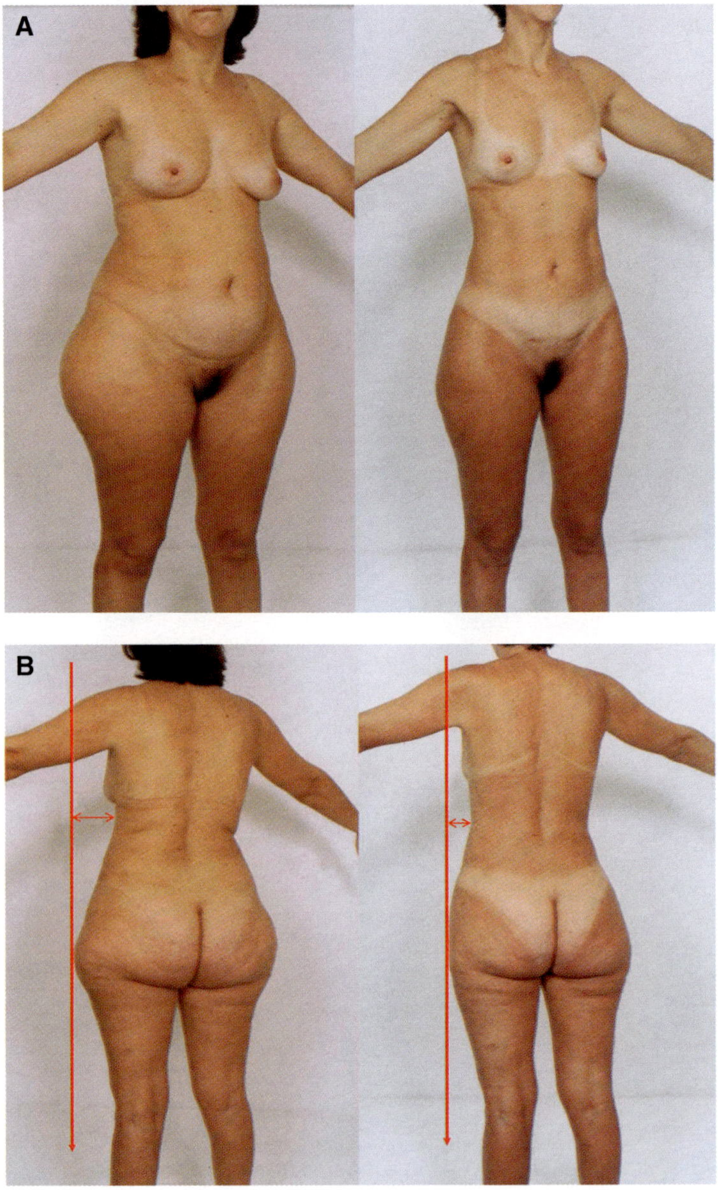

Fig. 10. Before (*A*) and 3 years after (*B*) VASER-assisted liposuction.

body core temperature at all times because of the wetting solutions [22]. The incidence of burns is not related to any UAL method itself but to its mistaken application. It seems that the VASER device in the hands of surgeons who are trained in UAL can produce excellent results with lower risk of complications than has been reported for earlier UAL equipment.

Summary

VASER is a fat pretreatment device based on the emission of pulsed or continuous ultrasound energy to emulsify fat before its aspiration by means of suction-assisted lipoplasty or power-assisted lipoplasty. If compared with previous generation UAL machines, it carries important technologic advances that focus on the safety and efficiency of the process. VASER is the result of improvements in surgical instrumentation and technique, proper use of wetting solutions, and knowledge about the best use of ultrasound for fat fragmentation. With its thinner cannulas and decreased use of ultrasonic energy, it allows greater emulsification of fat, creates more tunnels, diminishes the operative time, preserves vessels and nerves, and causes less pain and hematomas [8,13–17].

References

[1] Flynn TC, Coleman III WP, Field LM, et al. History of liposuction. Dermatol Surg 2000;26: 515–20.
[2] Pitanguy I. Trochanteric dystrophy. Plast Reconstr Surg 1964;34:280.
[3] Souza Pinto EB. Lipoaspiração superficial. Rio de Janeiro: Revinter; 1999.
[4] Fischer G. Liposculpture: the "correct" history of the liposuction. Part I. J Dermatol Surg Oncol 1990;16:1087–9.
[5] Avelar JM, Illouz YG. Histórico da técnica lipólise: lipoaspiração. In: Illouz YG, editor. Lipoaspiração. 1st edition. São Paulo: Hipócrates; 1986. p. 24–31.
[6] Jewell ML, Fodor PB, Souza Pinto EB, et al. Clinical application of VASER-assisted lipoplasty: a pilot clinical study. Aesthetic Surgery Journal 2002;22(2):131–46.
[7] De Souza Pinto EB, Saldanha OR, da Rocha RP, et al. Metodologia experimental para testar cânulas de lipoaspiração. Revista Soc Bras Cir Plast 2005;20(1):30–5.
[8] Zocchi M. New perspective in lipoplasty: the ultrasonic-assisted lipectomy (UAL). Presented at the Annual Congress of the French Society of Asthetic Surgery. Paris, May 1988.
[9] Scuderi N, Devita R, D'Andrea F, et al. Nuove prospettive nella liposuzione la lipoemulsificazone. Giorn Chir Plast Ricoster ed Estética 1987; 2:33–9.
[10] Coleman III WP, Brody HJ, Narins RS, et al. Update from the ultrasonic liposuction task force of the American Society for Dermatological Surgery. Dermatol Surg 1997;23:210–4.
[11] Lawrence N, Coleman III WP. The biologic basis of ultrasonic liposuction. Dermatol Surg 1997; 23:1197–200.
[12] Graf R, Auersvald A, Damásio RC, et al. Ultrasound-assisted liposuction: an analysis of 348 cases. Aesthetic Plast Surg 2003;27(2):146–53.
[13] Rohrich RJ, Morales DE, Krueger JE, et al. Comparative analysis of in vivo-treated adipose tissue. Plast Reconstr Surg 2000;105(6):2152–7.
[14] Beckenstein MS, Grotting JC. Ultra-sound assisted lipectomy using the solid probe: a retrospective review of 100 consecutive cases. Plast Reconstr Surg 2000;105(6):2161–74.
[15] Chang CC, Commons GW. A comparison of various ultrasound technologies. Clin Plast Surg 1999;26:261–8.
[16] Souza Pinto EB. Morphohistologic analysis of fat tissue in areas treated with lipoplasty. Aesthetic Surgery Journal 1991;22(6):513–8.
[17] Maxuel GP. Use of hollow cannula technology in UAL. Clin Plast Surg 1999;26:255–60.
[18] Rohrich RJ, Beran SJ, Kelken LM, et al. Extending the role of liposuction in body contouring with ultrasound-assisted liposuction. Plast Reconstr Surg 1998;101:1090–102.
[19] Gripaudo FR, Matarese RM, Macone A, et al. Effects of traditional and ultrasonic liposuction on adipose tissue: a biochemical approach. Plast Reconstr Surg 2000;106(6):197–9.
[20] Howard BK, Beran SJ, Kenkel JM, et al. The effects of ultrasonic energy on peripheral nerves: implications for ultrasound-assisted liposuction. Plast Reconstr Surg 1999;103(3):984–9.
[21] Trott SA, Rohrich RJ, Beran SJ, et al. Sensory changes after traditional and ultrasound-assisted liposuction using computer-assisted analysis. Plast Reconstr Surg 1999;103:2016–25.
[22] Ablaza VJ, Gingrass MK, Perry LC, et al. Tissue temperature during ultrasound-assisted lipoplasty. Plast Reconstr Surg 1998;102(2):534–42.

ELSEVIER
SAUNDERS

CLINICS IN PLASTIC SURGERY

Clin Plastic Surg 33 (2006) 117–127

Low-Level Laser-Assisted Liposuction: the Neira 4 L Technique

Rodrigo Neira, MD*, Luiz Toledo, MD, Jose Arroyave, BSc, MSc, TEM, SEM, Efrain Solarte, Dr, Rer, Nat, MSc, Carolina Isaza, MD, MSc, Oscar Gutierrez, MD, MSc, William Criollo, BSc, MSc, Hugo Ramirez, VMD, MSc, Maria I. Gutierrez, MD, MSc, PhD, Clara L. Ortiz-Neira, MD

Liposuction, a procedure that carves out body fat by suction and grafts fat in other places to recreate a harmonic, anatomic, and physiologic corporal shape, is an art. Although this procedure is the most commonly performed cosmetic surgery (384,686 procedures were performed in the United States in 2003) [1], it is not considered altogether benign [2]. In 2000, the mortality rate for patients having liposuction was similar to that for persons dying in motor vehicle accidents in the United States—about 20 in every 100,000 procedures done by physicians certified by the American Board of Plastic Surgery [3].

Liposuction causes severe trauma to the adipose tissue and crushes nerves, vessels, and connective tissue, generating a strong inflammatory response [4]. The patient undergoing liposuction is at risk for multiple problems, such as thrombosis, endothelial edema, fat embolism, immunocompromise, infection, local necrosis, transitory and definitive vascular damage, and lengthy healing processes. Hetter [4] described the surgical trauma in a classic lipoplasty as crush injuries and referred to these wounds as "the internal burn," stressing the loss of serum albumin as well as red cell mass and the release of intracellular products. These events initiate a giant inflammatory cascade that causes a marked fourth-space phenomenon during the first 3 days after surgery.

In an effort to mitigate the trauma of classic liposuction, surgeons have used external laser-assisted liposuction to reduce inflammation and control pain after surgery. This article describes low-level laser-assisted liposuction (LLLL), known as the Neira 4 L technique, a new procedure that our surgical team has developed to moderate the inflammatory response, reduce trauma to tissues, and promote subcutaneous wound healing after lipoplasty-assisted liposuction.

Department of Plastic Surgery, Maxillofacial and Hand Surgery, Pontificia Universidad Javeriana, Cali, Colombia
* Corresponding author. 103 Watermill Road, Greer, SC 29650.
E-mail address: rodrigoneiramd@aol.com (R. Neira).

doi:10.1016/j.cps.2005.09.005
plasticsurgery.theclinics.com

Mechanisms of action of low-level lasers

Effects of low-level lasers on the adipose cell membrane and mitochondria

Low-level laser irradiation modulates the attachment of cells in vitro by means of cytochrome C oxidase and activates the mitochondrial signaling pathway, which increases the effect of the laser on the cell membrane and the mitochondria [5] and the number of contacts of the endoplasmic reticulum with the mitochondria and plasma membrane [6]. Irradiation with a low-level laser increases ATP levels in cells cultivated in vitro, increasing the survival of the cell by increasing cell energy that could be necessary to repair and heal tissues after surgical trauma [7]. The increase in cellular ATP levels produced by monochromatic red light depends on the growth phase of the culture. ATP levels are insignificant in the lag phase of cultured cells, increase in the log phase, and reach a maximum (about 190%) in cells at the late logarithmic and early plateau phases [8,9]. Iaffaldano and coworkers [10] found increased ATP levels, electric potential across inner membranes, and action potential in the mitochondrial matrix, as well as small changes in the matrix configuration. Although increasing intracellular cAMP concentrations in vascular smooth muscle increases blood flow and promotes edema, increasing cAMP concentrations in the endothelium may suppress edema by enhancing the permeability barrier [11].

Radiation of cells with a low-level laser causes morphologic changes in the mitochondrial lymphocyte [12]. Because hemoglobin does not absorb in the red and near-infrared spectral region, light can penetrate deep into the living tissue.

At least three signaling pathways relate cell attachment, the respiratory chain, and the Na^+, K^+-ATPase, and N^+/H^+ exchanger activities [13]. Cu(A) and Cu(B) chromophores of cytochrome C oxidase may be involved as photoacceptors, and various signaling pathways between cytochrome C oxidase and cell attachment regulation are at work.

Effect of laser light on the body

Used in the treatment of a broad range of conditions, including acute and chronic pain and injured tissues, low-level laser therapy (LLLT) has improved wound healing, reduced edema, and relieved pain of various origins.

Inflammation

Low-level lasers have been used for many years to reduce inflammation. LLLT reversibly suppresses the action potentials elicited by bradykinin and blocks the conduction of nociceptive signals in primary afferent nerves [14]. At 4 J/cm^2, the anti-inflammatory effect is superior to that with 8 J/cm^2 [15]. LLLT is used to stabilize vascular endothelia to prevent tissue hypoperfusion through endothelial edema [16].

Pain

LLLT for pain involves suppression of late discharges in caudal neurons evoked by excitatory inputs from C-fiber afferents but not of early discharges evoked by impulses from A-fiber delta afferents [17]. These results suggest that low-level laser energy blocks the depolarization of C-fiber afferents and suppresses impulse conduction of unmyelinated A-fiber delta afferents in the peripheral sensory nerve, which causes pain. Kasai and coworkers [18] showed that LLLT acts as a reversible direct suppressor of neuronal activity.

In a study of the effect of low-power laser irradiation on pain using substance P in rat spinal dorsal root ganglion, Ohno [19] found a statistically significant difference in substance P–like immunoreactivity between the control group and stimulated group. These results suggest that laser irradiation suppresses excitation of the unmyelinated C-fibers in the afferent sensory pathway.

LLLT on local points in rats with arthritis relieved arthralgia, reduced swelling in the ankles, and produced instant analgesia [20].

Peripheral nerves

Irradiation with a low-level laser can prevent posttraumatic degeneration of peripheral nerves and postpone degeneration of the central nervous system [21]. Low-level laser energy inactivates the potential of the cell membrane, preventing the transmission of pain through afferent nerves after surgery, and acts on the demyelinated nerve to speed recovery. In one study [22], transcutaneous low-power irradiation with low-level lasers significantly increased the rate of regeneration of rat facial nerve after a crush injury when compared with that of the control group ($P<.01$).

In their classic study, Rochkind and coworkers [23] found that LLLT improved the recovery of injured peripheral nerves and the central nervous system, as well as the healing of cutaneous wounds and burns. LLLT applied to crushed injured nerves significantly increased the compound action potential in unirradiated tissue and irradiated tissue on the left side. Laser irradiation done on only the right side in bilaterally inflicted cutaneous wounds enhanced recovery on both sides ($P<.01$). In the nonirradiated control group, all rats sustained advanced necrosis of the feet and bilateral gangrene. These systemic effects have implications for the clinical application of LLLT and for basic research into the possible mechanisms involved.

Wound healing

Use of low-level lasers accelerates and improves wound healing and minimizes scarring. The mechanism of this phenomenon is unclear and still under investigation [24]. It is well known that cell-cell and cell-matrix adhesion is altered during wound repair [25]. The cell membrane may develop cellular adhesiveness, joining normal cells to each other when the membranes are exposed to the laser beam [26].

Biophysical effects of laser light on adipose cells

When our team studied the biophysical effect of low-level lasers on adipose cells, we found a transitory pore in the adipocyte membrane [27] and fat leaking from the inside of the cell into the interstitial space outside [28]. Moreover, laser light did not destroy the adipocyte when it mobilized the fat from the inside to the outside of the membrane [**Figs. 1–3**]. It kept the cell alive and in good condition, as confirmed with trypan blue staining and XTT [29].

Neira and colleagues, based on the work of Kolárová and coworkers [30], studied adipose-irradiated tissue samples for 2, 4, and 6 minutes with and without a tumescent solution. Scanning electron microscopy (SEM) and transmission electron microscopy (TEM) showed that, without laser exposure, normal adipose tissue appeared as a grape-shaped node [**Fig. 3**]. After 4 minutes of laser exposure, 80% of the fat was released from the adipose cells [**Fig. 4**]. At 6 minutes of laser exposure, almost all of the fat was released from the adipocyte [**Fig. 5**] [31]. The released fat collected in the interstitial space [32].

TEM images of adipose tissue taken at a magnification of 60,000× revealed a transitory pore

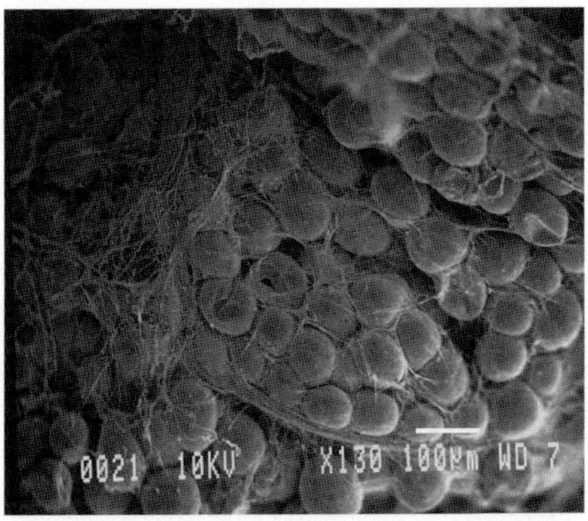

Fig. 1. Scanning electron microscope (SEM) image of normal adipose membrane of adipocyte. Some connective tissue is evident surrounding the adipose cells.

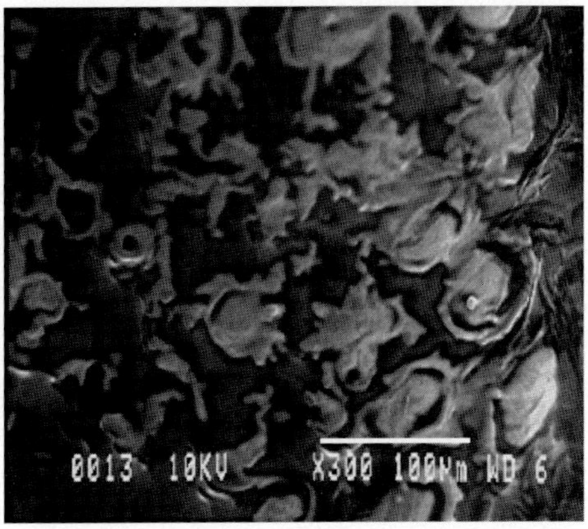

Fig. 2. Adipocytes after 4 minutes laser exposure. Some are deformed and have a crenate shape.

[**Fig. 6**]. Low-level laser energy opened this pore in the cell membrane, permitting fat to go from the inside to the outside of the adipose cell [**Fig. 4**]. The interstice and capillaries of the cell remained intact. By 4 minutes of exposure, partial disruption of the adipose cell was observed, but several cells maintained their properties and structure [32]. Adipose cells with and without laser exposure are shown in the same sample in **Fig. 7**.

When adipose cells were cultured until maturity and then irradiated with a low-level laser (637 nm) with an equivalent dose of 3.6 J/cm^2, the cells were semi-destroyed [31]. Five days after being recultured, the adipose cells were alive and had recovered their normal anatomy [29,31]. Although the initial results of further studies with light microscopy were not conclusive because of initial sample testing procedures, the case study was continued because the preliminary clinical evidence clearly warranted further investigation.

Both SEM and TEM were done on superficial and deep fat samples to establish whether cellular effects correlated with the penetration depth of the laser beam after application of the tumescent technique [33]. The analysis of fat samples indicated that tumescent infiltration facilitated laser beam penetration and movement of fat from inside to outside the cell. A detailed study of the adipose cell membrane with TEM confirmed the existence of the suspected pore [**Figs. 2,8**] [34].

When superficial and deep fat samples of laser-treated tissue taken from the infraumbilical area were studied [29], no major observable differences were found in the samples of adipose tissue exposed to laser radiation for 2 and 4 minutes without tumescence [31]. Laser penetration through the adipose tissue decreased when tumescent solution was not used, suggesting that the application of the tumescent solution is an important enhancement factor [35].

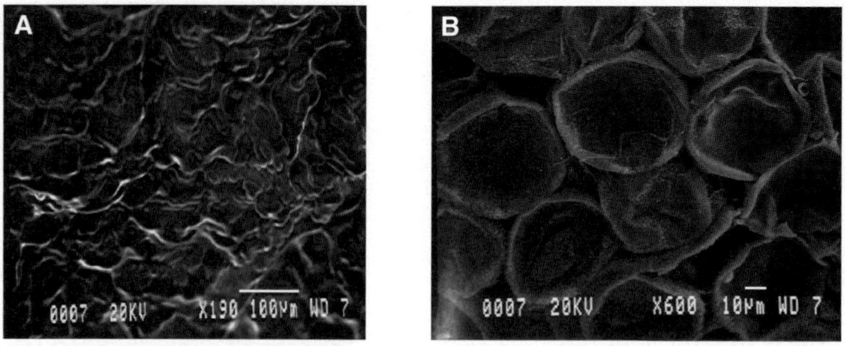

Fig. 3. (*A*) Adipose tissue after 6 minutes of laser exposure. Fat is outside the cell, and only membranes are seen. (*B*) The adipocytes have lost their fat and look deflate.

Without laser exposure, the adipose tissue remains intact; adipocytes maintain their round grapelike shape [see **Fig. 3**]. After 4 minutes of laser exposure, the membrane of the adipocyte is partially disrupted [**Fig. 4**], and 80% of the fat is outside the cell. Fat particles build up in the shape of a helmet on the cell. The membranes of adipocytes are partially disrupted, exposing fat bodies outside the cell [**Fig. 4**]. At 6 minutes of laser of exposure, SEM shows almost total disruption of the adipose cell membrane and evacuation of fat [**Fig. 5**]. The back fat sample shown in **Fig. 1** has increased connective and reticular tissue, explaining why is more difficult to take out.

Low-level laser-assisted liposuction

The procedure

The Neira 4 L procedure has been described previously [36]. In preparation for LLLL, the completely naked patient is washed with Isodine while standing up. The Isodine is sprayed on the body, including the hands and feet. Two blankets of sterilized rubber are placed on the operating table, one on top of the other, and covered with sterilized fields. The patient is then instructed to lie down on the operating table and given local sedation with propofol (fentanyl and or midazolam) intravenously.

An ultrawet infiltration is performed on the target areas [37]. The greater the hydration of the tissue, the deeper the transmission of the laser beam. When the tissue is not well hydrated, the beam will not reach the desired depth, and the results are not as good.

The surgeon makes 2 mm incisions with a No. 11 scalpel blade and introduces cannulas for infiltration. Almost simultaneously, the assistant begins to apply the laser continuously at 14 mW at a focal distance of 26 cm irradiating with two lines of light until a dose of 3.6 J/cm^2 is reached.

The assistant then applies laser radiation to the appropriate areas to extract fat, beginning with the left or right hemi-abdomen, for about 12 minutes. The infiltration may last 30 to 40 minutes, during which time the assistant simultaneously applies the laser to all of the tissues being infiltrated. This application saves time because the surgeon begins infiltration at the same time that the assistant begins to apply the laser. After completion of the

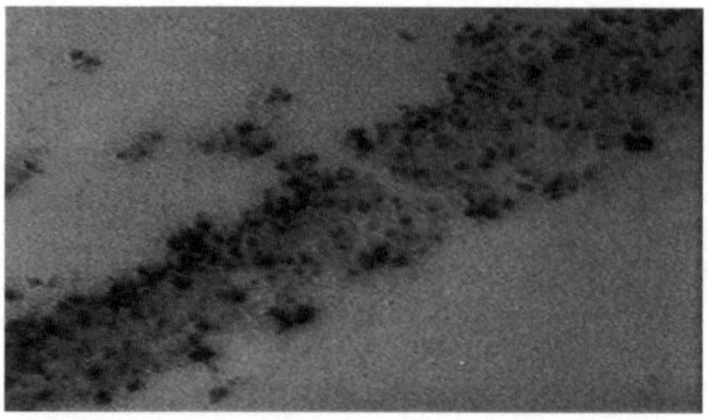

Fig. 4. Transmission electron microscopy (TEM ×60000) of the membrane after 6 minutes laser exposure. (Channel formation)

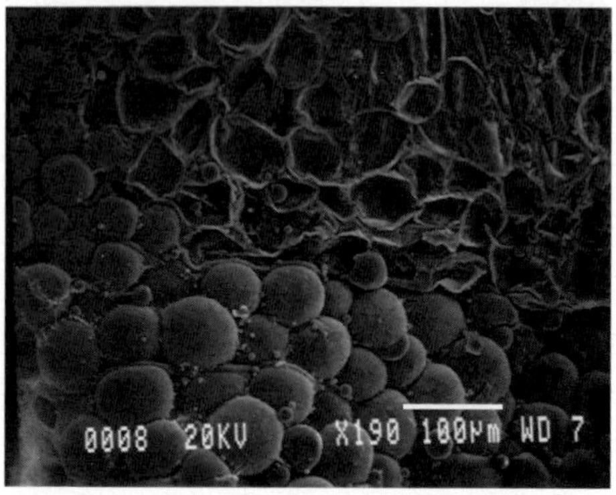

Fig. 5. Upper half of the image depicts "deflated" adipocytes. Lower half of the image demonstrates normal adipocytes.

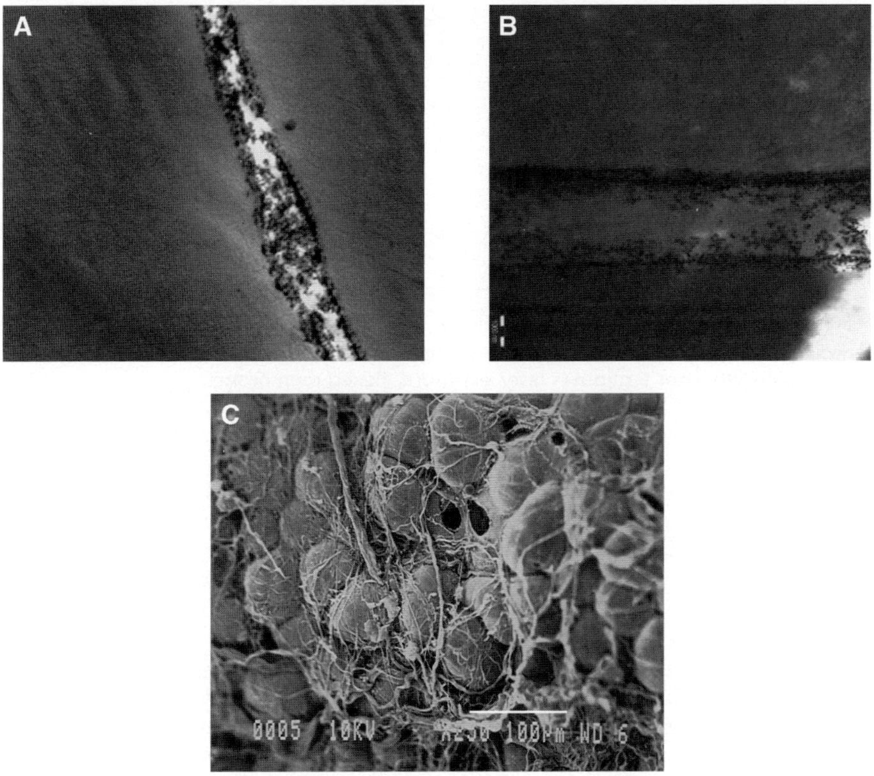

Fig. 6. Normal adipose membrane. (*A*) Transmission electron microscope (TEM) image without irradiation, original magnification ×400,000. (*B*) TEM image without irradiation, original magnification ×50,000. (*C*) Fat tissue from the back has more conjunctive and reticular tissue, explaining why it is harder to remove.

infiltration, about 10 to 12 minutes longer are needed to finish applying the laser to the tissue in target areas. Ultrawet infiltration is maximized in all tissues to ensure success of the procedure. Laser penetration and effectiveness are poorer in patients in whom tumescence is suboptimal [32,35].

As soon as infiltration and laser irradiation are completed, tunnels are started in the superficial layers of fat without suction. Fat is extracted later with a 3- or 4-mm cannula, a syringe, or regular wall vacuum without special machines. Deep fat is extracted carefully with the tip of the cannula just touching, or kissing, the deep fascia at all times so that no damage is done. Observations indicate that a smoother and more uniform surface is obtained this way [38–40].

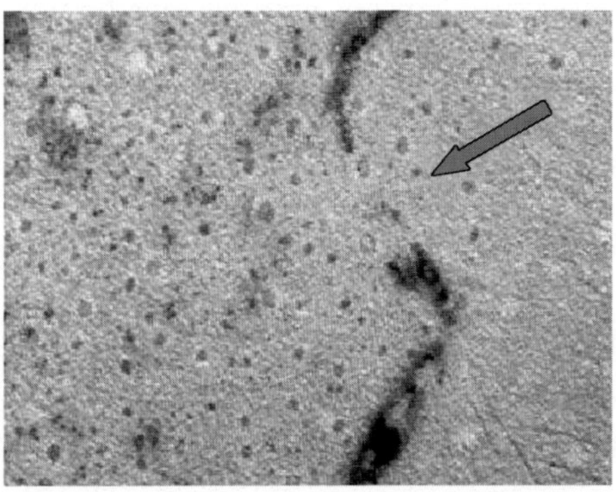

Fig. 7. 6 minutes laser exposure demonstrating interruption of the adipose cell membrane.

Fat is extracted from the superficial layer first. The surgeon then works downward toward the deep layer, where fat can be extracted with 2 and 3 mm cannulas without touching the skin. Fat is extracted with 3, 4, 5, and 6 mm Becker or Mercedes type cannulas. We always begin with 3 mm cannulas to remove superficial fat, and then use 4 and 5 mm cannulas to extract the fat more easily, especially in the dorsal area. Dorsal fat, in particular, is extremely reticular, dense, and hard, making it difficult to extract. The assistant can help keep the skin stretched to avoid damage. Because the fat is more liquefied, no nodules or condensed fat remains in the tissues undergoing fat extraction. Wounds are covered with Micropore rather than sutured, and the patient is completely wrapped in adult diapers, which are kept in place with a garment.

Three days after surgery, the laser can be applied for 3 minutes at 5 mW for each area to reduce the duration of inflammation. Massage can be initiated

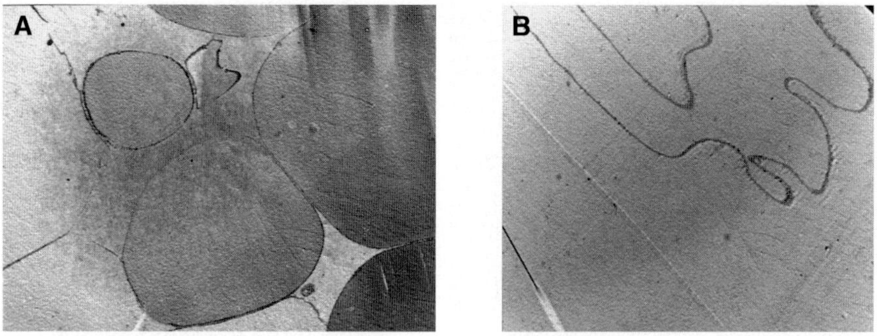

Fig. 8. (*A*) Transmission electron microscopy (TEM) showing adipocyte cell with well defined borders, no laser exposure. (*B*) TEM adipocyte after 6 minutes laser exposure, flexed membrane.

4 or 5 days after surgery. Improved skin retraction occurs within 3 months. Most patients express their satisfaction with the results obtained with this procedure [36].

Treatment of complications

Fluid in the lowest area of the abdomen during the first 3 days can be drained with a syringe and local anesthesia, or the flap can be squeezed and the liquid removed through the original surgical incision or with a needle and syringe. In general, fluid should be drained through the same incision or by syringe with local anesthesia. We have not seen real seromas in our patients.

Almost 20% of patients have pain, which can be controlled with nonsteroidal anti-inflammatory medication and codeine. Irregularities in the skin, which occur in 4% of patients, can be difficult to manage, but massage and the use of an external beam laser for a couple weeks may help. Itchiness can be treated with antihistamines and topical olive oil. Flap problems are treated with subcutaneous oxygen and 3 minutes of laser treatment over the area every day for 3 to 5 days. Edema of the hands and feet occurring 3 or 4 days after surgery is treated with furosemide 20 mg/day, PO for 2 to 3 days.

Infection, which occurs in 1% of patients, is more frequent in the sacral area. If infection is suspected, a hemogram, urinalysis, and hemodynamic evaluation should be done. If the results of these tests indicate infection, the wound may have to be drained. Antibiotics and culture are recommended if the infection is caused by *Staphylococcus*. Dicloxacillin 500 mg QID should be started. If the infection does not respond and the culture indicates no bacterial infection, which is rare, the patient should be monitored carefully within 8 hours, and vancomycin 1 g Q12H, ciprofloxacin 500 mg BID intravenously, should be started immediately. If *Escherichia coli* is found, oral ciprofloxacin (500 mg) should be started twice a day for 8 days.

Serosanguinous liquid that collects in the sacral area is usually extracted 1 week after surgery one or two times. Innovative adjuvant techniques for liposculpture have been used and have shown good postoperative results [36].

Discussion

The Neira 4 L technique offers a new less traumatic method of liposuction. The main goals of this technique are as follows:

- To protect the cells, especially the adipocytes, and the tissues around them
- To improve the defense mechanisms of receptor tissue
- To modulate the inflammatory response
- To improve the healing process
- To avoid creating a neuroaxonal lesion, preventing the development of neuralgias after surgery, decreasing postoperative pain, shortening recovery time, and decreasing the risk of side effects of surgical trauma

It is essential to reduce the surgical trauma to the patient or, at least, to improve their tolerance to the surgery and reduce pain. The Neira 4 L technique provides these benefits. Each new method or procedure comes with attendant expectations about its potential benefits. This article documents the scientific evidence that the Neira 4 L technique will make a valuable contribution to plastic surgery by decreasing the surgical risk, preventing side effects, and improving the quality of life for patients.

Summary

The Neira 4 L technique is less harmful to cells than ultrasound, the VASER, the power cannula, or lipoplasty-assisted liposuction, minimizing their destruction and death. Low-level lasers focus liposuction, protecting the patient's tissues, increasing

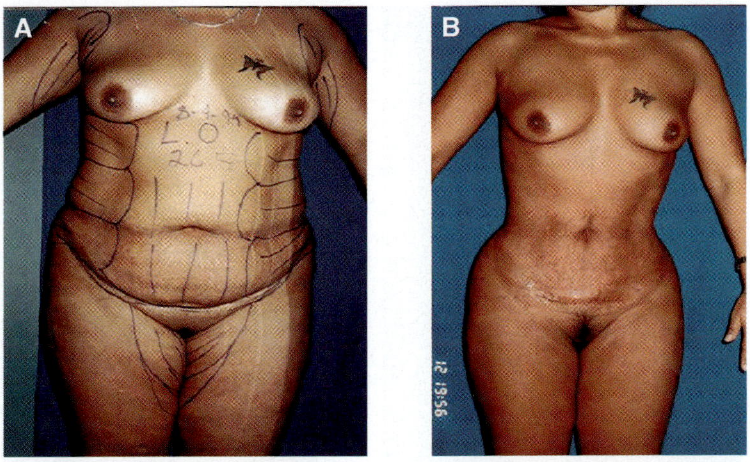

Fig. 9. Low-Level Laser Lipoplasty (LLLL) (Neira 4 L Technique). (*A*) Before and (*B*) after photos of a 26 year-old woman that had 9 liters of fat removed in one procedure.

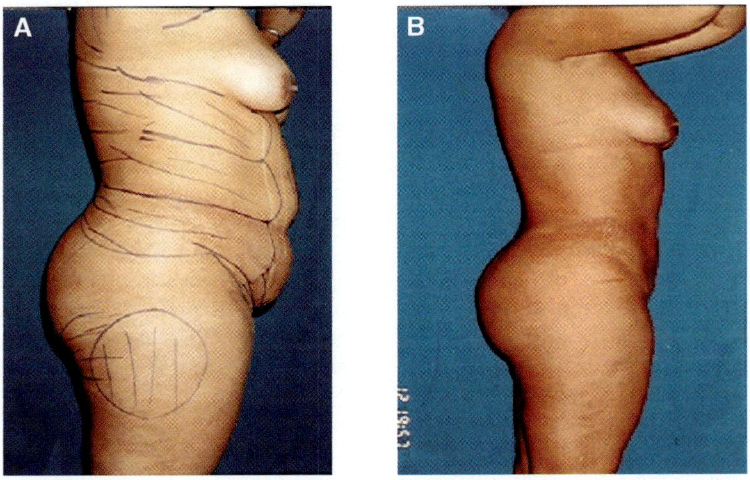

Fig. 10. Low-Level Laser Lipoplasty (LLLL) (Neira 4 L Technique). (*A*) Before and (*B*) after lateral views of a 26 year-old woman.

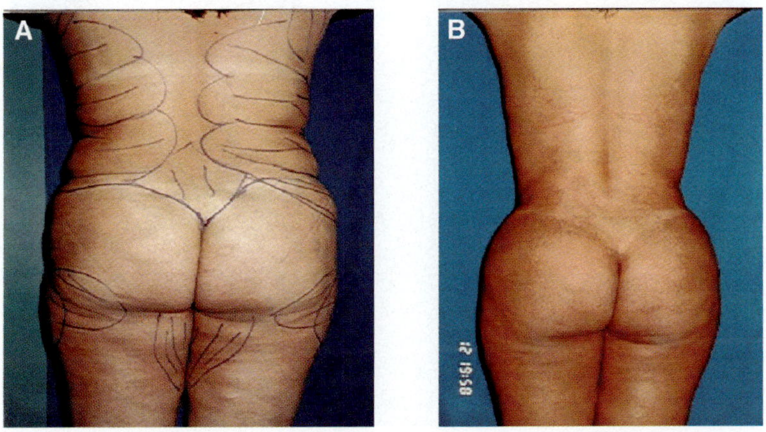

Fig. 11. Low-Level Laser Lipoplasty (LLLL) (Neira 4 L Technique). (*A*) Before and (*B*) after photos.

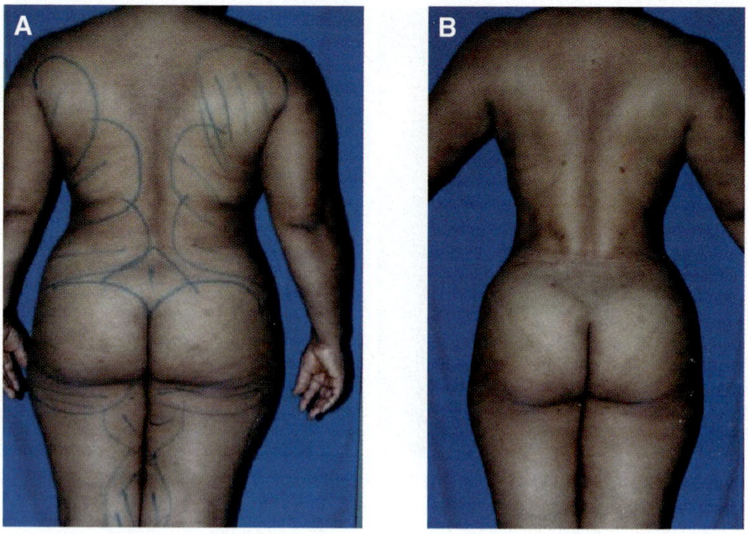

Fig. 12. (*A*) Before surgery and (*B*) after Neira 4 L Technique.

and activating cell mechanisms, and modulating the inflammatory response against surgical trauma. The main benefits of this procedure are improved tissue healing, decreased pain, minimal destruction of cells, improved cicatrization, improved nerve and vessel healing, and decreased risk of neuropathies.

The laser facilitates the formation of a transitory pore exclusively at the level of the adipocyte membrane and the release of fat by disrupting fat panicles and allowing the fat to leak from the cell into the interstitial space outside the cell. With use of ultrawet infiltration as an adjuvant, the remaining interstices are preserved.

This technique may be the precursor of other less aggressive plastic surgery procedures. Follow-up demonstrates adequate medium- and long-term body contouring. Clinical cases before and after LLLL are shown in Figs. 9–16. The patient is not exposed to

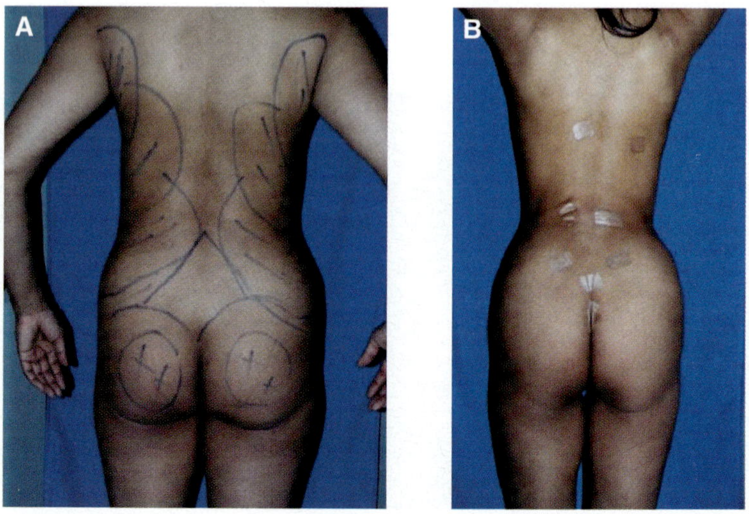

Fig. 13. Corporal liposculpture and gluteal Fat injection (*A*) before and (*B*) after surgery.

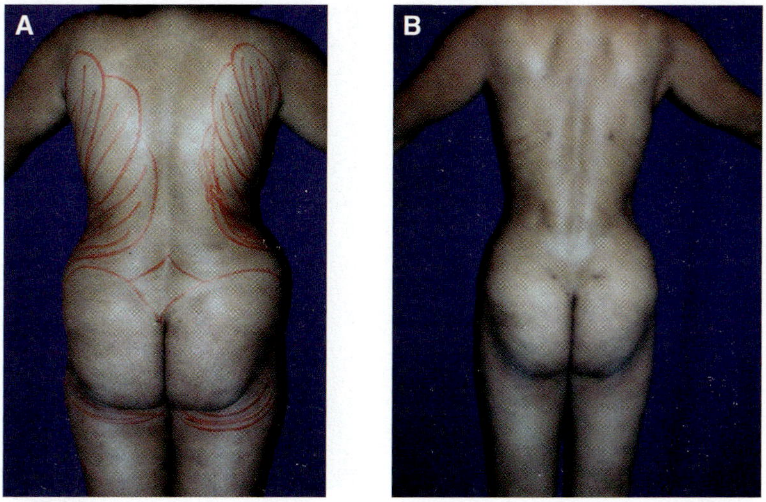

Fig. 14. (*A*) Before and (*B*) after gluteal sculpture, Low Level Laser Lipoplasty.

skin burns, cells are not killed, and adipose tissue is not damaged, which permits the use of irradiated tissue for fat grafts in other parts of the body. The time needed to extract fat seems to be reduced. Surgical trauma, postoperative edema and pain, and medical leave from work are diminished, as are ecchymosis, hematomas, and postoperative fibrosis. The resulting skin surface is even. The results are highly satisfactory for the patient and the surgeon. The technique is simple, easy to apply, and low cost, serving as an excellent adjuvant tool for the surgeon practicing liposculpture. Using LLLL, one may be able to carve the human body based on inspiration, imprinting the surgeon's love in pa-

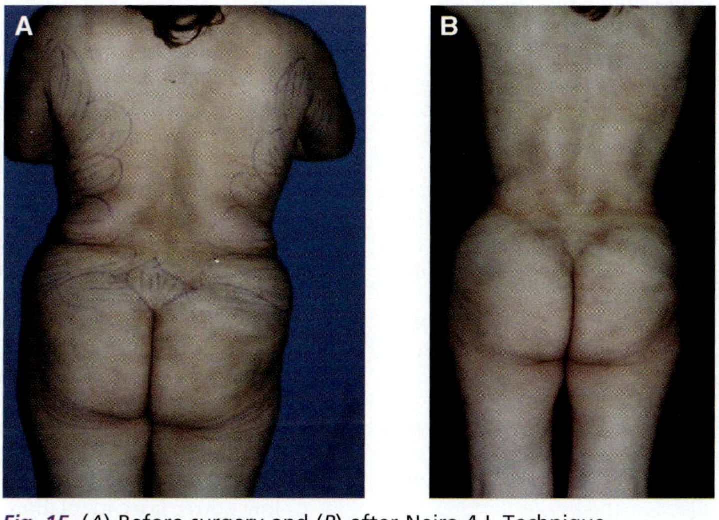

Fig. 15. (*A*) Before surgery and (*B*) after Neira 4 L Technique.

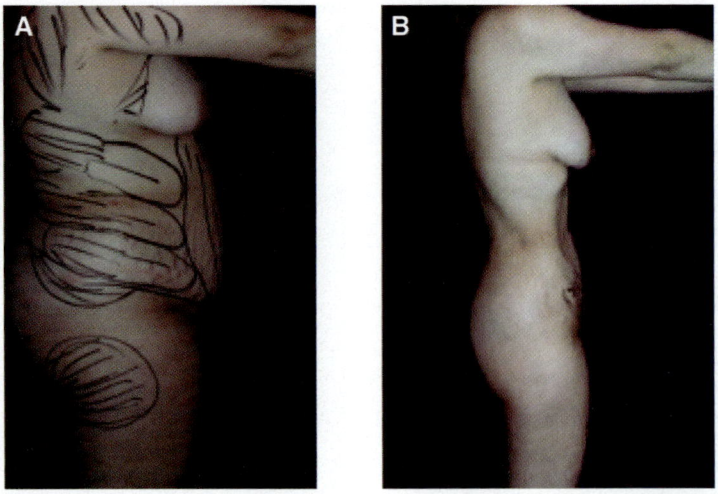

Fig. 16. (*A*) Before surgery and (*B*) after Neira 4L technique. 13 liters of fat were removed.

tients and creating a wonderful human art in plastic surgery.

Acknowledgments

All the surgeries were performed by Electric diode Erchonia laser 637 wave length. Thanks to Mr. Steve Shank for providing the Erchonia Laser machine to perform the surgeries.

References

[1] Sun Sentinel Press. December 14, 2004. Available at: imcvcar@sun-sentinel.com sun-sentinel.com.
[2] Rao RB, Ely SF, Hoffman RS. Deaths related to liposuction. N Engl J Med 1999;340(19):1471–5.
[3] Grazer FM, de Jong RH. Perioperative management of cosmetic liposuction. Plast Reconstr Surg 2000;105(1):436–46.
[4] Hetter GP. Blood and fluid replacement for lipoplasty procedures. Clin Plast Surg 1989;16(2):245–8.
[5] Karu TI, Pyatibrat LV, Afanasyeva NI. A novel mitochondrial signaling pathway activated by visible-to-near infrared radiation. Photochem Photobiol 2004;80(2):366–72.
[6] Manteifel VM, Karu TI. Increase in the number of contacts of endoplasmic reticulum with mitochondria and plasma membrane in yeast cells stimulated to division with He-Ne laser light. Tsitologiia 2004;46(6):498–505.
[7] Karu TI, Piatibrat LV, Kalendo GS. He-Ne laser radiation on the survival of HeLa cells subjected to ionizing radiation. Radiobiological 1992;32(2):202–6.
[8] Karu T, Pyatibrat L, Kalendo G. Irradiation with He-Ne laser increases ATP levels in cells cultivated in vitro. J Photochem Photobiol B 1995;27(3):219–23.
[9] Passarella S, Ostuni A, Atlante A, et al. Increase in the ADP/ATP exchange in rat liver mitochondria irradiated in vitro by helium-neon laser. Biochem Biophys Res Commun 1988;156(2):978–86.
[10] Iaffaldano N, Meluzzi A, Manchisi A, et al. Improvement of stored turkey semen quality as a result of He-Ne laser irradiation. Anim Reprod Sci 2005;85(3–4):317–25.
[11] Warren JB, Wilson AJ, Loi RK, et al. Opposing roles of cyclic AMP in the vascular control of edema formation. FASEB J 1993;7(14):1394–400.
[12] Karu TI, Piatibrat LV, Kalendo GS, et al. Changes in the amount of ATP in HeLa cells under the action of He-Ne laser radiation. Biull Eksp Biol Med 1993;115(6):617–8.
[13] Karu TI, Pyatibrat LV, Kalendo GS. Photobiological modulation of cell attachment via cytochrome C oxidase. Photochem Photobiol Sci 2004;3(2):211–6.
[14] Jimbo K, Noda K, Suzuki K, et al. Suppressive effects of low-power laser irradiation on bradykinin evoked action potentials in cultured murine dorsal root ganglion cells. Neurons Neurosci Lett 1998;240(2):93–6.
[15] Medrado AR, Pugliese LS, Reis SR, et al. Influence of low level laser therapy on wound healing and its biological action upon myofibroblasts. Lasers Surg Med 2003;32(3):239–44.
[16] Battal MN, Hata Y, Matsuka K, et al. Reduction of progressive burn injury by using a new nonselective endothelin-A and endothelin-B receptor antagonist, TAK-044: an experimental study in rats. Plast Reconstr Surg 1997;99(6):1610–9.
[17] Wakabayashi H, Hamba M, Matsumoto K, et al. Effect of irradiation by semiconductor laser on responses evoked in trigeminal caudal neurons by tooth pulp stimulation. Lasers Surg Med 1993;13(6):605–10.
[18] Kasai S, Kono T, Yamamoto Y, et al. Effect of low-power laser irradiation on impulse conduc-

tion in anesthetized rabbits. J Clin Laser Med Surg 1996;14(3):107–9.
[19] Ohno T. Pain suppressive effect of low power laser irradiation: a quantitative analysis of substance P in the rat spinal dorsal root ganglion. Nippon Ika Daigaku Zasshi 1997;64(5):395–400.
[20] Zhu L, Li C, Ji C, et al. The effect of laser irradiation on arthritis in rats. Zhen Ci Yan Jiu 1990;15(1):71–6.
[21] Belkin M, Schwartz M. New biological phenomena associated with laser radiation. Health Phys 1989;56(5):687–90.
[22] Anders MM, Borke RC, Woolery SK, et al. Low power laser irradiation alters the rate of regeneration of the rat facial nerve. Lasers Surg Med 1993;13(1):72–82.
[23] Rochkind S, Nissan M, Lubart R. A single transcutaneous light irradiation to injured peripheral nerve: a comparative study with five different wavelengths. Lasers in Medical Science 1989;4: 259–63.
[24] Capon A, Souil E, Gauthier B, et al. Laser assisted skin closure (LASC) by using 815-nm diode laser system accelerates and improves wound healing. Laser Surg Med 2001;28(2):168–75.
[25] Karu TI, Pyatibrat LV, Kalendo GS, et al. Effects of monochromatic low-intensity light and laser irradiation on adhesion of HeLa cells in vitro. Lasers Surg Med 1996;18(2):171–7.
[26] Karu TI, Piatibrat LV, Kalendo GS. The effect of He-Ne laser irradiation on the adhesive properties of the cell membranes. Int J Radiat Biol Med 1993;115(6):622–3.
[27] Neira R, Rebolledo AF, Solarte E, et al. Diffraction and dispersion of coherent light in adipose tissue. Revista Colombiana de Fisica 2002;33(1):191–5.
[28] Neira R, Arroyave J, Solarte E, et al. In vitro culture of adipose cells after irradiating them with a low level laser device. Presented at the II Congreso Bolivariano de Cirugia Plastica Reconstructiva, Peru, October 8–11, 2001.
[29] Neira R, Solarte E, Isaza C, et al. Effects of the electric laser diode beam on in vitro human adipose tissue culture. Presented at the II Congreso Bolivariano de Cirugia Plastica Reconstructiva, Peru, October 8–11, 2001.
[30] Kolárová H, Ditrichová D, Wagner J. Penetration of the laser light into the skin in vitro. Lasers Surg Med 1999;24:231–5.
[31] Neira R, Arroyave J, Ramirez H, et al. Fat liquefaction: effect of low-level laser energy on adipose tissue. Plast Reconstr Surg 2002;110(3):912–22.
[32] Solarte E, Isaza C, Criollo W, et al. In vitro effects of 635 nm low intensity diode laser irradiation on the fat distribution of one adipose cell. SPIE Proc 2002;4829(2):961.
[33] Reyes MA, Rebolledo AF, Montoya JA, et al. Dispersion de Luz Coherente Por Muestras De Tejido Adiposo. Revista Colombiana de Fisica 2001; 33(2):325.
[34] Solarte E, Gutierrez O, Neira R, et al. Laser-induced lipolysis on adipose cells. SPIE Proc 2004;5622:5–10.
[35] Solarte E, Reyes A, Montoya J, et al. Efectos de la Irradiation con luz LASER in los Espectros de Transmission de Diluciones de Adipocitos II. Revista Colombiana de Fisica 2002;34(1). Available at: http://calima.univalle.edu.co/revista/Eng/index.htm.
[36] Neira R, Ortiz C. Low level laser assisted liposculpture: clinical report of 700 cases. Aesthetic Surg J 2002;22(5):451–5.
[37] Neira R, Toledo L, Zafra D, et al. Serum lidocaine levels in low level laser assisted liposculpture: Neira 4L technique, ultrawet technique. Revista Colombiana de Cirugia Plastica 2003;9(1):38–47.
[38] Neira R, Arroyave J, Ramirez H, et al. Low level laser assisted lipoplasty: a new technique. Can J Plastic Surg 2002;10(3):131.
[39] Rebolledo AF, Reyes MA, Montoya JA, et al. Difraccion Y Dispersion De Luz Coherente Por Difractores Aleatorios y su Aplicacion a la Dispersion Por Tejido Adiposo. Revista Colombiana de Fisica 2002;34(10):191.
[40] Brown SA, Rohrich RJ, Kenkel J, et al. Effect of low-level laser therapy on abdominal adipocytes before lipoplasty procedures. Plast Reconstr Surg 2004;113(6):1796–804.

CLINICS IN PLASTIC SURGERY

Clin Plastic Surg 33 (2006) 129–163

Complications of Liposuction

Yves Gérard Illouz, MD

In 1977, I developed tunneling lipoplasty to reduce the invasiveness of body-contouring surgery [1,2]. I believed that this technique was simple, effective, devoid of major hazards, and reproducible. In my hands (and for several years I was the only person who used this technique), none of the adverse events that potentially are associated with tissue undermining occurred. I used a blunt cannula that spared the vessels and nerves to avoid bleeding, seromas, infection, and necrosis. To avoid "systemic" complications that are related to removal of a large amount of fat, I set the safety threshold at 3000 mm^3. Conversely, there clearly was a risk of unsatisfactory cosmetic outcomes, most notably at body sites that I subsequently described as "unforgiving." This preamble shows that adverse events that are associated with liposuction fall into two groups.

Surgical and systemic complications

Poor cosmetic outcomes

Surgical complications

Early attempts to remove body fat resulted in complications, some of which were devastating. Calf reduction surgery was first attempted in 1922 by Dujarrier, who removed a spindle-shaped piece of subcutaneous fat, and then closed the wound with a tension suture that caused compression of the femoral artery [3]. Necrosis developed, and amputation of the leg was required. This disaster prompted the first malpractice lawsuit in the history of cosmetic surgery. In 1972, Schrudde [4,5] described a procedure that involved the use of a uterine curette to scrape off subcutaneous fat [**Fig. 1**]. The results were poor, and the technique was abandoned. In 1977, Fischer [6] used a suction pump to remove fat from the saddlebag area. The fat was cut away from the overlying skin and underlying muscle using a large guided scalpel. The fat was minced by a powered blade that was reminiscent of a miniature guillotine before suction [**Fig. 2**]. In 1978, Kesselring and Meyer [7] used a sharp, double-bladed, large diameter, nonpowered curette [**Fig. 3**], which was connected to a suction pump, to remove fat that had been cut away from the over- and underlying tissues using long scissors. In 1981, Teimourian and Fisher [8] reported performing fat removal with a cutting instrument that was derived from the fascia lata stripper and was similar to the Kesselring curette.

With these techniques, cutting instruments are used to achieve complete detachment of the sub-

Department of Plastic and Aesthetic Surgery, Saint-Louis Hospital 14 Boulevard Suchet, 75016 Paris, France
E-mail address: ygillouz@hotmail.com

0094-1298/06/$ – see front matter
doi:10.1016/j.cps.2005.10.001
plasticsurgery.theclinics.com

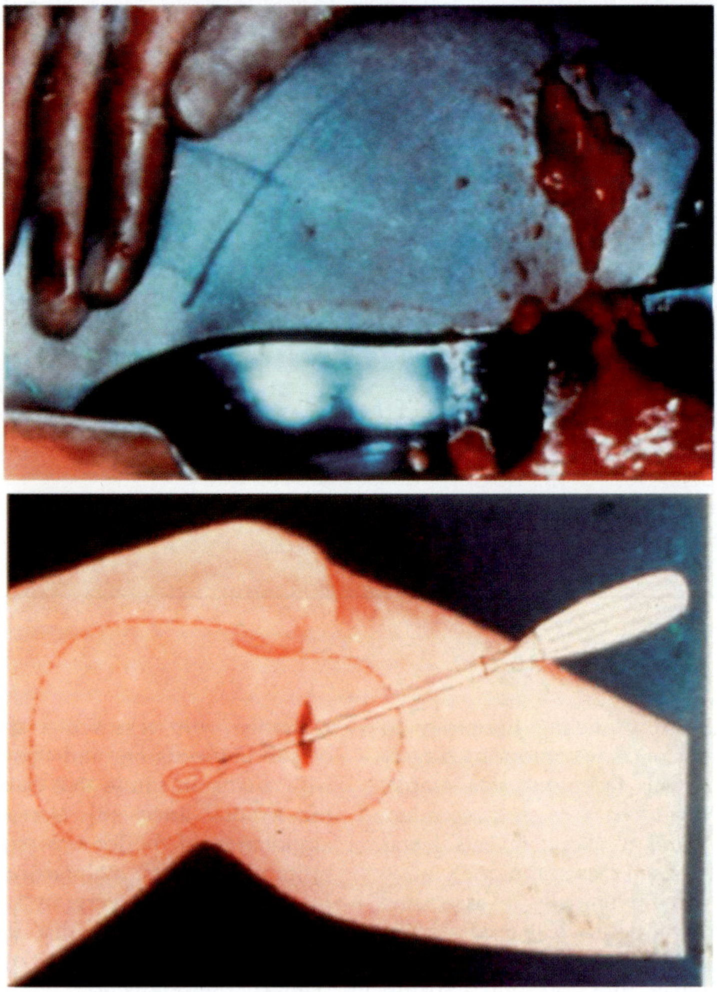

Fig. 1. The publication by Schrudde (1972) describing lipectomy using a uterine curette.

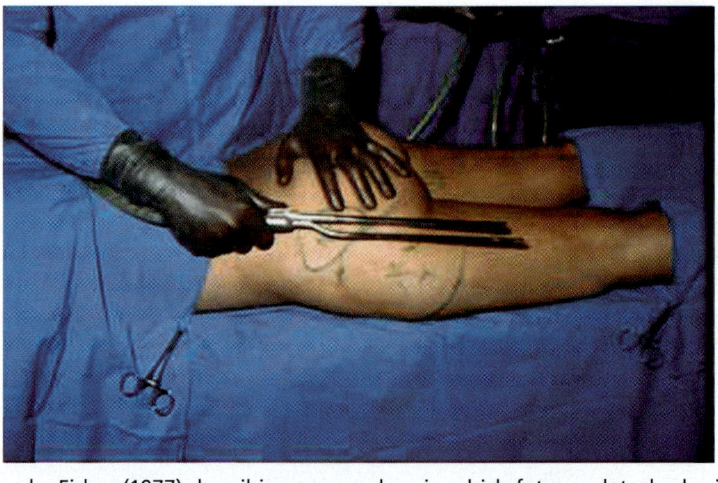

Fig. 2. The publication by Fisher (1977) describing a procedure in which fat was detached using a guided cutting blade, and then minced by a machine.

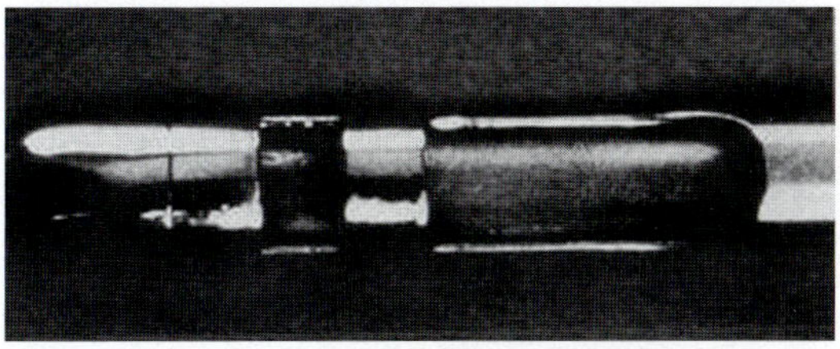

Fig. 3. The Kesselring (1978) curette with a 2-cm long cutting blade.

cutaneous fat layer; however, complete fat detachment can cause many complications, some of which are devastating. Complete fat detachment without visual guidance does not allow hemostasis, and can trigger a cascade of events that lead from hematoma or sero-hematoma to infection [9], necrosis, shock, and even death.

Serous fluid may collect in a cavity that is created by fat detachment [10]. The fluid fails to coagulate, and the collection recurs after aspiration. The cavity undergoes pseudoepithelialization (similar to the capsules surrounding breast implants), which precludes per primam wound healing. The skin slides over the cavity, and creates a hanging fold on the thigh [**Fig. 4**]. Surgery shows a bursalike structure of variable size [**Figs. 5 and 6**]. Severe bleeding is the rule during surgical correction. Painstaking efforts are needed to obtain harmonious approximation of the tissues.

Cutting-instrument procedures must be confined to small sites that receive a limited blood supply (eg, small saddlebag), because dividing major vessels results in necrosis [**Fig. 7**]. Thus, cutting methods cannot be used to contour the entire body. This is a major drawback compared with the technique that I developed. To reduce the risk of complications, liposuction must be performed without total fat detachment, creation of cavities, side-to-side cannula displacement, or uncontrolled cannula movements.

In 1977, I developed a new technique that was based on the observation that fat detachment was the starting point of all of the complications that were seen after liposuction or conventional saddlebag or abdominoplasty procedures. With this new technique, continuous fat detachment is replaced by discontinuous detachment to spare important subcutaneous structures (ie, blood vessels, lymphatics, nerves). A blunt cannula is used to create tunnels in the fat, which is pulled, rather than cut, away from the neighboring structures. With this technique, connections between the overlying and underlying tissues are preserved. These connections contain vessels that provide the skin with nutrients and contribute to skin elasticity.

The rate of surgical complications is extremely low with the Illouz technique [11]. A few cases of bleeding, seroma, infection, and abdominal perforation occurred at the beginning of the learning curve, but these complications were not seen later. The technique proved to be reliable and virtually risk-free. It rapidly gained widespread acceptance throughout the world as a means of contouring all sites of the female body. Surgical complications remained exceedingly rare until 1992, when several devastating events were reported, including shock, burns, necrosis, death on the operating table, and death during the postoperative course [12,13].

These catastrophic complications were unacceptable for a cosmetic procedure, and they negatively affected the reputation of liposuction. Most of

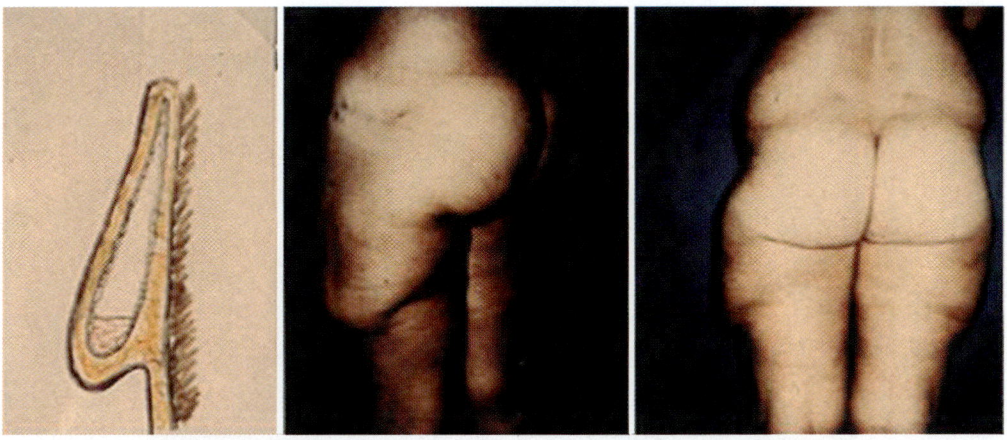

Fig. 4. Hanging folds. Cutting techniques create large cavities that fill rapidly with noncoagulable serous fluid. The effusion recurs after aspiration. As a result, the surfaces undergo epithelialization, which precludes per primam healing. These cavities are similar to the capsules that develop around breast implants. With time, the skin slides over the underlying tissues, and creates hanging folds.

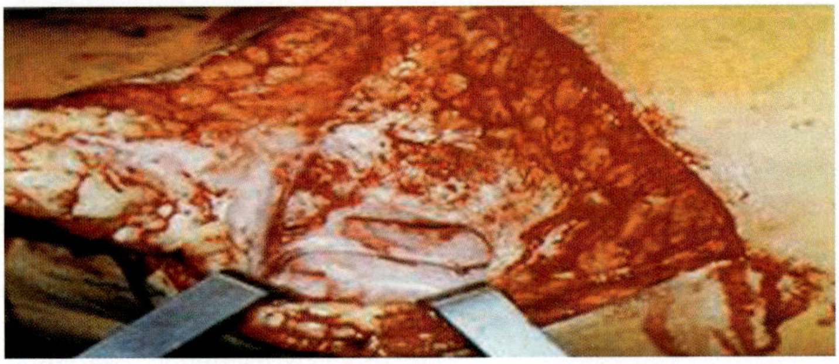

Fig. 5. Small epithelialized cavity discovered during surgery.

them occurred in the United States after the development of so-called "new" techniques [14], which were inappropriate modification of the Illouz technique, without regard for the restrictions that I set. These modifications included:

- The tumescent technique [15,16]
- Injection of an ice-cold solution
- Large-volume liposuction, which has been associated with severe shock, pulmonary embolism, and crush syndrome (exceedingly rare)
- Excessively tight compression garments, which were responsible for thrombus formation and pulmonary embolism
- Ultrasound-assisted liposuction, which can cause burns and necrosis
- Subdermal liposuction, which causes poor cosmetic outcomes rather than surgical complications, although necrosis from damage to the subcutaneous vascular arcade may occur when large sites are treated

The wet technique As early as 1977 to 1978, I recommended hydrodissection by injection of an aqueous solution [1]. Hydrodissection is used widely in plastic surgery. With my method, the amount to be injected was equal to the amount of fat to be removed (eg, removal of a saddlebag estimated at 300 mL called for injection of 300 mL of solution). The initial formula was as follows: to 1000 mL of isotonic saline, add 200 mL of distilled water and 1000 IU of hyaluronidase to ensure prompt diffusion. I later recommended the addition of 0.1 mg of adrenaline [17] and 500 mg of lidocaine when local anesthesia was desired [17].

With this technique, I consistently obtained a flowing fat suspension that contained no more than 5% blood [Fig. 8] [18]. In addition, the procedure was simple and minimally traumatic. In 1987, several dermatologists introduced modifications to convert liposuction into an office-based procedure, for doctors with no hospital privileges in the United States [19]. The Klein local formula anesthesia consisted of using large volumes of dilute anesthetic solution containing lidocaine (0.05%), epinephrine (1:1,000,000), and sodium bicarbonate (12.5 mEq/L). Because dermatologists were not allowed to keep patients overnight, one

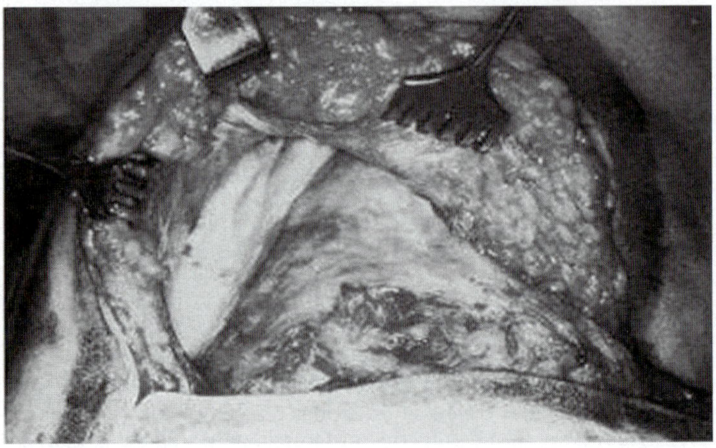

Fig. 6. Large epithelialized cavity that required removal to allow healing by approximation of raw surfaces. Cavity removal typically is associated with severe bleeding.

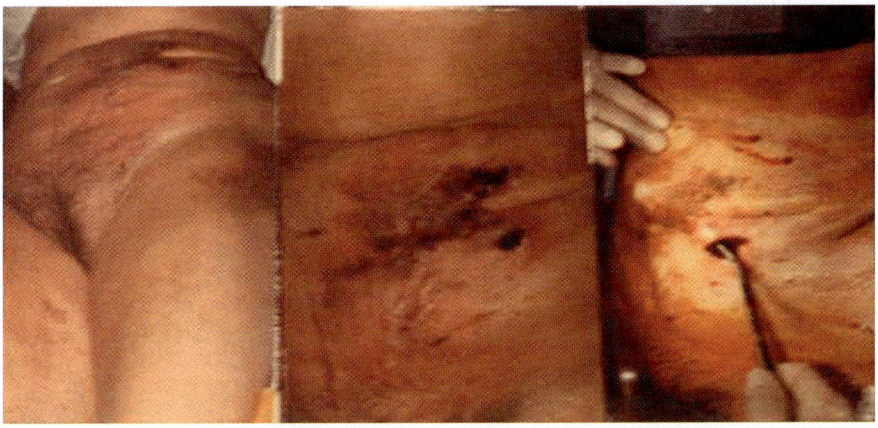

Fig. 7. Necrosis after uncontrolled scythelike movements of the cannula that were responsible for blood vessel damage.

of their goals was to ensure that patients could return home on the evening of the procedure. They used large amounts of solution to reduce pain and blood loss. In addition, they hoped that the abundance of fluid would allow them to remove larger amounts of fat on an outpatient basis. They used a ratio of 3:1 (eg, removal of 4 L of fat required the injection of 12 L of solution). The formula was similar to mine, with a small amount of bicarbonate added. Numerous studies sought to establish the safety of these massive amounts of fluid that contained unusually high doses of local anesthetics and adrenaline [20]. These studies failed to direct appropriate attention to idiosyncrasy, and to the cumulative effects of the fluid and vasoconstrictors. Complications occurred, such as acute pulmonary edema, which was fatal in a few patients [21]. I have identified a few dozen cases in the world.

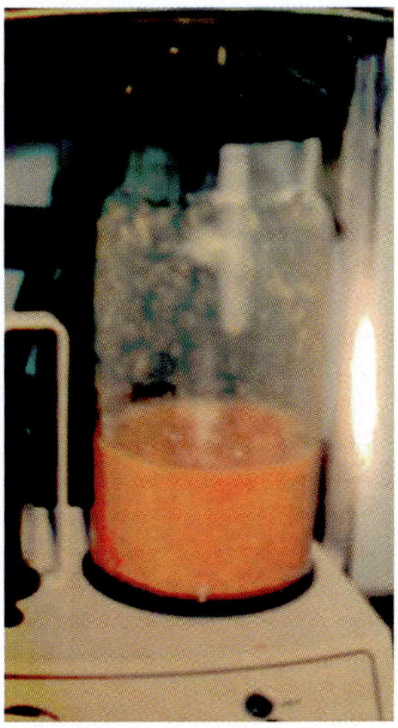

Fig. 8. Blood-free aspirate.

Recent comparative studies established that the best solution/fat ratio was 1:1 to 1.5:1 [22]. Smaller amounts of solution were not effective, and larger amounts failed to provide benefits and were associated with complications. Presently, the 1:1 to 1.5:1 ratio is accepted widely.

The adjective "tumescent" has become popular, and is used for all liposuction methods that involve injection of a wetting solution—as opposed to the dry technique, which is no longer used. Definitions for these terms vary in the medical literature. Many surgeons use "tumescent" to describe any kind of wet technique, whatever the quantity.

The four liposuction techniques include [23]:

Dry: no fluid is injected into the fat layer before suctioning. Approximately 25% to 45% of the aspirated volume is blood [24].

Wet: I pioneered this technique in the early 1980s. Before suctioning, 1 to 1 of saline distilled water and hyaluronidase solution is infused. The aspirated blood volume is decreased to 10% to 25% of the total aspirate. Hetter and Herhahn's [25] addition of 1 to 1,000,000 to the solution in 1983 reduced blood loss even more. Less than 5% of the aspirate was blood.

Superwet: this technique was devised in the late 1980s. It consists of an infusion of fluid containing epinephrine and low doses of local anesthetic in a 1:1½ ratio to the volume of expected aspirate. Blood loss was reduced to approximately 4% to 5% of the aspirated volume [26] like on the wet technique of Illouz.

Tumescent: Klein described this technique in 1987. Large volumes of saline containing 1:100,000 epinephrine and 0.05% lidocaine were injected subcutaneously before suctioning until the tissues were tense. The injected fluid volume could reach a 3:1 ratio, greater than what would be suctioned.

Injection of ice-cold solution Initially, injection of ice-cold solution was advocated; however, this technique induced tremor and shock, and some patients required major resuscitation [27]. In addition, using ice-cold solution failed to decrease the pain or the blood loss, because the time needed for suction was longer than the duration of the cold-induced response. Reactive vasodilation occurred, which induced a risk of bleeding.

Large-volume liposuction Large-volume liposuction with injection of massive amounts of solution was "marketed" by doctors who also advocated dry liposuction [28], injection of ice-cold solution, and even tumescent liposuction, despite the contradictions among these methods. Several doctors proudly stated that they removed up to 20 L or even 25 L of fat [29]. Complications were reported shortly after. A string of fatal events occurred, with several dozen deaths in all, most of them in the United States (the only country that publishes reliable statistics) [30].

How much fat removal is too much? In 1981, I stated that removing more than 3000 mL might carry a risk of severe systemic complications that require resuscitation and blood transfusion. Such complications would be unacceptable for a cosmetic procedure, particularly one that was intended to be simple; however, over the next 20 years, major improvements occurred in anesthesiology and in liposuction techniques. The absolute volume is no longer the only relevant factor. Factors that affect the risk of complications include the volume of fat removed, the surface area of the treated site, the amount of blood lost, and the patient's body weight.

A critical appraisal of all reported cases of deaths and nonfatal complications indicates that the amount of fat removed should not exceed 6% to 8% of the patient's body weight and 30% of the patient's body surface area. Blood loss should not exceed 1 unit, or at the most, 1.5 units. In addition, the patient should not be turned during the procedure [**Figs. 9 and 10**].

The amount of fat that can removed can be increased slightly when the fat is free of blood and comes from a single body site (eg, a massively adipose abdomen). When removal of a larger amount of fat is required, the procedure should be performed in two or three steps. Patients accept the need for several steps readily if they are informed properly [31,32]. They should be told that locally, removal of an excessive amount in a single step would not allow for appropriate redraping of the skin. They also should be told that regarding systemic complications, single-step removal of large volumes carries a major risk of blood transfusion, which can transmit the AIDS virus, hepatitis viruses, or other pathogens. Often patients are unwilling to consider autotransfusion

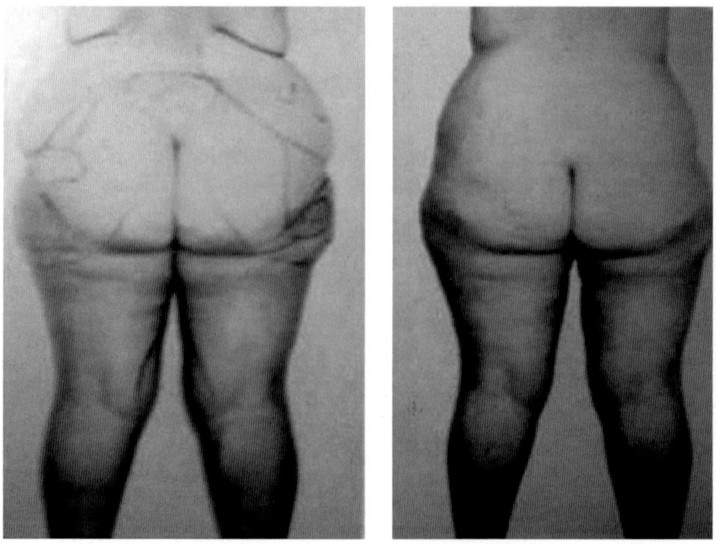

Fig. 9. Removal of 4 kg of fat followed by weight loss of 10 kg in a patient who had obesity.

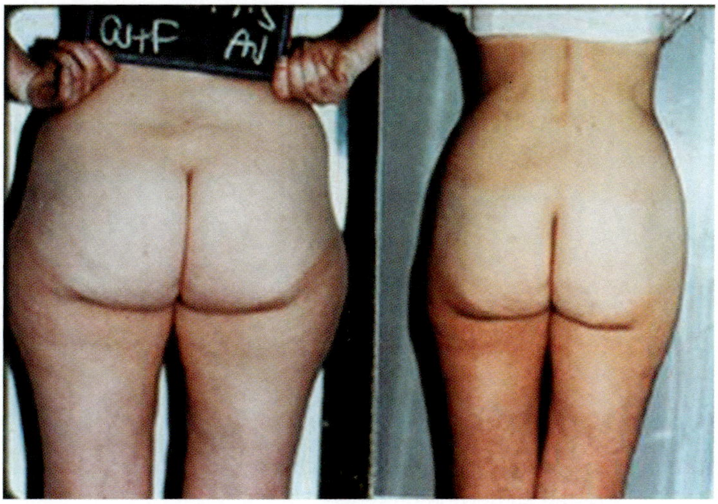

Fig. 10. Removal of 5 kg of fat followed by weight loss of 9 kg.

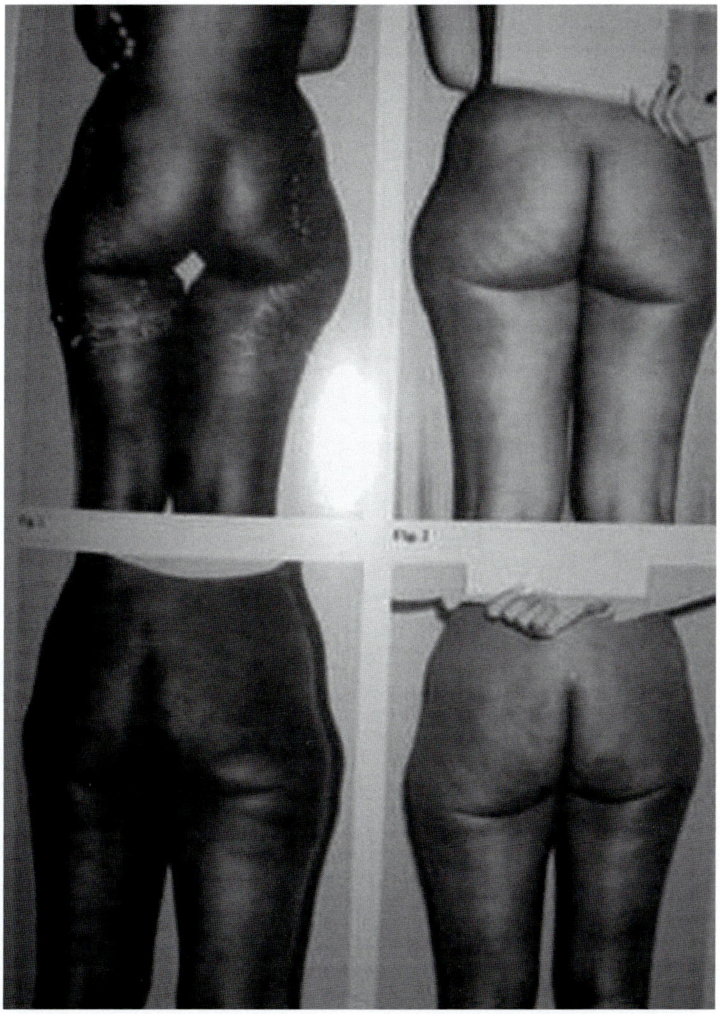

Fig. 11. Two-step liposuction procedure. Step 1 (top), removal of 3 kg of fat; step 2 (bottom), removal of 3 kg of fat 6 months later. Sustained improvement after 9 years.

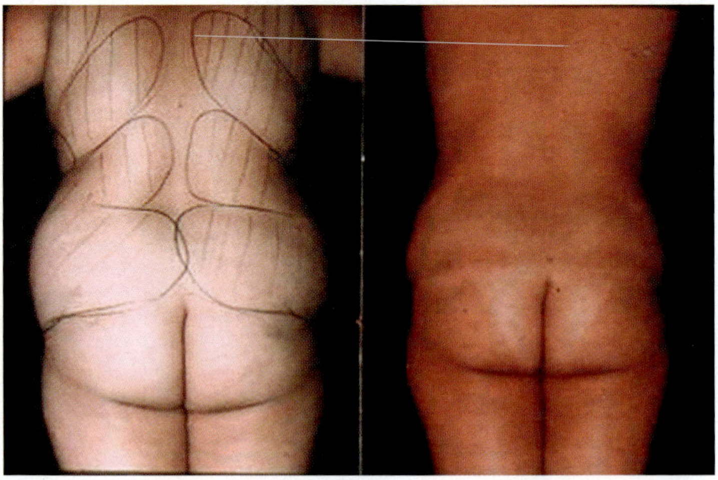

Fig. 12. Two-step liposuction procedure.

for a cosmetic procedure, and their perception of autotransfusion as appropriate for major surgery tends to dampen their enthusiasm for liposuction. These rules produce very good results [**Figs. 11 and 12**] [1].

Causes of severe morbidity and death Crush syndrome first was described in the United Kingdom during the London blitz. In individuals who had no visible injuries, but who had been trapped under fallen masonry, release from the rubble was followed within a few hours by shock with severe hypotension, anuria, coma, and death in the absence of treatment. During liposuction, the numerous tunnels that are created through the fat constitute a mechanism of subcutaneous injury that is similar to crush syndrome. Third-space fluid loss, which is responsible for an abrupt decrease in blood volume may occur, and produces severe symptoms [33]. Hemoglobin is released into the bloodstream. Classic crush syndrome is characterized by muscle tissue disintegration with release of myoglobin, which is toxic for the renal glomerule. Although this is a key difference from liposuction, uncontrolled cannula movements may cause muscle injury, and creation of numerous crisscrossed tunnels may produce large cavities that expand the third space [34]. Treatment consists solely of massive fluid resuscitation to restore the blood volume. Physicians should be alert to the possibility of crush syndrome in patients who have oliguria, because progression to anuria may be rapid. Prophylactic fluid management before, during, and after the procedure is crucial [35].

Burn syndrome may develop when a large surface area is treated [36]. Surface area affects the risk of burn syndrome, the complications, and their severity.

Edema of the lungs may develop when a large amount of fluid is injected subcutaneously or intravenously [37]. The total volume injected should be computed.

Hypothermia can cause severe disorders [38]. Ice-cold fluids increase the risk of hypothermia. Ideally, injected solutions should be warmed to the temperature of the body. Excessive cooling of the operating room may cause hypothermia in the patient (surgeons often feel hot and request temperatures that are too cold for the patients).

Fortunately, fat embolism is uncommon [38]. The underlying mechanism is chemical, rather than mechanical. Severe shock results in the release of catecholamines, which cleave triglycerides into smaller molecules that are capable of crossing the capillary wall. A mushlike substance, which is composed of fatty acids, may be visible in the lungs or brain. The excess of circulating fatty acids causes acidosis and vasoconstriction of the pulmonary arteries, with increased capillary permeability. Often, the presenting symptom is respiratory distress of sudden onset; however, the only diagnostic manifestation, lipiduria, may not be present [39]. Treatment consists of resuscitation to correct the shock. Intravenous alcohol administration has not been proved to be effective (F.M. Grazer, MD, Board Certified Plastic Surgeon, personal communication, 1989).

Tight compression garments and thromboembolism During the first few years, I used semicircular compressive dressings that were made from strips of elastic bandage. I placed the first strips vertically to lift the skin over the thigh. On top of this, I placed horizontal strips to reduce the edema, bruising, and pain. Thromboembolism that was due to deep vein thrombosis did not occur with these semicircular bandages. In addition, I allowed the patients to ambulate early—1 day or even 6 hours after the procedure. The pain that was caused by removal of the dressings sometimes was more severe than the pain that was due to the procedure itself [Fig. 13].

The introduction of compressive garments for use after liposuction has been associated with pulmonary embolism that is due to thrombosis of the lower limb or iliac vein, which is caused by excessive pressure on the proximal thigh and pelvis [40]. Pressure within the veins is 24 mm Hg. Compression with less than 18 mm Hg is ineffective, and pressures of 22 mm Hg or more can cause thrombosis [41]. Few garments produce compression forces in the 18 to 22 mm Hg range. In addition, treatment sites have complex shapes; a garment may be too loose in one place and too tight in another [Fig. 14]. I have adopted a prudent and empiric approach. I ask the patient to bring three sizes of compressive undergarments. It is extremely difficult to put a compressive garment on in the operating room while the patient is lying on the table; the conjoined efforts of up to three people may be needed. In addition, a patient who is still under the effect of the anesthesia cannot complain if the garment is too tight. Therefore, I wait until the patient is fully awake, able to stand, and capable of putting on the garment herself, with the help of a nurse. I ask whether the garment is too tight and, if needed, I recommend a larger size or make cuts in the garment (often at the calf or ankle). The patient can return the unused sizes to the pharmacist. She is told that edema or pink discoloration of the foot within the first few days requires immediate removal of the garment and a visit to the surgeon. None of my patients has experienced thromboembolism. A single patient who had a history of varicose veins complained of leg pain; however, a Doppler study found no evidence of venous obstruction. No compressive garment is better than an ill-fitting compressive garment.

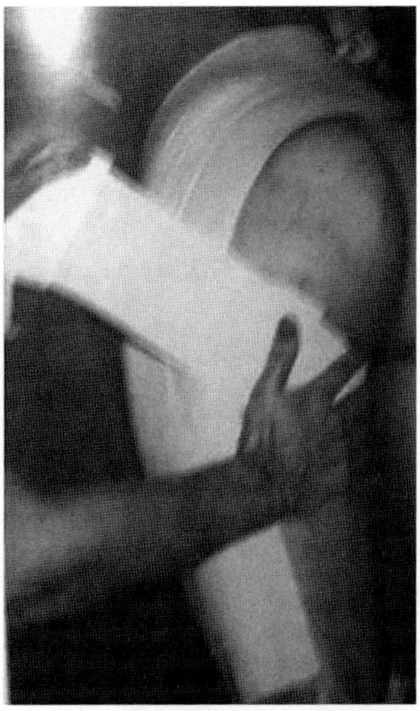

Fig. 13. Semicircular bandages used initially by the author. The bandages did not cause venous compression. No cases of pulmonary embolism occurred.

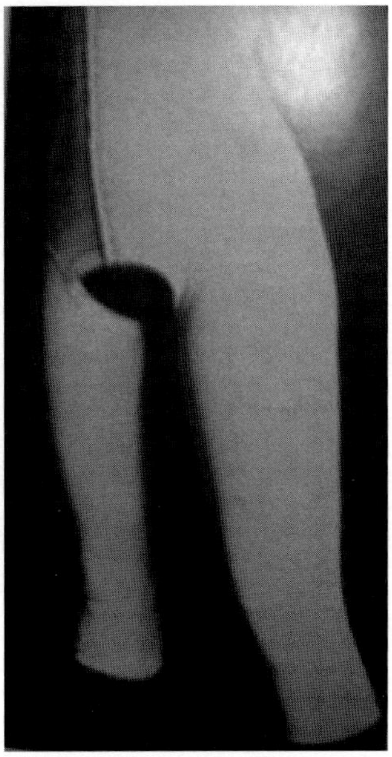

Fig. 14. Currently used compressive garments should be fitted with care to avoid venous compression.

Ultrasound I started to study ultrasound in 1988 after seeing an ophthalmology device that simultaneously pulverized and aspirated the lens. I asked the manufacturer (Cataract Center, San Diego, California) to make a device that would have the same effect on fat. The device, called Ultravac, was ready that same year. I tested it for 1 year, often in the presence of numerous observers. I was impressed by how easier and softer the procedure was in addition to producing good results. I was always in favor of the idea, but was afraid of the heat of the machines and the present results. Now, 15 years later, I have not changed my mind; the devices on the market are either dangerous or useless.

The main advantages of ultrasound are selectivity for adipose tissue and an ability to pulverize fat in vitro. These effects are replicated in vivo, provided the tissue is immersed in aqueous fluid. Dry tissue fragments, however small, are "burned" immediately [42]. Studies have shown that contact with the hypodermis can cause a burn in-

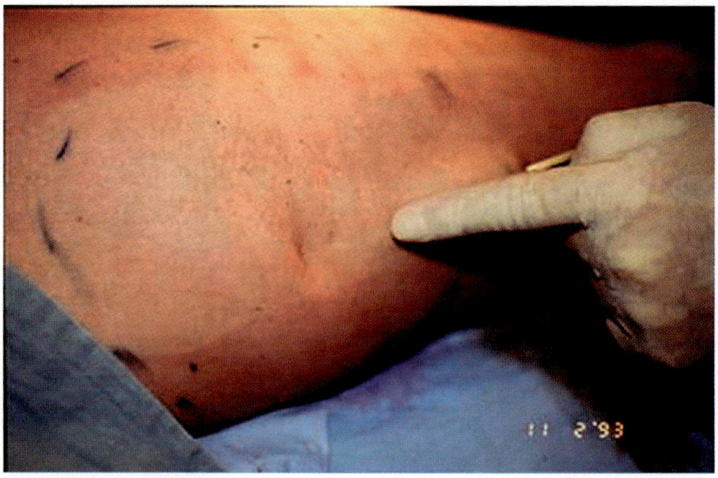

Fig. 15. Small burn caused by the ultrasound probe after more than 10 seconds of contact with the dermis.

jury [43]. In one study, various ultrasound devices were compared with conventional liposuction [44]. In each patient, the same surgeon used ultrasound-assisted liposuction on one side and conventional liposuction on the other. Postoperative pain, bruising, and edema were similar on the two sides. The only difference was a substantial increase in operating time with ultrasound—nearly twice the time required for the conventional procedure. Long-term outcomes were identical with the two techniques.

These data raise the issue of the potential benefits of ultrasound. Ultrasound may be useful for treating fibrotic tissue (touch-ups in men) or the breasts (gynecomastia or selective destruction of intraglandular fat in the female breast) [45]; however, these limited benefits fail to compensate for the major disadvantages which include:

Burns, ranging from small entry-site burns [**Fig. 15**] to extensive burns

Extensive necrosis on the seventh postoperative day as a result of injury to the perforating arteries or superficial arcades. Both complications have been reported by experienced surgeons who specialized in the use of ultrasound [**Figs. 16 and 17**] [41].

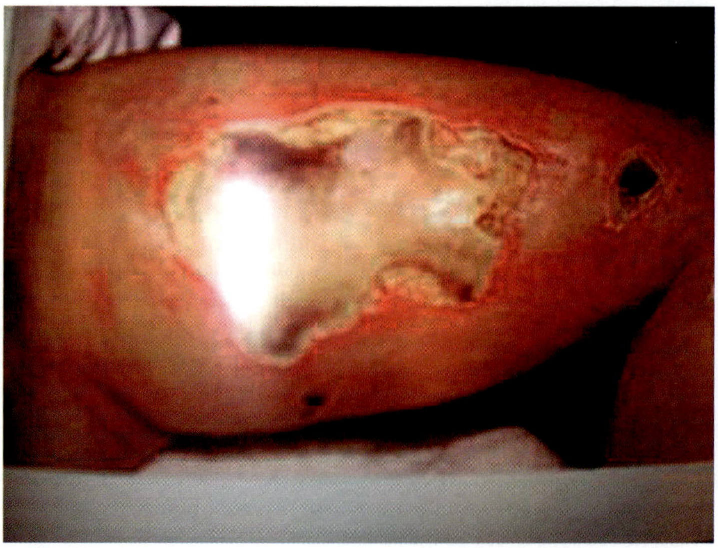

Fig. 16. Extensive necrosis caused by destruction of the perforating arteries during ultrasound lipoplasty.

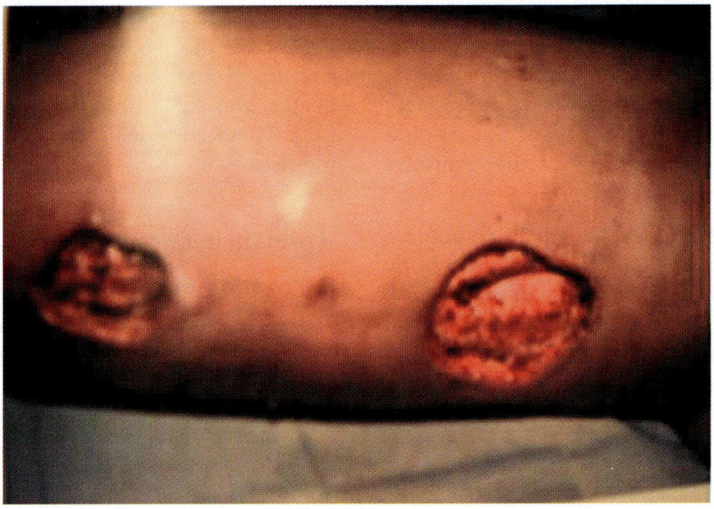

Fig. 17. Foci of necrosis caused by ultrasound-induced burns.

Superficial ultrasound application can leave residual abnormalities [Fig. 18]:

- Hyperesthesia, which is extremely unpleasant and long-lasting (often 2 years), ascribable to ultrasound-induced damage to the phospholipids in protective nerve sheaths
- Redness and cyanosis of the treated sites and lower limbs, caused by injury to the superficial capillaries
- Permanent pigmentation related to subdermal tattooing

The advantages of ultrasound are outweighed by the considerable risks. Furthermore, even if these risks could be eliminated, the limited advantages would not justify the longer time and the higher cost that is needed for ultrasound-assisted liposuction, compared with conventional liposuction.

Superficial liposuction Superficial liposuction was introduced by Gasparoti in 1992 [46]. Initially, fat was removed from the subdermal area; however, the complications that were generated by this technique have led to a consensus that 5 mm of tissue should be left under the dermis. Subdermal fat removal can cause local damage to the blood vessels. Although necrosis does not occur consistently, livid or purplish discoloration of the skin with a visible network of blood vessels may develop [47]. These changes are more prominent in the dependent position. The patients report discomfort, often with pain and a sensation of heaviness in the leg.

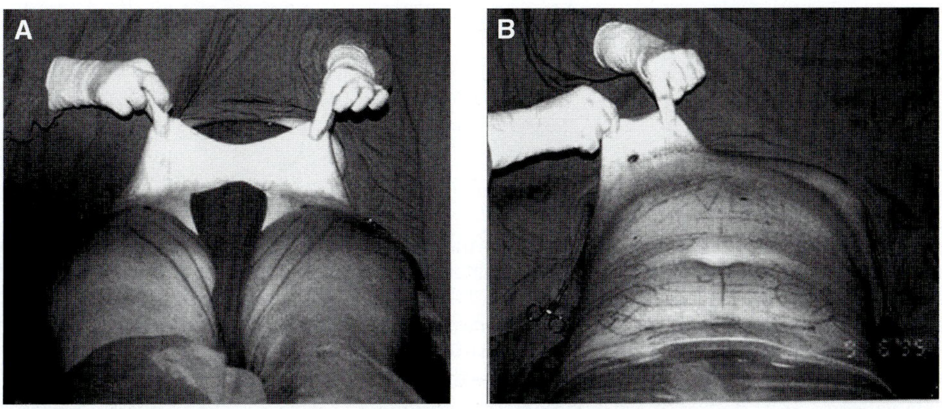

Fig. 18. (*A,B*). Subdermal ultrasound-assisted fat removal. This technique causes numerous complications that are due to destruction of the subcutaneous capillaries and sensory nerve myelin sheaths. The complications include cyanosis and dysesthesia (burning or electric sensations) with unbearable pain in response to the lightest touch.

The symptoms are severely incapacitating and extremely unsightly.

At the 2005 Congress of EPRAS in Vienna, Gasparotti's assistant (who presented Gasparotti's paper for him) admitted that 8 mm of fat should be left under the skin, a thickness that I always have advocated.

Combinations of risk factors Clearly, high-volume liposuction that exceeds 7% of the patient's body weight, and that is performed using an ultrasound-assisted technique, with subdermal fat removal and injection of large volumes of ice-cold solution that contains high doses of epinephrine, in an operating room that is too cold, with an operating time that is longer than 3 hours, and turning of the patient on the table results in an extremely high risk. Combinations of risk factors can explain the deaths that have been reported with liposuction [48]. These combinations do not add, but multiply risks.

Cosmetic sequelae

Description of cosmetic sequelae

The most common and least serious cosmetic sequelae consist of harmonious undercorrection; asymmetry; residual bulge [Fig. 19], large- or small-step contour deformity, common over the ankles; and

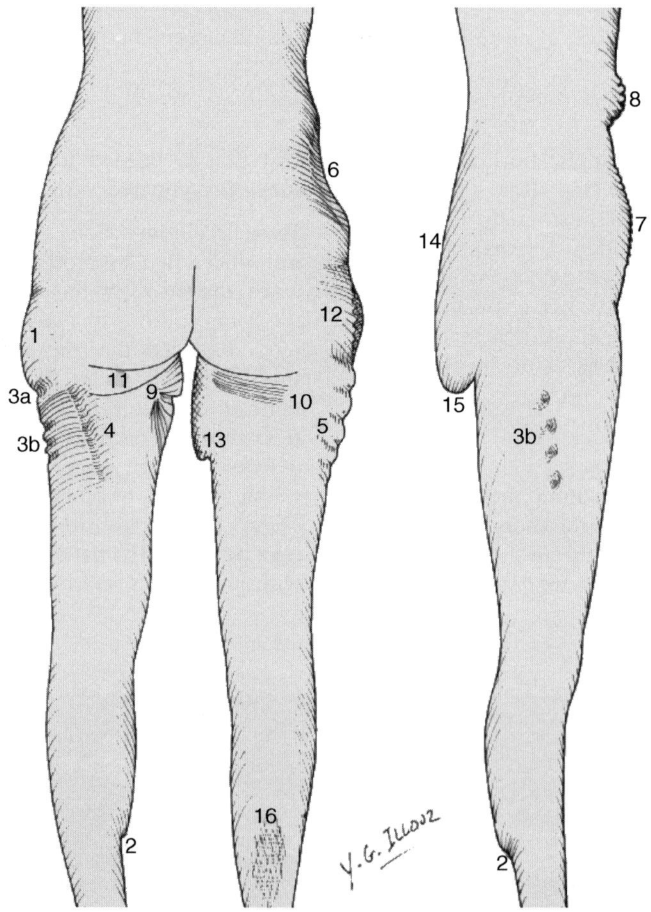

Fig. 19. Schematic representation of the various defects that may result after adipoaspiration. **1** – Residual bulge; **2** – Stair-step deformity, frequent in the ankles; **3a** – Solitary dimple; **3b** – Multiple dimples, with gaps often seen along the fascia lata; **4** – Furrow; **5** – Waves; **6** – Crater; **7** – 'French pastry' wrinkling often seen on the abdomen; **8** – Padded, matresslike wrinkling resulting from infraclinic seroma formation, almost exclusively seen in the upper abdomen; **9** – Adhesion to deep, musculoaponeurotic structures that retracts the overlying region; **10** – 'French pastry' wrinkling because of minimal skin excess of a neighboring region after correction of an LFD; **11** – Double gluteal fold ('banana'); **12** – False bulge because of accordionization of excess skin; **13** – Ptosis or 'sliding' as a result of a neglected seroma; **14** – Flat buttocks after overcorrection and disregard of the 'Bermuda Triangle'; **15** – Gluteal ptosis after adipoaspiration of the inferior segment and overcorrection; **16** – Residual pigmentation frequently seen in the dependent regions (ankles) and areas where the skin is particularly thin.

Box 1: More serious cosmetic sequelae

Dimple or dimples in a crenellated, checkerboard, or waffle pattern [Fig. 20]
Groove [Fig. 21] or multiple grooves, either parallel to one another or in a fanlike arrangement [Fig. 22]
Simple or high-volume overcorrection, which may produce a cavity [see Fig. 23] or poor cosmetic results [Fig. 24]
Wrinkles, which may be layered, parchment-like, padded, or serrated [Fig. 22]
A variable combination of the above-listed sequelae that produces a moonscape appearance [see Fig. 20]
Excess skin, of variable size [see Fig. 21]
Tissue collapse [see Fig. 19]
Postoperative "banana roll" [see Fig. 19]
Double fold [see Fig. 19]
Ptosis, which is common after excessive removal of fat from the buttocks

pigmentation, common over the calves. The more serious cosmetic sequelae are shown in Box 1.

Causes and evaluation of cosmetic sequelae

The situation is fairly simple. First, the anatomic characteristics of the subcutaneous fat should be borne in mind. Under the dermis, the superficial fat is divided by vertical septa that are anchored on either side to the dermis and to the fascia superficialis [Figs. 25A, 25B and 26]. At some sites, sharply demarcated "steatomas" are found under the fascia superficialis. They are divided by horizontal septa, and extend down to the muscle fascia. This deep fat produces unsightly deformities, and is the main target for removal by liposuction. Superficial liposuction, in which the cannula comes into contact with the dermis [Fig. 27], creates a surface dent or divot. Upon physical examination, the dent persists in the supine position. Similarly, subdermal liposuction that uses small cannulas causes wrinkling by destroying or damaging the subcutaneous septa, which (in my opinion) are responsible for skin contraction [see Fig. 28]. Deep liposuction damages the muscle and fascia, and causes retractile fibrosis with adhesion of the skin to the underlying tissue [see Fig. 27]. Muscle contraction worsens the deformities. In patients who have redundant skin before liposuction, the procedure worsens the skin excess. Similarly, excess skin will be present when the characteristics of skin retraction are not taken into account (ie, when tall narrow bulges are removed [Fig. 29]). The deformities persist in the supine position.

Minimizing the risk of cosmetic sequelae

The surgeon must be alert to the pitfalls that exist at each step of the liposuction procedure.

Careful patient selection

Careful patient selection is essential. Answers to the following questions should be sought when examining the patient:

Is the amount of subcutaneous fat sufficient to warrant liposuction? False bulges should be differentiated from fat deposits [Fig. 30].
Look for redundant skin, which may be marked or latent, based on the skin retraction principle or on comparison of the standing and supine positions.
Predict the future postoperative appearance using the retraction test, contraction test, or lift test.
Assess the treatment sites according to their specific challenges [Fig. 31].
Perform tests to evaluate quantity, quality, and the prognosis [2].
Examine the gluteal fold for an incipient double fold, to avoid creating a "banana roll" [Fig. 32].

Use appropriate instruments

Blunt cannulas, made of titanium to ensure sliding without friction, should be preferred. The holes should be limited number in and appropriately placed, sufficiently far from the tip to avoid suction of subdermal fat [see Fig. 27; Fig. 33]. The antiripple cannula has side holes that ensure surface suction,

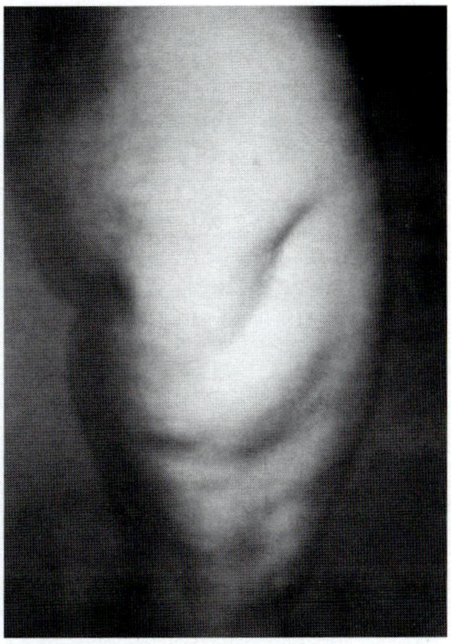

Fig. 20. Complications: irregularities, adhesion, dimples, and waviness.

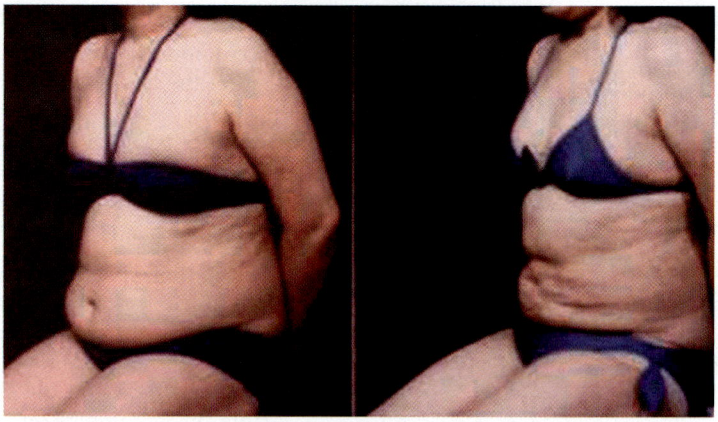

Fig. 21. Waviness and irregularities after superficial suction.

and thereby, remove residual trabeculae between tunnels and simultaneously suction superficial and deep fat. Therefore, a single cannula is sufficient (or almost sufficient) for the entire procedure. Flexible cannulas [see Fig. 33] can be wrapped around curves to avoid the creation of deformities at points or lines that snag the cannula. I described these distinctive deformities in my book [1].

Use proper technique

Inject fluid in a 1:1 ratio.

Stay within the proper plane, in the middle of the fat layer, to allow fat-to-fat healing, because this is the only situation that does not cause sequelae.

Leave a 5-mm layer of fat under the skin and a 5-mm layer on the fascia.

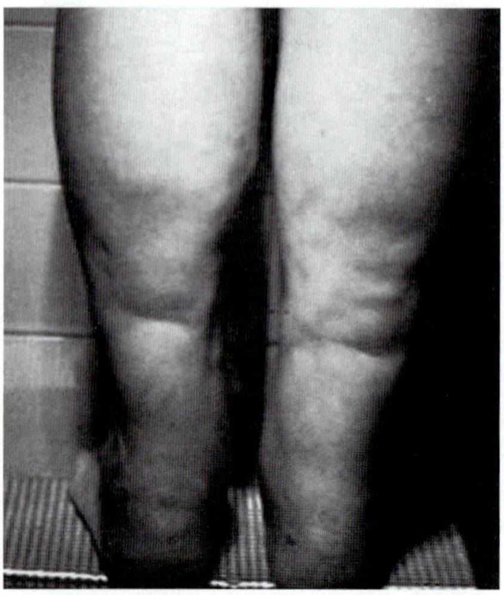

Fig. 22. Parallel grooves at the ankle caused by excessively superficial suction.

Do not use the "superficial technique." Do not remove the subdermal fat, because this causes surface dents, destroys the septa (which I believe are crucial to skin retraction), and may result in necrosis if the terminal superficial arcade is damaged.

The contour should be undercorrected to allow for postoperative fat lysis and skin retraction, which amplify the result and cannot be evaluated on the operating table.

Work methodically, patiently, and carefully.

Avoid structures that snag the cannula, chiefly the fascia lata, but also the Achilles tendon, umbilicus, and so forth.

Provide adequate postoperative care

A compressive garment that is too tight or that applies uneven pressure can cause folds or adhesions, most notably over the abdomen when the patient bends forward. To avoid this, check that the garment does not roll up. If creases are visible at the 8-day follow-up visit, remove the garment. Early removal of the garment has no negative effects. Early on, when I used only elastic bandages, a few patients removed the bandages themselves to relieve itching; the only effect was a slight delay in the resolution of postoperative edema and bruising that did not affect the final result. A good operation with no compressive garment is better than a mediocre operation followed by prolonged use of a compressive garment that simply masks the defects. I recommend use of a compressive garment 24 hours a day for the first week, and then during the day or night for the next 2 weeks. This duration is more than sufficient.

Minor complications should lead to appropriate treatment. Hematomas and seromas should be drained carefully until they dry up. They may

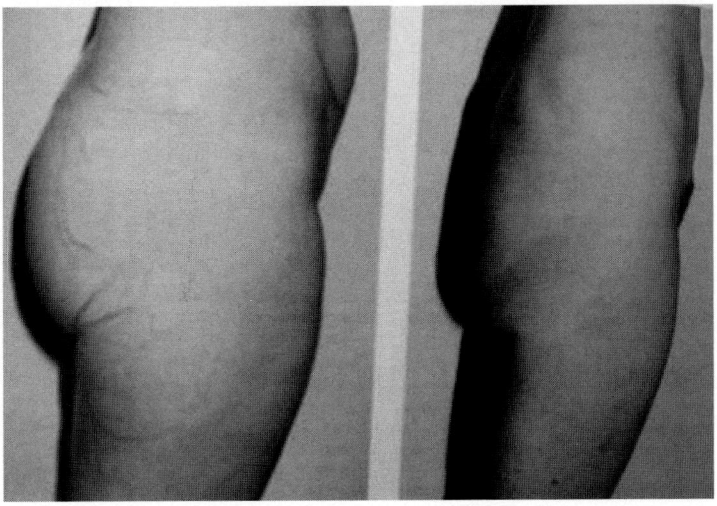

Fig. 23. Overcorrection with suction of the "Bermuda triangle" producing flat buttocks.

leave a wrinkled padded area, which is common at the abdomen above the umbilicus, but often escapes notice.

Instruct the patient to protect the site from sunlight until all bruises or other postoperative marks have resolved. Ultraviolet radiation converts hemoglobin in bruised areas to hemosiderin, which produces virtually permanent pigmentation.

Correcting cosmetic sequelae

Easily corrected sequelae

Touch-up liposuction allows correction of sequelae that are characterized by excess residual fat, such as bulges, undercorrection, step deformity, or true asymmetry (as opposed to congenital asymmetry or asymmetry that is due to scoliosis). A 6-month wait allows complete resolution of the edema, as well as recovery of tissue flexibility at the treated site. The patient's cooperation should be obtained (ask the patient to draw her "bulge"), and the final marking should be done in the standing position [41]. Active cooperation ensures that the patient shares in the responsibility for the touch-up.

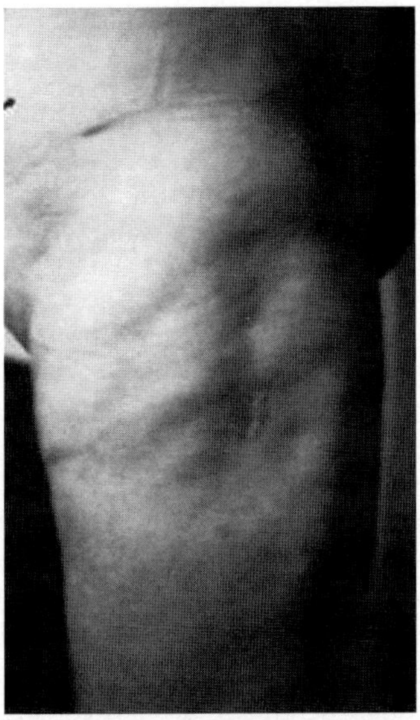

Fig. 24. Wrinkles and excess skin after superficial suction.

Hyaluronidase or a "diffusing" agent can be injected subdermally at the site to ensure gradual fading of the residual pigmentation. Hydroquinone bleaching creams can be applied to the site.

Challenging cases

Excess skin If the excess is small enough to be objectively and subjectively acceptable to the patient, no treatment is needed, because improvement may occur over time. If the excess skin persists, the patient can be asked to put on some weight. When a small excess is unacceptable to the patient, perform a small incision for local resection of the epidermis and dermis. For major excess of skin, remove the redundant skin.

When excess skin is present only below the umbilicus, perform a lip-shaped plasty [**Fig. 34 and 35**] [41], which maintains a satisfactory distance between the umbilicus and the pubic triangle [**Fig. 36**]. The "lazy M" incision becomes more horizontal at the time of suturing and completely horizontal during the postoperative course [**Figs. 27 and 37**].

When excess skin is present over the entire abdomen, to minimize challenges and complications, I developed an en bloc abdominoplasty technique that does not require undermining. In my opinion,

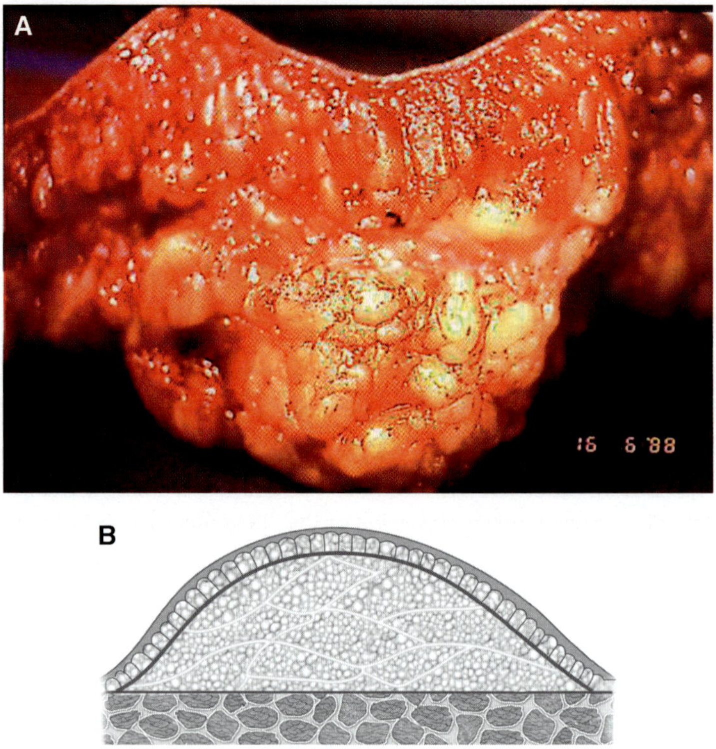

Fig. 25. (*A,B*). Subcutaneous fat anatomy. Superficial layer (skin to fascia superficialis), divided vertically. Deep layer (fascia superficialis to muscle fascia), divided horizontally.

undermining generates a cascade that explains all of the complications including sero-hematomas, infections, necrosis, and shock. The lower flap is removed en bloc, together with the umbilicus, and a neo-umbilicoplasty is performed. Pleasing proportions are obtained; the distance between the neo-umbilicus and the pubis is satisfactory, and the pubic triangle is an isosceles triangle with a side length of 10 cm [see **Figs. 34–42**].

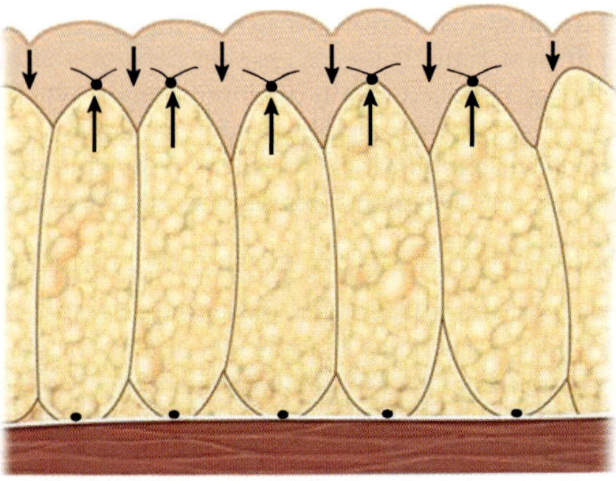

Fig. 26. Diagram showing that cellulite is related to fat hypertrophy responsible for a pressure increase that causes bulging (orange-skin appearance). (*From top to bottom*) Dermis, Vertically elastic septa that seem responsible for skin retraction, Fascia superficialis, Muscle.

At the inner thigh, simple removal of a skin wedge in the groin carries two major risks: downward displacement of the scar to a position where it is visible and opening and deformity of the vulva as a result of traction.

In 1988, Lockwood [49] developed a technique in which the lower flap is secured to an extremely strong ligament that is part of the fibrous sheath that surrounds the pubis (ligament of Colles, or infrapubic ligament of Rouvière). This method considerably diminishes the risk of descent of the scar and the opening of the vulva.

In 1990, I developed the "thong technique" [50], which produces a short scar that is hidden in the pubic triangle and pubic hair. The excess skin on the inner thigh is corrected by rotating the flap and performing a triangular plasty to correct dog ears [**Figs. 43–46**].

At the anterior thigh, the lower flap can be secured to the inguinal ligament to prevent or to delay recurrent skin sagging [**Fig. 47**]. At the pelvis, in general, circumferential treatment is needed that involves the inner, anterior, and outer thighs.

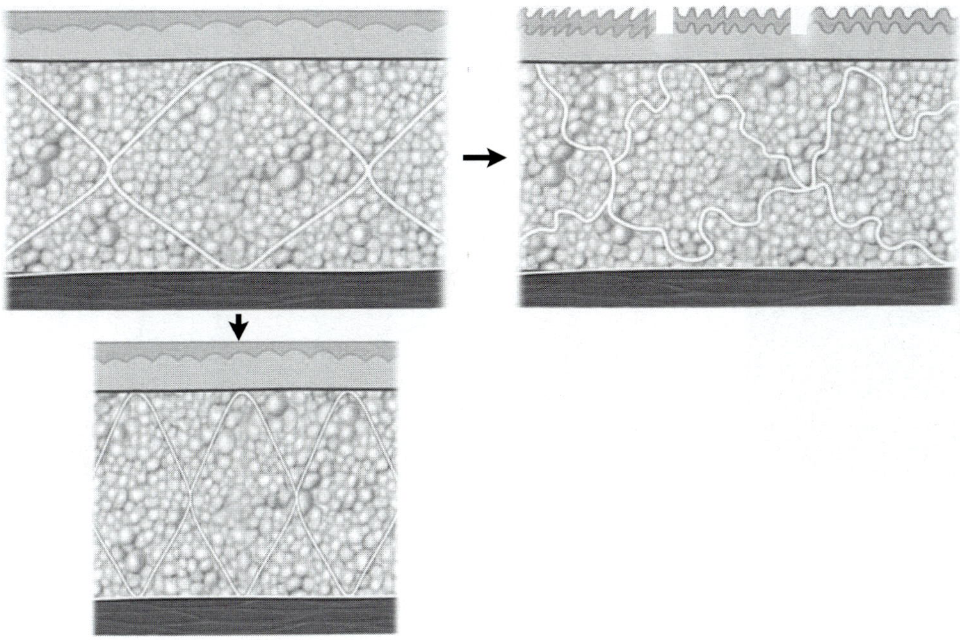

Fig. 27. If the subdermal baffle system is destroyed by superficial suction, the skin cannot retract normally, and wrinkling occurs.

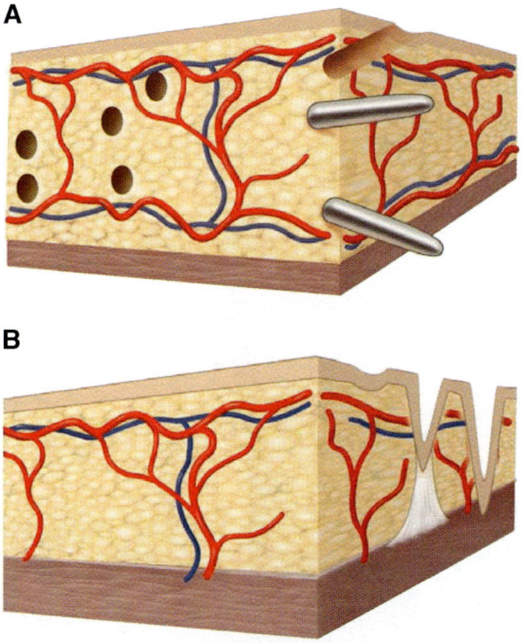

Fig. 28. Mechanisms underlying cosmetic sequelae. (*A*) Middle: appropriate fat removal from the middle of the fat layer. Suction near the skin produces a dimple. Suction near the muscle causes injury to the muscle and fascia. (*B*) Muscle injury leads to fibrosis that causes adhesions.

Contour irregularities: filling procedures The course of action depends on whether the floor of the dent is above or below the ideal line [see **Fig. 48**]. If it is above the ideal line, remove the fat in the residual lumps; if it is above and below the ideal line (the most common situation), remove the residual lumps and inject fat into the remaining dents; and if it is below the ideal line, inject fat.

The number of available allogenic products for injection is increasing at a fast pace, which indicates that none is fully satisfactory. Each product has its drawbacks [**Figs. 49 and 50**] [51,52].

Fat that is aspirated from the patient [**Figs. 51–57**] [53–56] is the only product that carries no risk of allergy or rejection; however, partial or complete reabsorption tends to occur. Reabsorption is more marked at the body than at the face. Multiple sequential injections can be performed to combat this problem, and ultimately, achieve virtually complete filling [see **Fig. 57**]. The face is a favorable site for volume restoration [see **Figs. 54–57**].

My experience and my laboratory experiments with fat cultures led me to conclude that 100% filling cannot be achieved at the body with a single injection [57]. Fat injections can induce complications, such as calcification of fat injected into a breast [**Fig. 58**].

Deep depressions Deep depressions are caused by adhesions. The need for patience should be explained to the patient; deep depressions can

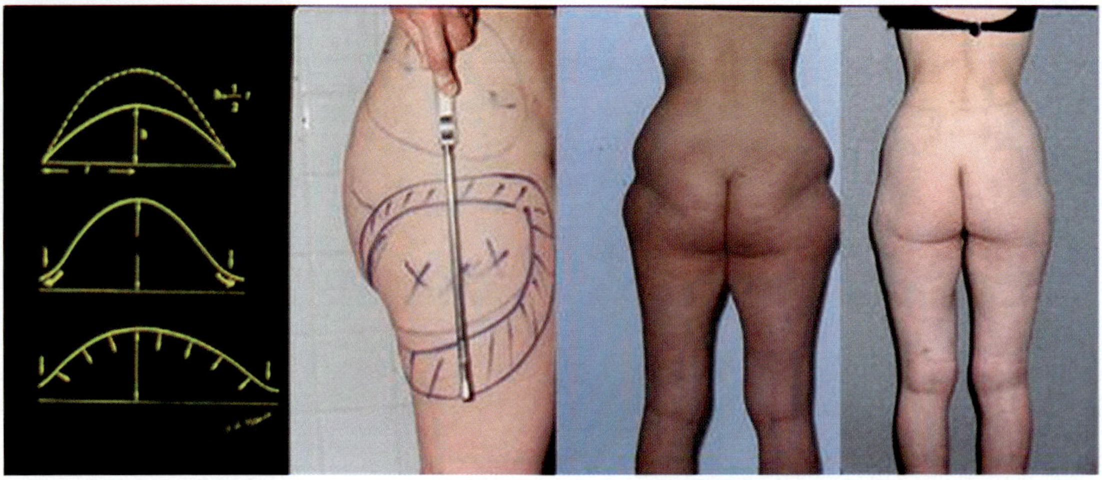

Fig. 29. Evaluating the potential for skin retraction. The Illouz Law: to ensure satisfactory skin retraction, the height of the bulge should not be greater than one half of the radius of the bulge. If the bulge is tall, improve the ratio by undermining the surrounding tissue to increase the diameter.

improve or worsen over time. The contour deformity requires 1 year to become established. Use deep massage to release the adhesions or external ultrasound and lytic injections after an accurate topographic evaluation or perform a minor surgical procedure with a small incision to attempt to release the tissue planes using a fork-shaped Toledo cannula or a curved-blade scalpel [Fig. 59]. In patients who have severe adhesions that persist despite the above-described treatments, perform

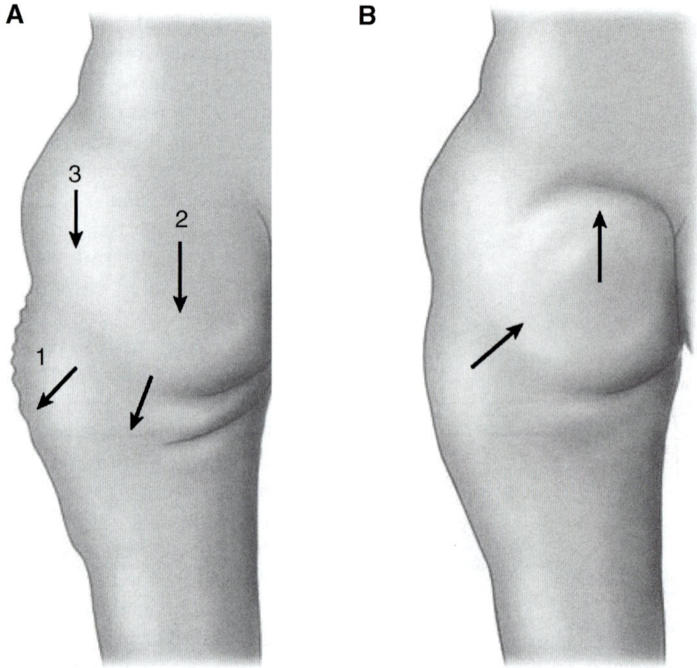

Fig. 30. (*A,B*). False bulge in the saddlebag area. Three factors are involved: the weight of the buttock (2) reverses the direction of the buttock fold, and creates a false saddlebag (1); the weight of the hips (3) has a similar (although less marked) effect; and infraclinical accordion skin folds may simulate a saddlebag. The Illouz test for detecting a false bulge consists of contracting the gluteal muscles to return the fat deposits to their normal position. When a false bulge is found, the underlying abnormality should be corrected (ie, remove fat from the buttocks or hips).

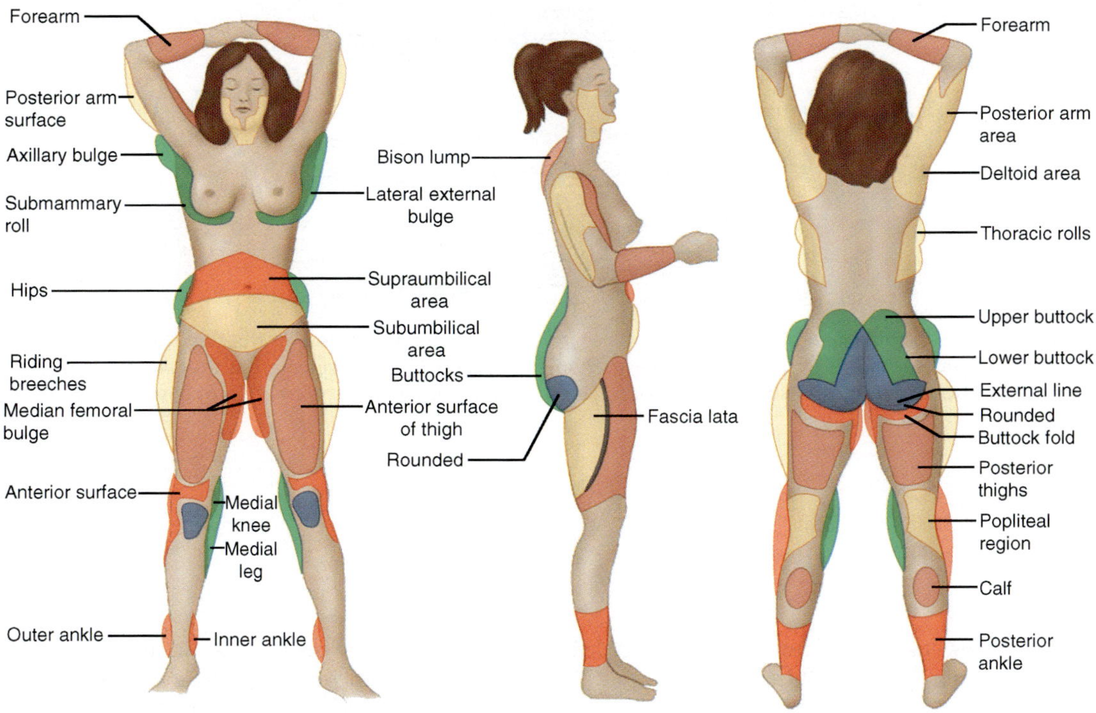

Fig. 31. Classification of body sites based on the risk of poor cosmetic outcomes, according to the author. Green: forgiving sites, where small mistakes may be tolerated. Yellow: less forgiving sites. Orange: challenging sites. Red: unforgiving sites: even small mistakes cause unfavorable outcomes. Blue (the Illouz Bermuda triangle): sites that carry a high risk of unfavorable outcomes (ie, flat buttocks in females) [see **Fig. 23**].

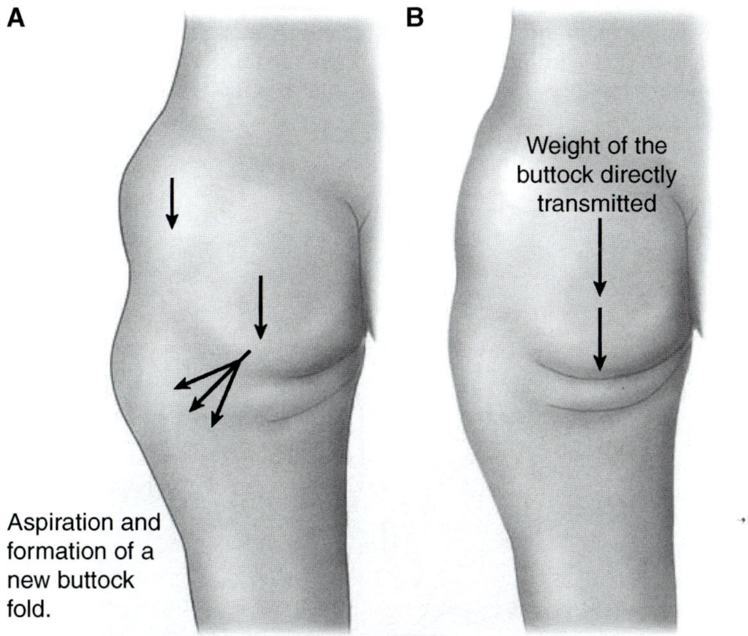

Fig. 32. (*A,B*). Mechanism underlying production of a banana roll. When a saddlebag is increased by the weight of the buttock or hips and exhibits an incipient double fold, excessive fat removal allows direct transmission of the weight of the tissues, which produces a large double fold or a banana roll.

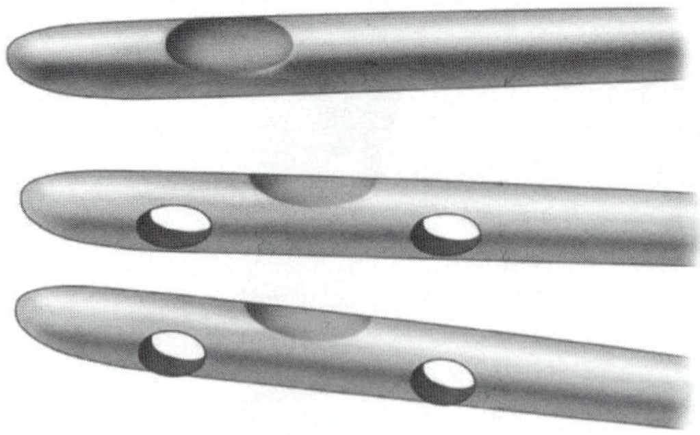

Fig. 33. Titanium cannula designed by the author. Note the single ventral hole and the two holes on each side, each with a diameter of less than 2 mm. The ventral hole ensures deep suction, whereas the lateral holes ensure superficial suction. The cannula is flexible and bends easily. The design avoids the creation of crisscrossing tunnels.

plane-by-plane tissue reconstruction, if needed with fat injection [see Fig. 59].

Other contour irregularities Orange-peel skin (cellulite) is not eliminated by liposuction or any other treatment. Cellulite is caused by hypertrophy of the superficial fat layer (with vertical anchorage in women, Fig. 60), which is under the dependence of estrogen [57]. In laboratory experiments, we found that adding β-estradiol to fat cell cultures resulted in fourfold increases in the rate and magnitude of growth [41]. In male transsexuals and patients who have prostate cancer, estrogen administration can induce the development of orange-peel skin [58]. Orange-peel skin also occurs in men who have testosterone deficiency (eg, due to Klinefelter syndrome). Conversely, androgen therapy or androgen-secreting tumors lead to the resolution of cellulite in women. Androgen deficiency seems to be the main causative factor.

A forked curette has been used to sever the dimple-causing septa. Severing all of the septa cannot be achieved by this method. This is fortunate, because destruction of the blood vessels within the septa would lead to necrosis. Severing the septa eliminates the effect rather than the cause, and the cellulite recurs promptly after reabsorption of the edema [Fig. 61].

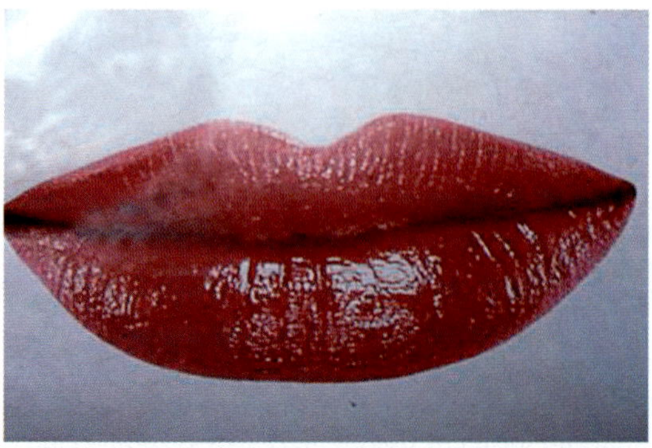

Fig. 34. Lazy M abdominoplasty.

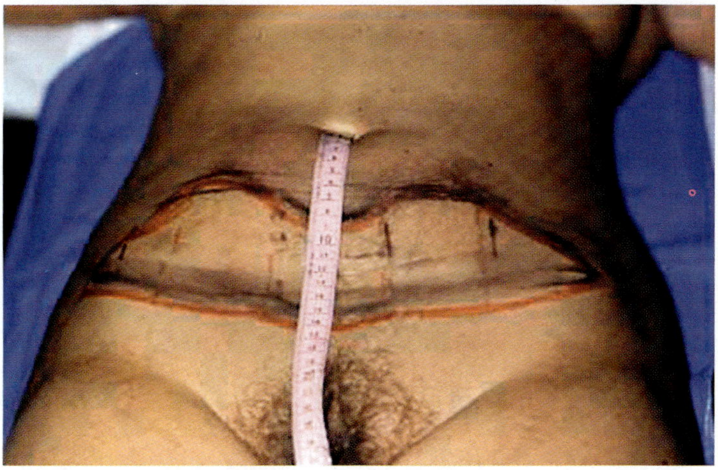

Fig. 35. Lazy M abdominoplasty.

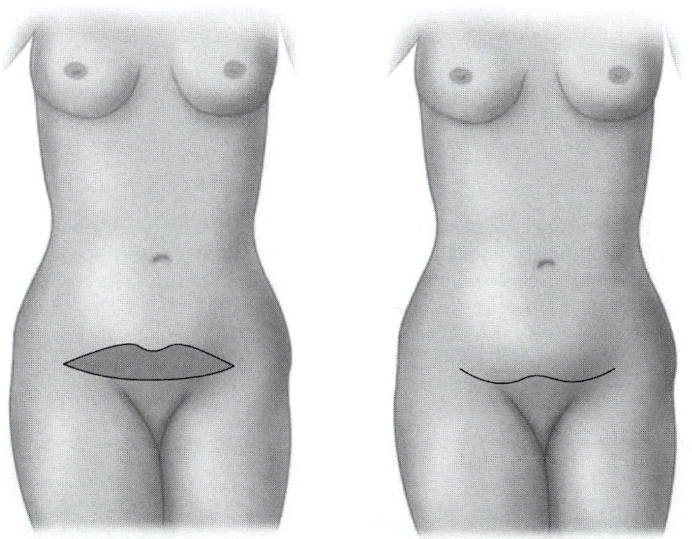

Fig. 36. The lazy M incision moves to a more horizontal position.

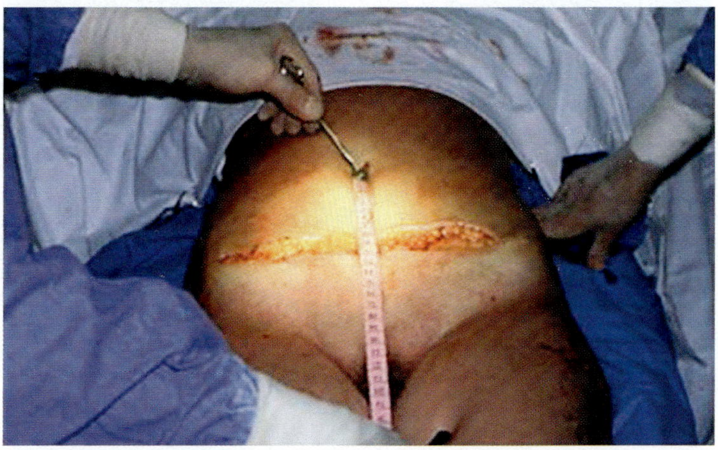

Fig. 37. The lazy M incision moves to a more horizontal position.

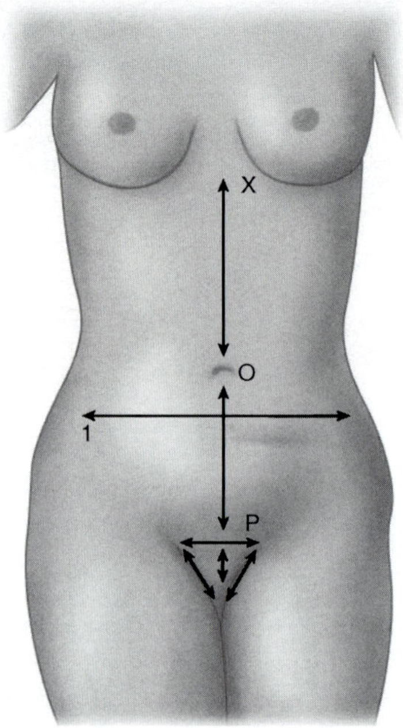

Fig. 38. Diagram showing the appropriate location of the umbilicus. The Illouz "theorem": OP = 1/2 XP – 10% XP, where O is the position of the umbilicus and XP is the distance from the xyphoid to the pubic triangle. The pubic triangle should be an isosceles triangle, ideally with 10-cm long sides; the sides never should be shorter than 7 cm. The OP must never be less than 10 cm or more than 13 cm.

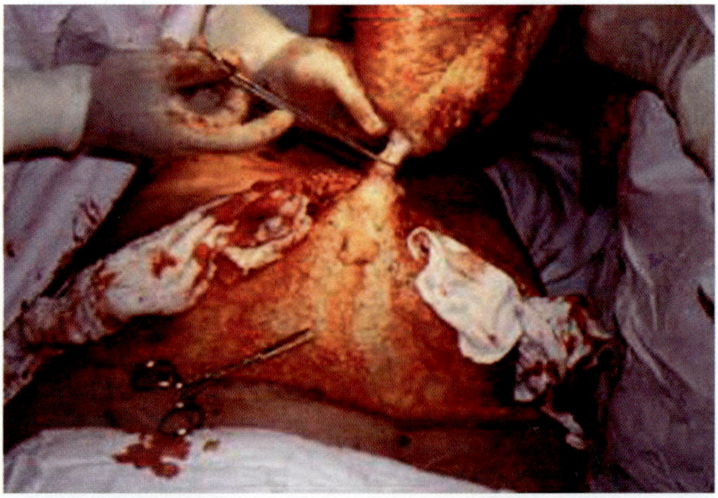

Fig. 39. En bloc abdominoplasty. Suction of fat from the upper flap and en bloc resection of the lower flap, including the umbilicus, which is marked before the procedure. The umbilical tether is severed during the procedure.

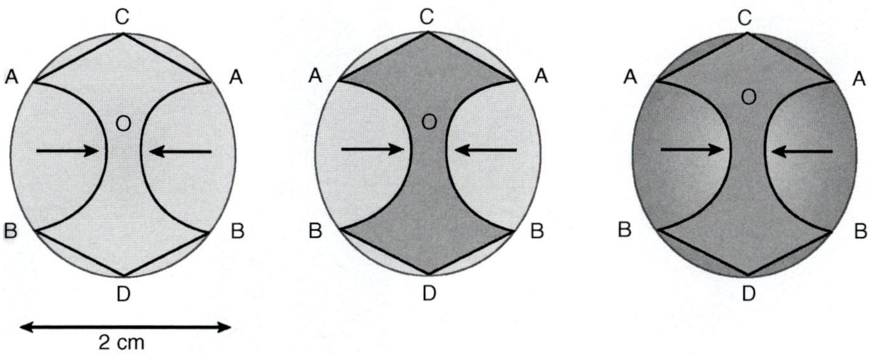

Fig. 40. The Illouz technique for constructing a neoumbilicus, with two reversed Cs ("Chanel" umbilicus).

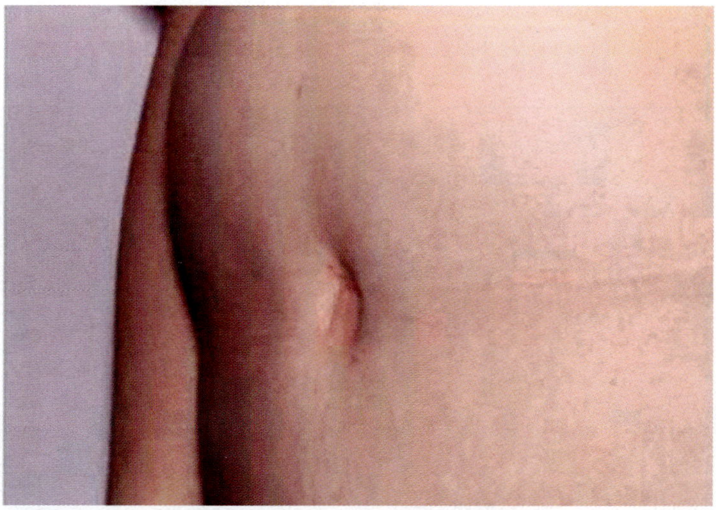

Fig. 41. Close-up view of a "Chanel" umbilicus 6 months after the procedure. The scar is inside the umbilicus and the invagination is of good quality.

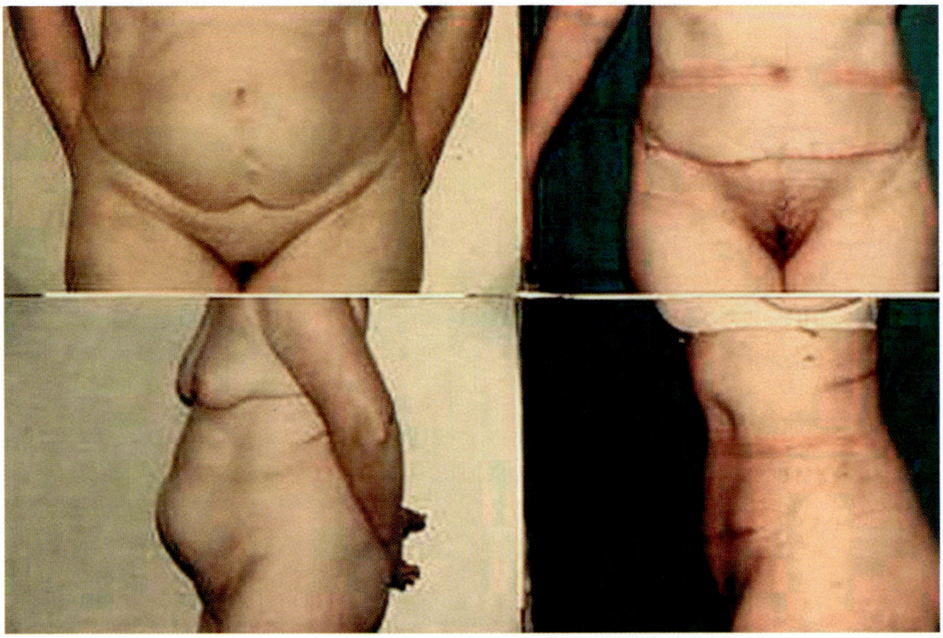

Fig. 42. Result of the Illouz en bloc abdominoplasty with a vertical neoumbilicus producing a youthful appearance.

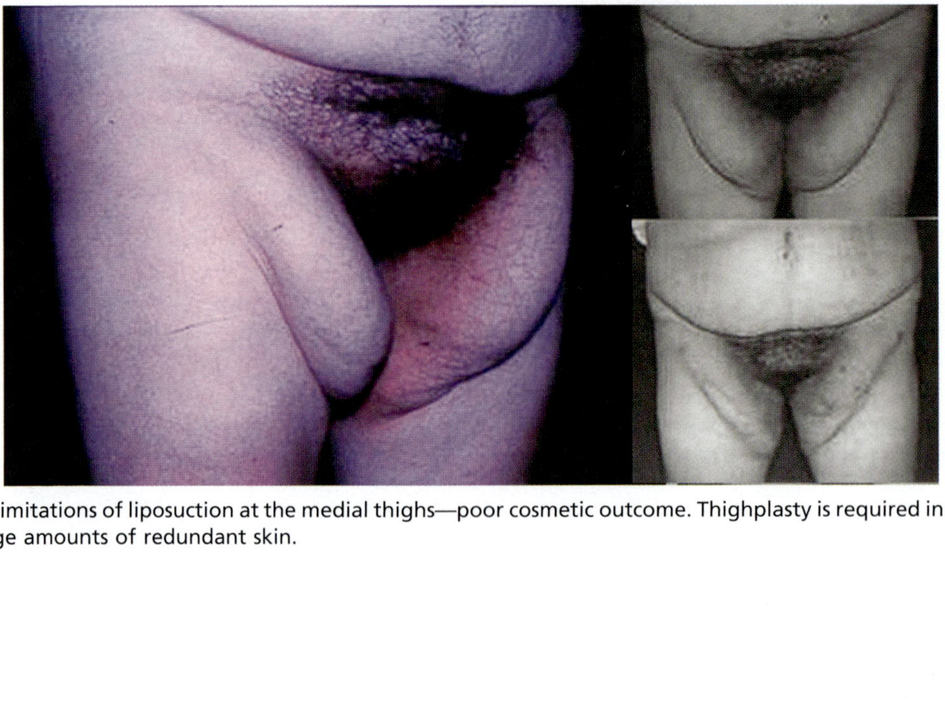

Fig. 43. Limitations of liposuction at the medial thighs—poor cosmetic outcome. Thighplasty is required in patients with large amounts of redundant skin.

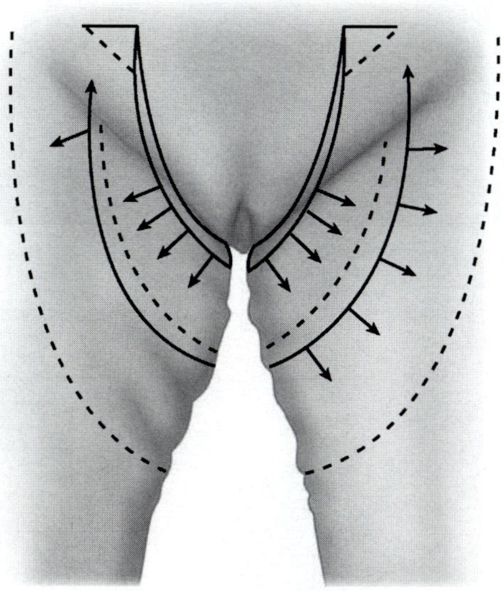

Fig. 44. Diagram of the medial thighplasty procedure developed by the author.

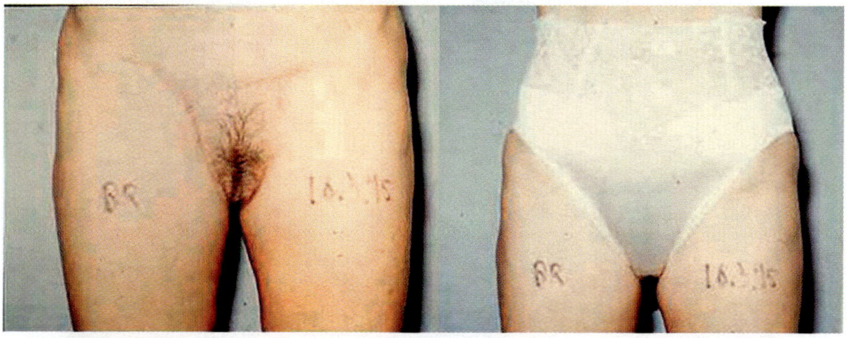

Fig. 45. Result of medial thighplasty after 3 months. The scar is hidden by the pubic hair and undergarment.

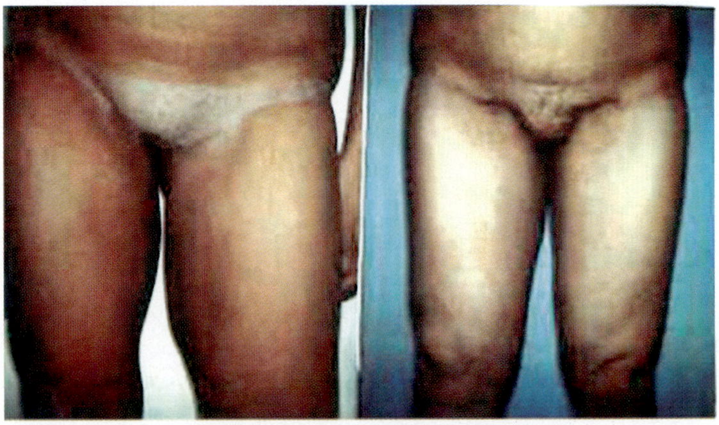

Fig. 46. Result of medial thighplasty after 3 months. The scar is hidden by the pubic hair and undergarment.

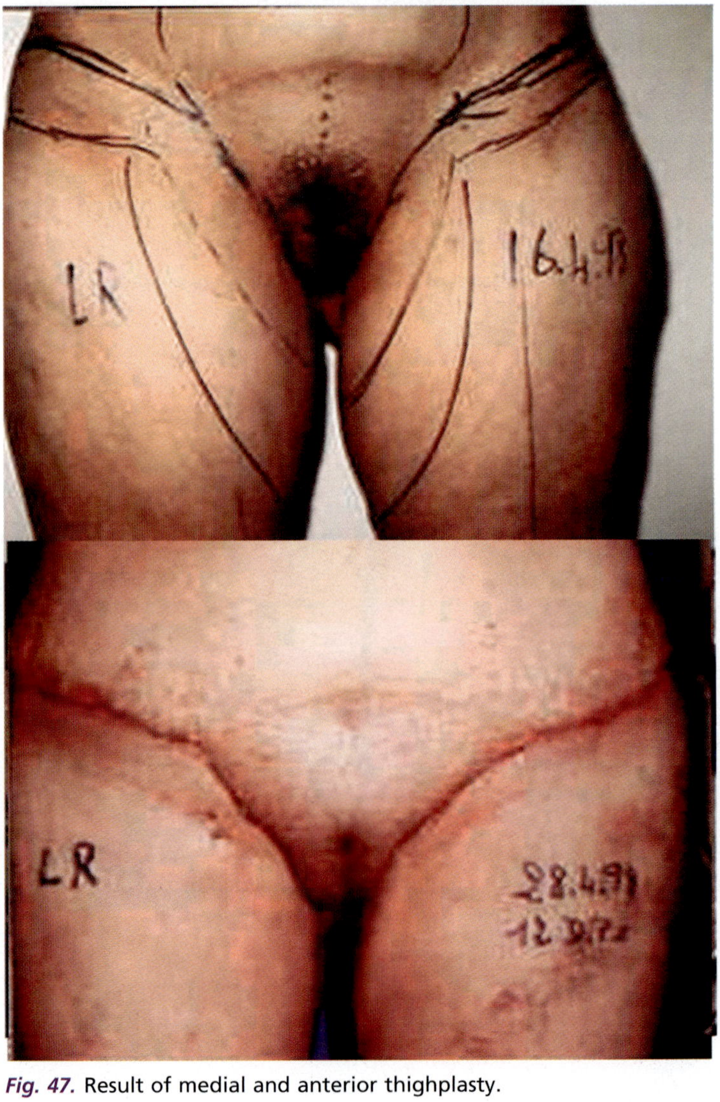

Fig. 47. Result of medial and anterior thighplasty.

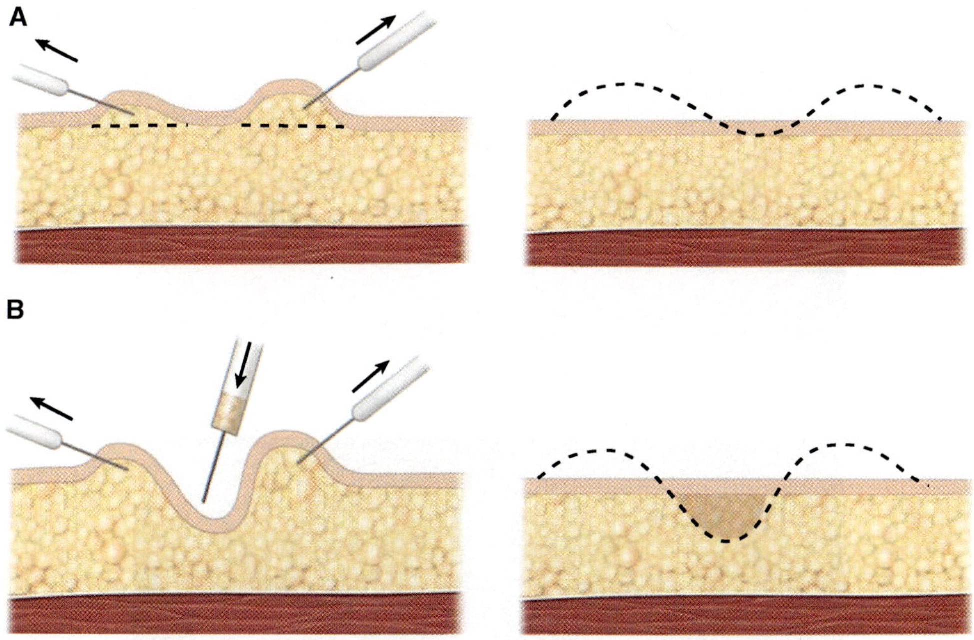

Fig. 48. How to correct a dent. (*A*) When the floor of the dent is located above the ideal line, between two bulges, remove the fat from the bulges. (*B*) When the floor of the dent is under the ideal line, remove the fat from the bulges and inject fat into the remaining dent.

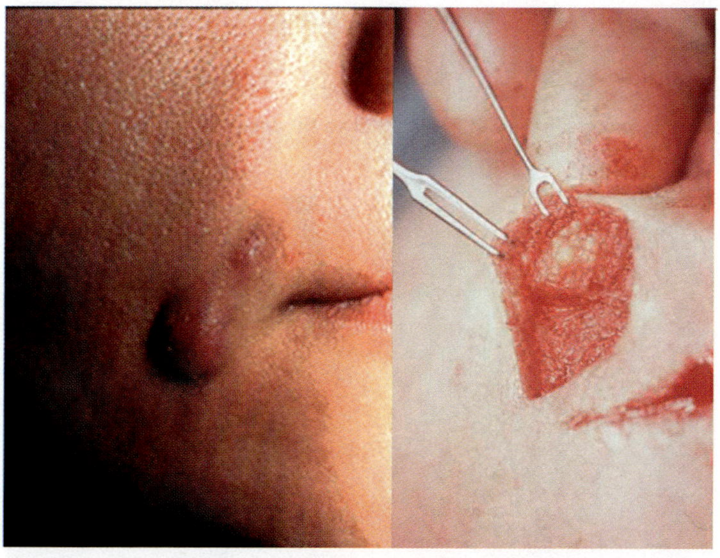

Fig. 49. Large granuloma induced by an Artecol injection.

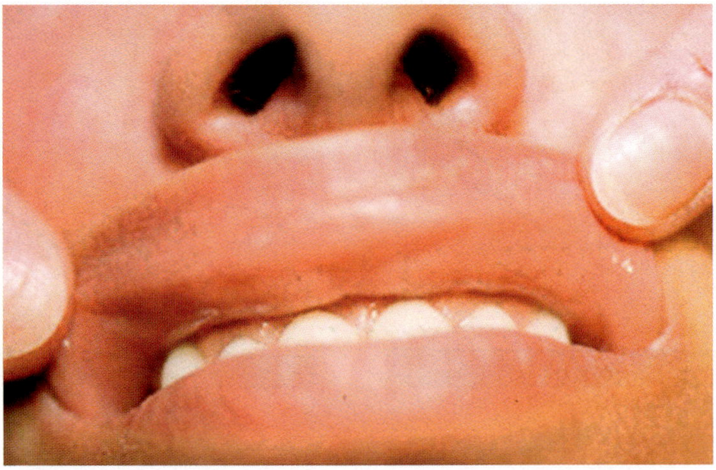

Fig. 50. Gore-Tex visible in the upper lip.

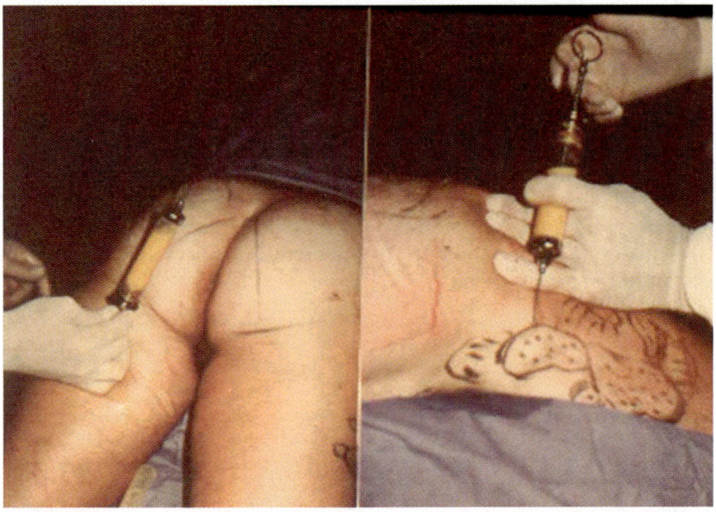

Fig. 51. First procedure performed by the author in 1983 to fill depressions that were produced by liposuction.

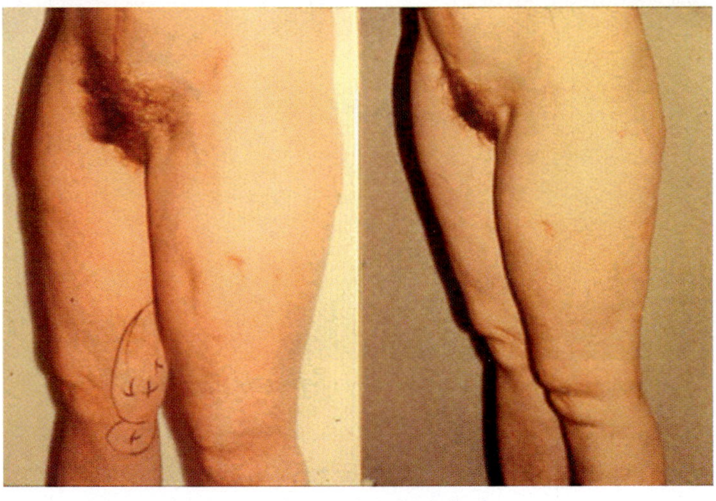

Fig. 52. Results of filling at the medial thigh [53].

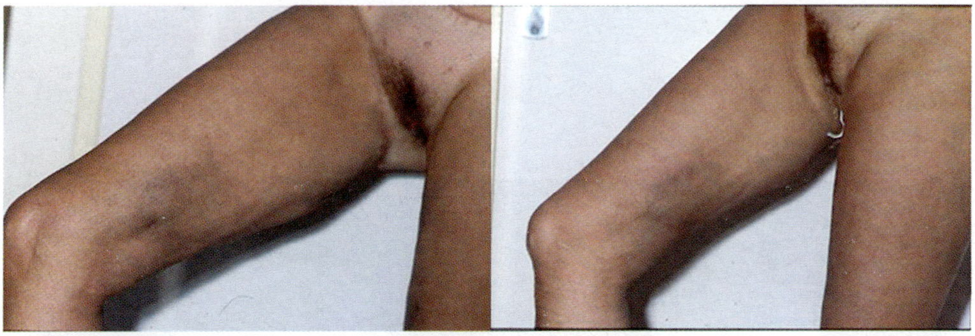

Fig. 53. Results of filling at the medial thigh (Illouz 84).

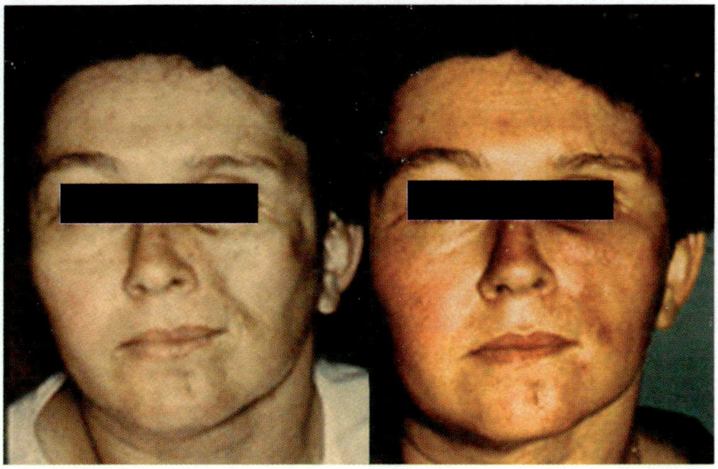

Fig. 54. Romberg syndrome: single fat injection (40 mL) under local anesthesia in 1985. Sustained good result 2 years later.

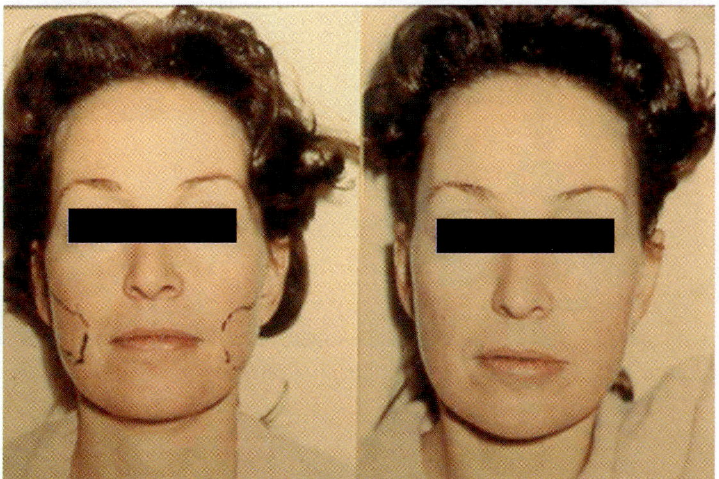

Fig. 55. 1984: 1-year result after filling of naturally occurring depressions to rejuvenate the face.

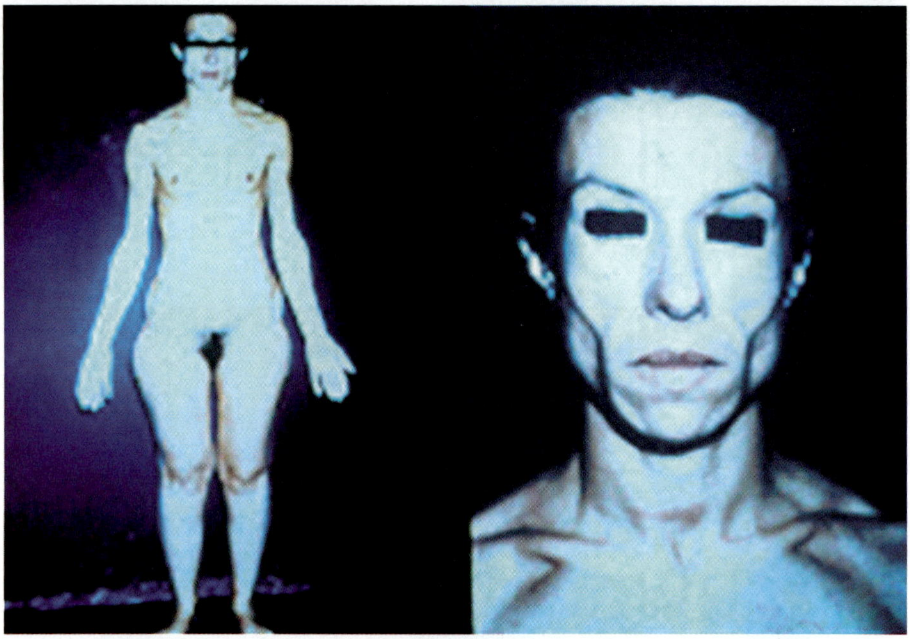

Fig. 56. Barraquer-Simmons syndrome: subcutaneous fat atrophy in the upper half of the body, with a skeleton face, hypertrophy in the lower half of the body, with a large saddlebag. Fat taken from the saddlebag was injected into the face.

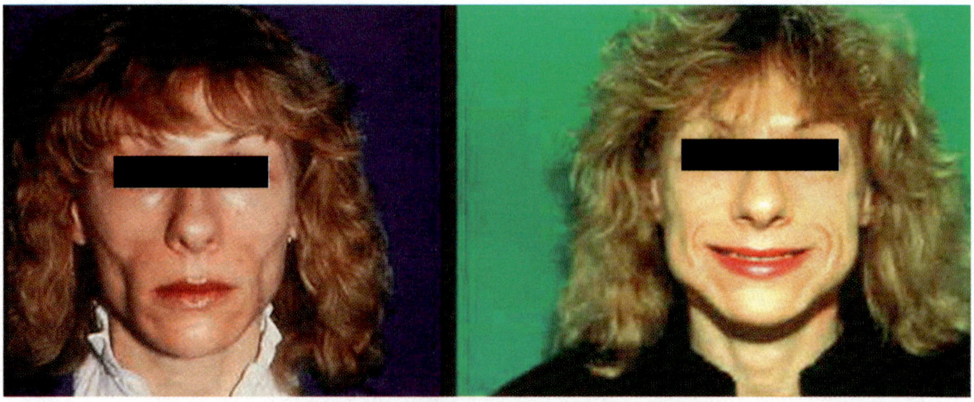

Fig. 57. Stable result 3 years after three injections in a patient who had Barraquer-Simmons syndrome.

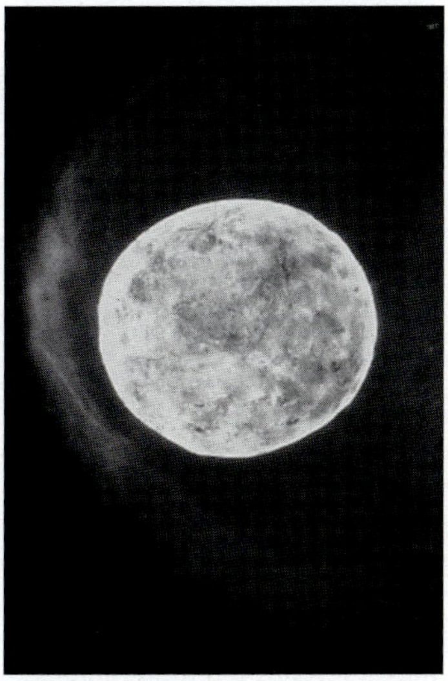

Fig. 58. Calcifications 3 years after injection of 40 mL of fat into a breast.

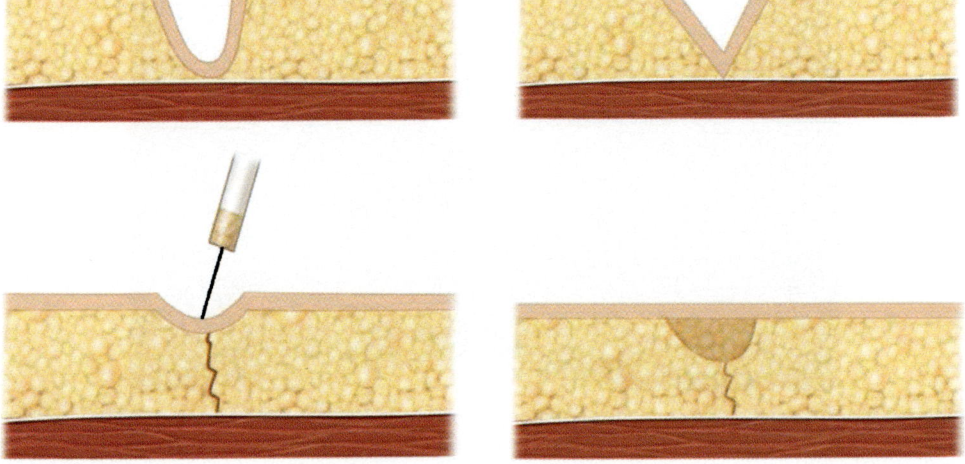

Fig. 59. Treatment of adhesions—suction of residual bulges, release of adhesions using a Toledo cannula, and fat injection into residual dents.

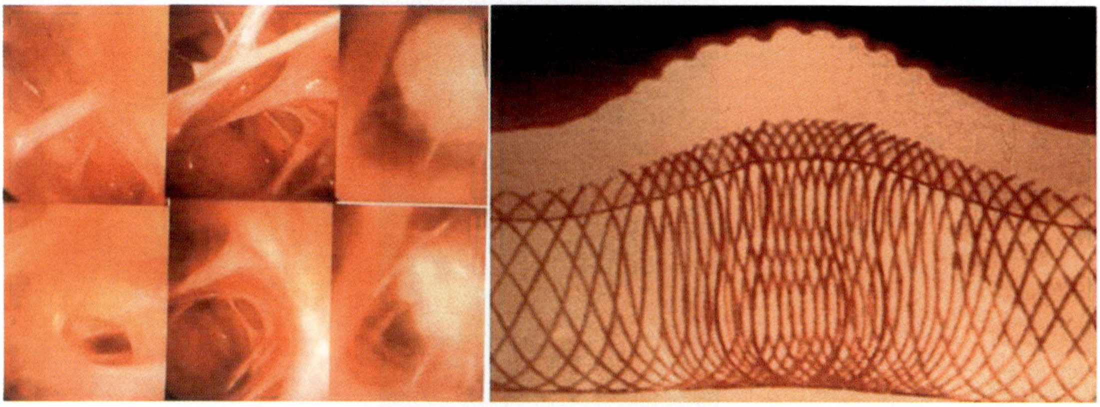

Fig. 60. Endoscopy after liposuction showing intact septa that carry blood vessels. The septa extend from the dermis to the fascia superficialis and cause the orange-peel appearance of the skin. Endoscopic view: a cannula hole larger than 2 mm in diameter can destroy the subdermal conjunctive tissue, and therefore, is inappropriate for superficial suction.

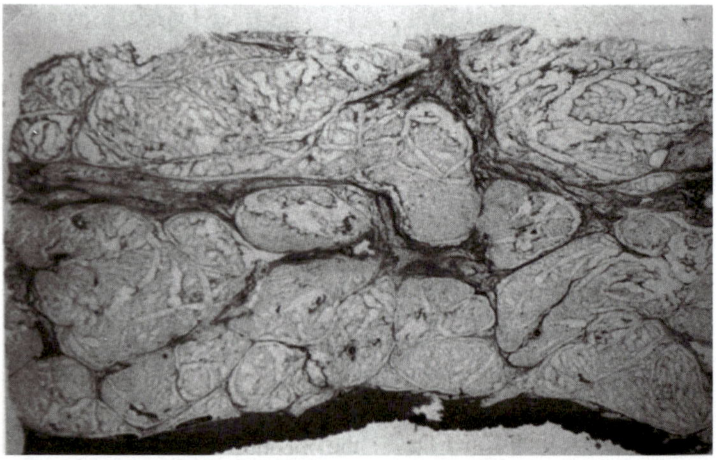

Fig. 61. Biopsy 6 months—deep and superficial suction severing the septa in an attempt to eliminate the orange-peel appearance of the skin. Recurrence of the vertical separations in the superficial layer with a return of the orange-peel appearance.

Summary

Remain within the limits determined by the technique, which has limitations that I have tried to quantify; the patient, because obesity, hypertension, diabetes, and other morbidities create specific limitations; and the surgeon, who should be aware of the boundaries to his or her expertise.

To minimize the systemic complications, the surgeon should minimize:

The amount of solution injected (1:1 ratio)
The nature of the solution (room temperature, containing a vasoconstrictor)
The amount of fat removed: no more than 6% to 8% of the patient's body weight
The amount of blood lost (400 mL)
The surface area of the treatment site: no more than 30% of the body surface area
The duration of the procedure: try not to exceed 3 hours
Turning: avoid turning a fragile or obese patient on the table, because severe shock has been reported after sudden changes in the direction of application of gravity to the body, which causes an abrupt change in fluid compartments. Furthermore, dissection of the carotid artery has been reported after inappropriate lateral movements of the neck.

To minimize cosmetic sequelae, the surgeon should minimize:

The diameter of the cannulas: the smaller the diameter, the closer the surgeon can move toward the surface to shape the contour without removing the subdermal fat
Cutting capacity: use a blunt, round-tipped cannula whose holes have rounded edges
The number of holes: according to the Poiseuille law, O = D, which means that the sum of the diameters of the holes should be equal to the diameter of the cannula. An excessively large number of large holes decreases suction power and may render the cannula ineffective.
Trauma, most notably the number of to and fro movements of the cannula (the antiripple cannula requires fewer movements)
Crisscrossing, because this creates cavities that may heal in a haphazard manner or not at all
Suction too close to the surface or too close to the muscle
Use of machines that may be difficult to control or of limited usefulness (eg, ultrasound machines, "laser," rotating blades, vibrators)

Stop in time to avoid complications, the surgeon should not complicate the technique.

References

[1] Illouz YG. A new technique for localized fat deposit. Paris: Les Nouvelles Esthetiques; 1978.
[2] Illouz YG. Une nouvelle technique pour les lipodystrophies localisées. La Revue de Chirurgie Esthétique de Langue Française 1980;6(19): 10–2 [in French].
[3] Comiskey C. Cosmetic surgery in Paris in 1926: the case of the amputated leg. J Women's History 2004;16(3):30–54.
[4] Schrudde J. Liperexis in the correction of local adiposity. Presented at the First Congress of the International Society of Aesthetic Plastic Surgery, Rio de Janeiro. 1972.
[5] Schrudde J. Lipexhaerese zur beseitigung der lokalen adipositas. Plastiche chirurgie des kopf - und halsbereichs und der weiblichen brust. Stuttgart (Germany): Thieme; 1975 [in German].
[6] Fisher GM. Revised technique for cellulites fat reduction in riding breeches deformity. Cosmetic Surg 1977;2:4.
[7] Kesselring UK, Meyer R. Suction curette for removal of excessive local deposits of subcutaneous fat. Plast Reconst Surg 1978;62:305.
[8] Teimourian B, Fisher JB. Suction curettage to remove excess fat for body contouring. Plast Reconstr Surg 1981;68(1):50–8.
[9] Schrudde J. Lipexheresis (liposuction) for body contouring. Clin Plast Surg 1984;11(3): 445–56.
[10] Ersek RA, Schade K. Subcutaneous pseudobursa secondary to suction and surgery. Plast Reconstr Surg 1990;85(3):442–5.
[11] Hetter GP, Herhahn F. Experience with the Illouz technique of blunt suction lipectomy in North America. Aesth Plast Surg 1983;7:69.
[12] Grazer FM, de Jong RH. Fatal outcomes from liposuction: census survey of cosmetic surgeons. Plast Reconstr Surg 2000;105(1):436–46 [discussion 447–8].
[13] The American Society of Plastic Surgery Lipoplasty Task Force Report 1998.
[14] Lehnhardt M, Homann HH, Druecke D, et al. [No problem with liposuction?] Chirurg 2003; 74(9):808–14.
[15] Klein JA. The tumescent technique for liposuction surgery. Am J Cosmet Surg 1987;4:263.
[16] Klein JA. Anesthesia for liposuction in dermatologic surgery. J Dermatol Surg Oncol 1988; 14(10):1124–32.
[17] Hetter GP. The effect of low-dose epinephrine on the hematocrit drop following lipolysis. Aesthetic Plast Surg 1984;8(1):19–21.
[18] Illouz YG. Princípios básicos da técnica da lipoaspiração. In: Avelar J, Illouz YG, editors. Lipoaspiração. São Paulo (Brazil): Hipócrates.
[19] Klein JA. Anesthesia for liposuction in derma-

tologic surgery. J Dermatol Surg Oncol 1988; 14(10):1124–32.
[20] Ostad A, Kageyama N, Moy RL. Tumescent anesthesia with a lidocaine dose of 55 mg/kg is safe for liposuction. Dermatol Surg 1996;22(11): 921–7.
[21] Richling N, Friedrich E, Deutinger M, et al. Surgical reduction of fat surplus leading to pulmonary embolism. Wien Klin Wochenschr 2004; 116(24):854–7.
[22] Rohrich RJ, Kenkel JM, Janis JE, et al. An update on the role of subcutaneous infiltration in suction-assisted lipoplasty. Plast Reconstr Surg 2003;111(2):926–7 [discussion 928].
[23] Samdal F, Amland PF, Bugge JF. Blood loss during suction-assisted lipectomy with large volumes of dilute adrenaline. Scand J Plast Reconstr Surg Hand Surg 1995;29(2):161–5.
[24] Fournier PE, Otteni FM. Lipodissection in body sculpturing: the dry procedure. Plast Reconstr Surg 1983;72(5):598.
[25] Hetter GP, Herhahn F. Experience with "lipolysis": the Illouz technique of blunt suction lipectomy in North America. Aesthetic Plast Surg 1983;7(2):69–76.
[26] Samdal F, Amland PF, Bugge JF. Blood loss during liposuction using the tumescent technique. Aesthetic Plast Surg 1994;18(2):157–60.
[27] Toledo LS, Regatieri FLF, Carneiro JDA. The effect of hypothermia on coagulation and its implications for infiltration in lipoplasty: a review. Aesthetic Surgery J 2001;21(1):40–4.
[28] Fournier PE, Otteni FM. Lipodissection in body sculpturing: the dry procedure. Plast Reconstr Surg 1983;72(5):598.
[29] Alegría Perén P, Barbara Gómez J, Guerrero-Santos J. Total corporal contouring with mega-liposuction (120 consecutive cases). Aesthetic Plast Surg 1999;23(2):93–100.
[30] de Jong RH, Grazer FM. "Tumescent" liposuction alert: deaths from lidocaine cardiotoxicity. Am J Forensic Med Pathol 1999; 20(1):101.
[31] Schmidt P, Dettmeyer R, Alpers K, et al. B. Madea Septisch-toxischer Schock nach Liposuktion Rechtsmedizin 2001;11(6):275–9.
[32] Greenberg G. Lipoplasty: the informed consent and medicolegal considerations. Clin Plast Surg 1989;16(2):375–9.
[33] Beck-Schimmer B, Pasch T. Tumescent technique for local anesthesia. Anasthesiol Intensivmed Notfallmed Schmerzther 2002;37(2):84–8.
[34] Dolsky RL. Blood loss during liposuction. Dermatol Clin 1990;8(3):463–8.
[35] Trott SA, Beran SJ, Rohrich RJ, et al. Safety considerations and fluid resuscitation in liposuction: an analysis of 53 consecutive patients. Plast Reconstr Surg 1998;102(6):2220–9.
[36] Hetter GP. Blood and fluid replacement for lipoplasty procedures. Clin Plast Surg 1989;16(2): 245–8.
[37] de Jong RH, Grazer FM. Perioperative management of cosmetic liposuction. Plast Reconstr Surg 2001;107(4):1039–44.
[38] Fourme T, Vieillard-Baron A, Loubieres Y, et al. Early fat embolism after liposuction. Anesthesiology 1998;89(3):782–4.
[39] Kenkel JM, Lipschitz AH, Luby M, et al. Hemodynamic physiology and thermoregulation in liposuction. Plast Reconstr Surg 2004;114(2): 503–13 [discussion 514–5].
[40] Schraibman IG, Lewis B, Parmar JR. Clinical comparison of elastic supports for venous diseases of the lower limb and thrombosis prevention. Phlebologie 1982;35(1):61–71.
[41] Illouz YG, De Villers YT. Body sculpting by lipoplasty. New York: Churchill Livingstone; 1989.
[42] Mourad PD, Crum LA. A review and examination of ultrasound for lipoplasty. Clin Plast Surg 1999;26(3):409–22.
[43] Grolleau JL, Rouge D, Chavoin JP, et al. Severe cutaneous necrosis after ultrasound lipolysis. Medicolegal aspects and review. Ann Chir Plast Esthet 1997;42(1):31–6.
[44] Fodor PB, Watson J. Personal experience with ultrasound-assisted lipoplasty: a pilot study comparing ultrasound-assisted lipoplasty with traditional lipoplasty. Plast Reconstr Surg 1998; 101(4):1103–16 [discussion 1117–9].
[45] Walgenbach KJ, Riabikhin AW, Galla TJ, et al. Effect of ultrasonic assisted lipectomy (UAL) on breast tissue: histological findings. Aesthetic Plast Surg 2001;25(2):85–8.
[46] Gasparotti M. Superficial liposuction: a new application of the technique for aged and flaccid skin. Aesthetic Plast Surg 1992;16(2):141–53.
[47] Porto da Rocha R, Porto da Rocha EL, de Souza Pinto EB, et al. Cutis marmorata resemblance after liposuction. Aesthetic Plast Surg 2005;29(4): 310–2.
[48] Yoho RA, Romaine JJ, O'Neil D. Review of the liposuction, abdominoplasty, and face-lift mortality and morbidity risk literature. Dermatol Surg 2005;31(7)(Pt 1):733–43 [discussion 743].
[49] Lockwood TE. Fascial anchoring technique in medial thigh lifts. Plast Reconstr Surg 1988;82(2): 299–304.
[50] Illouz YG. En bloc abdominoplasty: a new, safer and more esthetic technique. Ann Chir Plast Esthet 1990;35(3):233–42.
[51] Ersek RA, Gregory SR, Salisbury AV. Bioplastique at 6 years: clinical outcome studies. Plast Reconstr Surg 1997;100(6):1570–4.
[52] Wang J, Fan J, Nordstrom RE. Evaluation of lip augmentation with Gore-Tex facial implant. Aesthetic Plast Surg 1997;21(6):433–6.
[53] Illouz YG. L'avenir de la réutilisation de la graisse après liposuccion. La Revue de Chirurgie Esthétique de Langue Française 1984;9(36):13–4 [in French].
[54] Illouz YG. L'avenir de la réutilisation de la graisse après liposuccion (suite). La Revue de Chirurgie Esthétique de Langue Française 1985;10(38):19–22 [in French].

[55] Illouz YG. De l'utilisation de la graisse aspirée pour combler les defects cutanés. Rev Chir Esthét Lang Fran 1985;10(40):13–9 [in French].
[56] Illouz YG. Note to the editor. The fat cells graft, a new technique to fill depressions. Am Soc Plast Reconstr Surg 1986;J78:122.
[57] Gruber CJ, Wieser F, Gruber IM, et al. Current concepts in aesthetic endocrinology. Gynecol Endocrinol 2002;16(6):431–41.
[58] Nurnberger F, Muller G. So-called cellulite: an invented disease. J Dermatol Surg Oncol 1978; 4(3):221–9.

ELSEVIER SAUNDERS

CLINICS IN PLASTIC SURGERY

Clin Plastic Surg 33 (2006) 165–168

Index

Note: Page numbers of article titles are in **boldface** type.

A

B

doi:10.1016/S0094-1298(05)00132-X
plasticsurgery.theclinics.com

M

Changing Your Address?

Make sure your subscription changes too! When you notify us of your new address, you can help make our job easier by including an exact copy of your Clinics label number with your old address (see illustration below.) This number identifies you to our computer system and will speed the processing of your address change. Please be sure this label number accompanies your old address and your corrected address—you can send an old Clinics label with your number on it or just copy it exactly and send it to the address listed below.

We appreciate your help in our attempt to give you continuous coverage. Thank you.

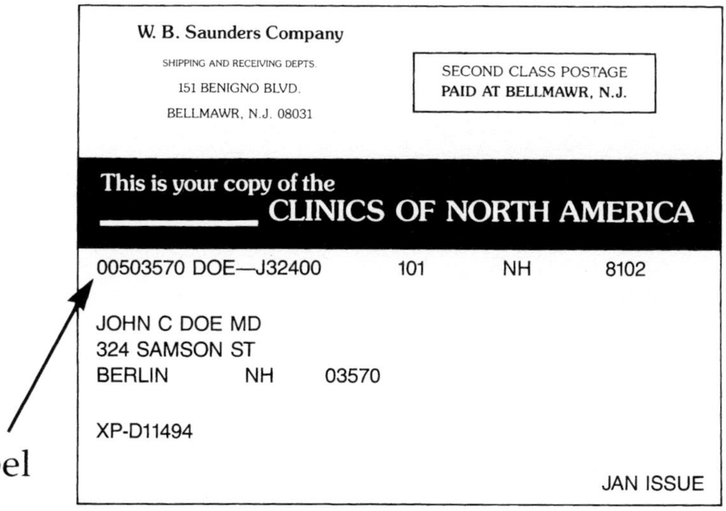

Your Clinics Label Number

Copy it exactly or send your label along with your address to:
W.B. Saunders Company, Customer Service
Orlando, FL 32887-4800
Call Toll Free 1-800-654-2452

Please allow four to six weeks for delivery of new subscriptions and for processing address changes.